The Minor Illness Manual

This sixth edition of the best-selling *The Minor Illness Manual* has been completely revised and updated to include the latest clinical guidance and prescribing information, with a reworked introductory chapter reflecting the changing demands of primary care and a new chapter added on COVID-19 and pandemics.

The simple, clear and easy-to-use format gives primary care professionals – including doctors, nurses, pharmacists, physician associates and paramedics – speedy access to evidence-based guidance for dealing quickly and appropriately with the wide-ranging situations they are likely to encounter in their daily practice.

The Minor Illness Manual

Sixth Edition

Gina Johnson MSc MB BS MRCGP
General Practitioner

Ian Hill-Smith BSc MB BS MRCP FRCGP MD
General Practitioner

Chirag Bakhai BSc MB BS MRCGP DRCOG DGM MBA
General Practitioner

Bhavina Khatani BSc MSc MB BS MRCGP
General Practitioner

CRC Press
Taylor & Francis Group
Boca Raton London New York

CRC Press is an imprint of the
Taylor & Francis Group, an **informa** business

Sixth edition published 2024
by CRC Press
2385 NW Executive Center Drive, Suite 320, Boca Raton, FL 33431

and by CRC Press
4 Park Square, Milton Park, Abingdon, Oxon, OX14 4RN

CRC Press is an imprint of Taylor & Francis Group, LLC

© 2024 Gina Johnson, Ian Hill-Smith, Chirag Bakhai and Bhavina Khatani

Fifth edition published in 2019
Fourth edition published in 2012

ISBN: 978-1-032-54694-0 (pbk)
ISBN: 978-1-032-61652-0 (ebk)

DOI: 10.1201/9781032616520

Typeset in Minion Pro
by Evolution Design & Digital Ltd (Kent)
Printed in Great Britain by Bell and Bain Ltd, Glasgow

Contents

Preface to the sixth edition

In 1997, *The Minor Illness Manual* emerged as a groundbreaking resource at the forefront of a revolutionary concept — the prospect of non-doctor-led services in primary care. Fast forward to its sixth edition, with over 30,000 copies sold, the manual stands as a testament to the remarkable growth and new opportunities arising from the expansion of professional roles in an ever-evolving landscape.

Navigating this complex terrain requires acquiring new proficiencies in the assessment, prescribing, and referral of acute undifferentiated illness. This edition of *The Minor Illness Manual* acknowledges the challenges posed by distinguishing major from minor illnesses, and aims to equip healthcare professionals with the necessary skills to manage a wide range of conditions safely and effectively. Our evidence-based practical advice is meticulously crafted to steer you through the process of diagnosis, knowing what not to miss, understanding when to seek help, and formulating an appropriate management plan. Recognising the diverse settings in which this manual is utilised, we have adapted our referral guidance to ensure its broad applicability.

As healthcare continues to evolve *The Minor Illness Manual* remains a reliable and indispensable companion, providing essential insights and strategies to empower you to deliver the highest standard of care.

Gina Johnson
Ian Hill-Smith
Chirag Bakhai
Bhavina Khatani

Acknowledgements

We would like to thank our highly skilled minor illness nurses, both past and present (especially the pioneer, Rhona Rollings). We are grateful to the many people from diverse healthcare professions who have attended our courses and seminars, who have taught us so much, and also to the staff at Kingfisher Practice, for their support over many years. We give especial thanks to Jill Fenwick, our very capable NMIC administrator from 2006 to 2023.

We acknowledge the excellent work of the Clinical Knowledge Summaries team in gathering together the evidence for the management of a wide range of conditions and would like to thank them for their patience in responding to our queries and comments.

We also thank our patients for allowing us to learn from their experiences of minor illness.

About the authors

National Minor Illness Centre (NMIC) Three of the authors have previously worked together in Kingfisher Practice, an NHS general practice near Luton Airport. In 1996, the practice designed an innovative educational programme for nurses on the management of minor illness, and in 2007, the National Minor Illness Centre (NMIC) was developed as an educational component to the practice. NMIC has received commissions from Health Education England and the Centre for Postgraduate Pharmacy Education to provide bespoke training. Over 3000 healthcare professionals (nurses, pharmacists, health visitors, paramedics, physician associates and others) have attended our NMIC courses; the NMIC Diploma is a nationally recognised qualification.

Dr Gina Johnson graduated from Guy's Hospital in London in 1979 and worked as a general practitioner in Luton from 1983 to 2017. She has always been actively involved in primary care audit and research, and has published articles on a wide range of topics. She is very aware of the limitations of Western medicine, which led her to study for an MSc in medical anthropology in 2002. She is a medical acupuncturist and has an interest in holistic care.

Dr Ian Hill-Smith started publishing research papers while studying for his first degree in anatomy, before graduating in medicine from University College London, in 1980. He is both a member of the Royal College of Physicians and a fellow of the Royal College of General Practitioners. He is fascinated by fundamental science and how it can be applied to medical practice, particularly how medicines can be prescribed to best effect, which was the subject of his research MD. His previous local and national roles have led to the development of a primary care prescribing formulary, reduced medicines wastage and courses on medicines optimisation. Currently he is a member of the expert panel advising on the clinical management of common infections for the National Institute for Health and Care Excellence (NICE) and works as an out-of-hours general practitioner and general practitioner trainer.

Dr Chirag Bakhai discovered his affinity for teaching while at university. Now, as a general practitioner, Strategic Lead for Long Term Conditions for an Integrated Care Board, and with regional and national leadership roles, he supports education and quality improvement at scale. He has designed and implemented programmes, interventions and innovations to help identify and address learning needs for healthcare professionals and has delivered teaching across the country, as well as influencing policy and driving efforts to improve care, support self-management and reduce inequalities.

Dr Bhavina Khatani is a general practitioner based in Hertfordshire. She acquired her interest in teaching at a young age, designing and delivering language classes to children during her teens. She has loved teaching ever since! In 2021, she gained a Masters in Health Education and joined the NMIC team. Her particular areas of interest are medically unexplained symptoms, including chronic pain, and the complex biopsychosocial factors underlying people's experiences.

CHAPTER 1

Introduction

GENERAL ADVICE

History

- Listening is the greatest skill; try not to interrupt the person's story
- What is their agenda?
- Be sensitive to nuances of how symptoms are described – they signpost the best way ahead
- When visible, the person's body language may give useful clues
- Open questions may reveal hidden concerns
- Most diagnoses are made on the history – 'Listen to the patient: they are telling you the diagnosis'

Examination

- As well as helping to make (or rule out) a diagnosis, examination provides key information for assessing how unwell the person is
- May reveal important signs but will also serve to reassure the person
- It invades their personal space – be aware of this, but implied consent is usually all that is needed

Tests

- Not usually helpful in minor illness
- Only useful if the management depends on the result
- May give false-positive results and cause unnecessary concern
- May be misleading – for example by identifying bacteria that are harmless commensals

Self-care

- Discuss the options and agree the proposed plan of management with the person
- For a choice to be genuine, the person needs to be informed about the options
- Safety-netting: explain the likely progress and ask the person to contact the most appropriate NHS service if the situation worsens, or fails to improve within a specified time, or if new symptoms start. Aim to be as specific as possible, based on the diagnosis, the evidence and your knowledge
- Handouts or sending links by text message may help people to retain information, for example, nhs.uk, patient. info, *When Should I Worry* leaflet or TARGET toolkit (see References)

Prescription

- Always check with the British National Formulary (BNF) or British National Formulary for Children (BNFC) – these may be accessible directly through your clinical IT system
- Be aware of local guidelines (so long as they are up to date) as patterns of antibiotic resistance vary nationally

Caution

- Although guidelines support clinical judgement, they can never replace experience and intuition
- Know the unique limits of your own competence and never exceed them
- Always seek help if you feel concerned
- Be alert for red flags

Red flags are factors that suggest a serious condition rather than a minor illness. Unless you are very experienced, the presence of a red flag requires referral of the person to an experienced colleague. To help you to decide on the best course of action, which depends on your expertise and place of work, we have given a brief indication of the possible serious diagnoses and appropriate management. We are aware that some of the suggested pathways may currently only be accessed via a doctor. We also recognise the challenge of finding the best course of action for a person who is remotely assessed. Consider potential delays before further assessment and treatment can begin; see if they can be avoided. One example is when urgent admission to hospital is indicated and there is no immediate risk to life; if a friend or relative is available to drive the person to hospital then that may be quicker than waiting for an ambulance to attend.

HIGH-RISK GROUPS FOR INFECTIONS

Immunosuppressed

Recovery from infection relies on a competent immune response. This can be impaired by medication or medical conditions (Box 1.1), making the past medical history an essential part of every consultation.

BOX 1.1   MORE COMMON CAUSES OF IMMUNOSUPPRESSION TO VARYING DEGREES (EXAMPLES, NOT AN EXHAUSTIVE LIST, WITH COMMON ONES IN BOLD)

Medication

- Antithyroid (e.g., carbimazole) – most people have no immunosuppression, but rarely the drug can cause severe bone marrow impairment
- Azathioprine
- **Biologic drugs** (e.g., infliximab, rituximab)
- **Chemotherapy** – and up to 6 months after
- Ciclosporin
- **Corticosteroid** (e.g., prednisolone) – will lead to a degree of immunosuppression in everyone, but mild with low doses and short courses
- **Disease-modifying antirheumatic drug** (DMARD) (e.g., methotrexate)
- **Non-steroidal anti-inflammatory drug** (NSAID) – weak immunosuppressant action that increases the risk of secondary infections where the skin is not intact
- Tacrolimus

Medical conditions

- **Diabetes** – especially if not well controlled (Box 1.2)
- **Human immunodeficiency virus** (HIV) infection
- Inherited immunodeficiency
- Leukaemia
- Lymphoma
- Malnutrition
- Neutropenia
- **Pregnancy**
- **Prematurity** – up to the age of 2
- **Sickle cell anaemia**
- **Splenectomy**

For information on checking for suspected diabetes, see Box 8.3.

BOX 1.2 PEOPLE WITH DIABETES

Even if diabetes is normally well controlled, it is associated with a greater risk of severe infections. Furthermore, infections themselves may trigger hyperglycaemia, which can acutely impair the immune response. There is a risk of diabetic ketoacidosis in those who are more susceptible (mainly people with type 1 diabetes but also some people with type 2 diabetes, particularly those who have not stopped taking their sodium-glucose linked transporter type 2 (SGLT2) inhibitor when unwell). All people with diabetes should have a care plan that tells them what to do if unwell ('sick-day rules'). The details will vary, but the principles are:

- Stop taking medications such as metformin (risk of lactic acidosis) and SGLT2 inhibitors (risk of diabetic ketoacidosis) when unwell. These can be restarted a few days after recovery
- Do not automatically reduce insulin or medications for diabetes (other than metformin and SGLT2 inhibitors) just because you are not eating much
- Keep eating as much as you are able. If you are unable to eat, drink something nutritious
- Have lots of sugar-free drinks (with sugary drinks included if blood sugars are low)
- If you think you are becoming dehydrated, seek help immediately
- If you test your blood glucose levels, do so more frequently
- If you have been advised to check for ketones, do so if your blood glucose is >17 mmol/l or you feel thirsty/breathless; a blood ketone result of >3 mmol/l requires admission urgently under Medical/ Paediatrics (probable diabetic ketoacidosis)

Frailty/long-term conditions

- Frailty describes a lack of resilience due to having less 'in-built' reserves, often due to a combination of ageing and multimorbidity. This can make people vulnerable to sudden changes in health from even seemingly minor infections
- Older adults are generally at higher risk of poor outcomes with infections than younger adults (e.g., during the first wave of the COVID-19 pandemic, those aged ≥80 were 70 times more likely to die after a positive test than people aged <40)
- Significant heart, lung, kidney, liver or neuromuscular disease all result in higher risks associated with infection

MEDICATION ADVICE

Dose of medication

The appropriate adult dose of medication for a condition is given in the text of this book. For the latest information, see the BNF and, for children, the BNFC.

Risk alerts for medications

Table 1.1 lists abbreviations found after drug names in the text where there is a significant risk of adverse events. Any drug may have potential for multiple interactions, but the majority are not clinically significant. The tags provide warnings where there is a significant risk and may vary depending on the context. For example, oral prednisolone is suitable for use in asthma for a pregnant woman where the benefit outweighs the risk, but not when it is being considered as an option to treat hay fever.

Manufacturers often advise against the use of a medication in pregnancy or breastfeeding when there is insufficient evidence of safety. Independent information sources, such as the BNF, UK Teratology Information Service (UKTIS) and Drugs and Lactation Database (LactMed) may advise that there is no evidence of harm. A balance needs to be struck to avoid denying pregnant or lactating women helpful medication whilst maintaining adequate safety for the fetus or infant.

It should be remembered that the elimination of many drugs can be affected by renal or hepatic impairment. If the person has either, check the dose of the drug in the relevant section of the BNF/BNFC.

These symbols are designed to alert you quickly and simply to prescribing issues which are common and important (Table 1.1). They cannot cover all possibilities; further information on prescribing is available in the BNF, the BNFC and the Prescribing Insights Members' section of our website.

Table 1.1 Prescribing symbols used in this book

P	**Pregnancy** risk (N.B. the woman may not yet realise that she is pregnant). Use an alternative medication known to be safe in pregnancy. If they are allergic to penicillin, alternatives include erythromycin or cefalexin (as it shares some molecular structure with penicillins, cefalexin should not be used if the person has had an anaphylactic reaction to any penicillin). Erythromycin is preferred to clarithromycin if a macrolide is needed. Information sources: BNF or UKTIS
B	**Breastfeeding** risk. The drug affects breastfeeding or is secreted in milk and is not suitable for the baby. Use an alternative medication known to be safe in breastfeeding. Information sources: BNF or LactMed
C	**Children**. The medication is either harmful to children or has a limited licence; for example, the medicine may only be licensed for children over a certain age. Information source: BNFC
I	**Interactions** likely. For example, macrolides such as clarithromycin inhibit the liver enzymes that metabolise drugs. This can result in an accumulation of another drug to potentially toxic levels. Many drugs can be affected (e.g., amlodipine, colchicine, simvastatin, ticagrelor and warfarin), so always check the BNF for any interaction before prescribing. If a macrolide is needed but clarithromycin is precluded because of interactions, consider azithromycin, which has fewer interactions because it does not interact significantly with the hepatic cytochrome P450 system. Information sources: BNF, emc, Flockhart Table
Q	**QT interval** prolonged. Avoid for anyone with a known long QT interval, or an unknown QT interval plus a family history of unexplained sudden death, or for anyone already taking another drug that prolongs the interval. A long interval between the Q and T waves on an electrocardiogram (ECG) indicates an increased risk of cardiac arrhythmias that can cause sudden death. Information sources: SADS or CredibleMeds

Websites
- BNF: bnf.nice.org.uk
- BNFC: bnfc.nice.org.uk
- CredibleMeds: www.crediblemeds.org
- emc: www.medicines.org.uk
- Flockhart Table: drug-interactions.medicine.iu.edu
- LactMed: www.ncbi.nlm.nih.gov/books/NBK501922/
- SADS: www.sads.org.uk
- UKTIS: www.uktis.org
- NMIC Resource: www.minorillness.co.uk/content/insights/

Every drug mentioned in this book has its own entry in our Prescribing Insights in the Members' section online. The voucher code in the front of this book gives you 6 months' free access. For further information and an example, refer to the end of Chapter 14.

REFERENCES

Patient Info. https://patient.info/

Royal College of General Practitioners (RCGP). 2021. TARGET antibiotics toolkit hub. https://elearning.rcgp.org.uk/course/view.php?id=553

Public Health England. 2020. Disparities in the risk and outcomes of COVID-19. https://assets.publishing.service.gov.uk/government/uploads/system/uploads/attachment_data/file/908434/Disparities_in_the_risk_and_outcomes_of_COVID_August_2020_update.pdf

When Should I Worry? 2016. www.whenshouldiworry.com *A booklet for parents about respiratory tract infections in children.*

TIPS ON REFERENCES

If you are interested in reading any of the references in this book, we have often provided a 'doi' number which will find the relevant website without too much typing. Alternatively, you could download the Google Lens app onto your phone and use it to capture the text and take you to the relevant web page. Using the Google Lens app's Homework function, crop the text until only the https://doi reference is displayed, then click Search.

CHAPTER 2

Fever and sepsis

FEVERISH ILLNESS

Sometimes fever alone is the presenting problem; it almost always signifies infection. In UK primary care, this is more likely to be viral than bacterial. A careful history can usually identify the probable source, but sometimes this is not obvious. Be aware that although most people with a flu-like illness may indeed have a simple viral infection, there are many uncommon diseases that can cause the same initial symptoms. Ask open questions to see if there could be an alternative source of infection (such as the urinary tract). This is particularly important if the history has some odd features, or if the symptoms have been present for >5 days. Fever in children is considered separately later in this chapter.

SEPSIS

RED FLAG CONDITION

BOX 2.1 SEPSIS

Sepsis is 'life-threatening organ dysfunction due to a dysregulated host response to infection'. It is hard to spot in primary care because it is rare and often presents at an early stage.

You may get the impression from the news that sepsis often affects young people. But 75% of sepsis-related deaths in England are in people aged ≥75 (Singer et al., 2019). In a Welsh study, 70% of those who died from sepsis had a 'do not attempt cardiopulmonary resuscitation' (DNA-CPR) order in place (Kopczynska et al., 2018).

Many of the 'red flags' given for different conditions in this book indicate a significant risk of sepsis. For more information, see NICE guideline NG51 (2024) and the Sepsis Toolkit of the Royal College of General Practitioners (RCGP, 2022).

Consider sepsis if the patient appears very unwell. Fever is usually present, but the very young, old or frail may have a normal temperature. Low temperature ≤36°C and altered mental state are also warning signs, especially if there are risk factors for sepsis:

- Age <1 year or >75
- Frailty
- Immunosuppression (see Chapter 1)
- Surgery or other invasive procedure in past 6 weeks
- Pregnancy (or recent termination/miscarriage)
- Breach of skin (e.g., cut, burn or skin infection)
- Intravenous drug misuse
- Indwelling lines or catheters
- Urinary retention >18 hours

History

- Duration
- High-risk group (see Chapter 1)
- New joint or muscle pain, especially in children and young people
- Headache/photophobia/drowsiness/confusion
- Rigors/shaking (increased risk of bacterial infection)
- Prostration (i.e., unable to stand up, difficulty in walking)

- Any symptoms to localise the infection:
  - Sneezing/nasal discharge
  - Sore throat
  - Earache
  - Cough
  - Skin wounds: recent operation, bites or cuts
  - Rash
  - Vomiting/diarrhoea
  - Pain (usually at the site of infection but occasionally referred elsewhere)
  - Urinary symptoms
  - Pregnant/lactating
- Travel to tropical region in last 12 months
- Exposure to rats' urine (e.g., in sewers or rivers)
- Vaccination status

Examination (modified as suggested by symptoms)

- In all people with fever:
  - Mental state – drowsiness or confusion?
  - Temperature (taking into account any recent antipyretic)
  - Heart rate
  - Respiratory rate
  - Capillary refill time (CRT) in children aged <12 years/BP in adults and older children
  - Oxygen saturation, if respiratory infection or sepsis are suspected
- Hydration
- If no focus of infection is apparent, consider examining:
  - Ears
  - Throat
  - Cervical lymph nodes
  - Chest (auscultation and percussion)
  - Gait and coordination
  - Breasts, in a lactating woman
  - Any painful area (e.g., abdomen)
  - Skin: any wounds or breaks? Look carefully for a rash (if present, does it blanch? Note that, although important to consider, the chance of a child with fever and non-blanching rash having meningococcal septicaemia is now <1% [Waterfield et al., 2020])

Tests

- If the cause of fever is not obvious, dipstick the urine for nitrites, leucocytes and blood (to avoid contaminating the whole sample, pour a little urine on the test strip). Note that most strips are incompatible with bottles containing boric acid
- However, do not diagnose a urinary tract infection on the basis of a positive dipstick in people aged >65 (see Chapter 9)
- Send midstream urine (MSU) for culture in a feverish person if dipstick test is positive, or any urinary symptoms
- Consider testing capillary blood glucose (in a person not known to have diabetes, a result >7.7 mmol/l may indicate sepsis)
- If available, consider testing capillary blood lactate (a result >2 mmol/l is suggestive of sepsis)
- People who have been identified in the highest-risk groups for adverse outcomes with COVID-19 should have access to lateral flow tests. If COVID-19 is suspected and the initial test is negative, they should then be advised to perform three tests over 3 days

- If the person travelled to a tropical area in the last 12 months, consider sending thick and thin blood films for malaria parasites, and a full blood count (FBC). If the first malaria test is negative, repeat the blood film after 12 to 24 hours. If the second test is negative, repeat the blood film again after a further 24 hours

Self-care

- If cause is apparent, give appropriate treatment
- Assume a viral cause if no other clues, fever <5 days' duration and generally well
- Advise adequate fluid intake (1.5 to 2 litres a day including food for an adult, plus extra for any fluid loss such as sweating [Wise, 2022])
- Maximise sleep and avoid over-strenuous activity
- Reduce anxiety about fever by explaining that it is produced by the body in response to an infection to boost the effective immune response (Wrotek et al., 2021)
    - Fever itself does not cause any harm and may aid recovery. It is important to make people/parents aware that the fever caused by an infection is not dangerous but is 'a sign that the immune system is busy'
    - It is not necessary to lower a fever; the relevant indication for paracetamol or ibuprofen in the BNFC is limited to 'pyrexia with discomfort'
    - The height of the fever does not predict the seriousness of the illness; in adults, the higher the body temperature the **lower** the mortality with sepsis (Rumbus et al., 2017) or bacterial infection (Yamamoto et al., 2016)
- Advise on what to do if symptoms worsen, change or persist: 'safety-netting'. Explain the warning signs of sepsis and any relevant complication, give a link or a handout, and advise the person to stay with someone who can check on them regularly
- If the person has diabetes, explain 'sick-day rules' and optimise/maintain glucose control (see Box 1.2 in Chapter 1)

BOX 2.2 FEVER IN PREGNANCY

It has previously been recommended that a pregnant woman with a fever should take regular paracetamol because of concerns that a fever may adversely affect the fetus. This is a difficult issue; there are (unsurprisingly) no relevant randomised controlled trials, and observational studies are inherently unable to disentangle the effects of the infection itself from the effects of the resulting fever (Graham, 2020).

Some specific infections are known to carry an increased risk of miscarriage (e.g., mumps, rubella, parvovirus, pityriasis rosea). These infections apart, feverish illness in pregnancy is not associated with an increased risk of miscarriage or stillbirth (Andersen et al., 2002). And a Danish study of over 77,000 women (Sass et al., 2017) found no evidence of an increased risk of congenital malformations.

Paracetamol has been generally regarded as safe in pregnancy and is now in common use. The percentage of women who reported taking paracetamol during pregnancy increased from 1.3% in 1985 to 42% in 2015 (Zafeiri et al., 2022). However, concerns have been raised that prenatal exposure to paracetamol may increase the risk of neurodevelopmental disorders (Bauer et al., 2021). The Summary of Product Characteristics (SmPC) data sheet for paracetamol was therefore amended in 2019 to state: 'Paracetamol can be used during pregnancy if clinically needed however it should be used at the lowest effective dose for the shortest possible time and at the lowest possible frequency' (emc, 2023).

To this, NMIC would add:

1. The risk of malformations resulting from any medication taken in pregnancy is greatest in the first trimester

2. In pregnancy there is no evidence of benefit from lowering a fever, and so the only evidence-based indication for paracetamol is pain

---

Antipyretics

- Antipyretic medicines cannot prevent febrile convulsions (Hashimoto et al., 2021)
- The distress of an unwell child may be unrelated to the fever (Corrard et al., 2017)

- The aim of giving an antipyretic should be to improve a child's overall comfort rather than focusing on the normalisation of body temperature (Sullivan et al., 2011)
- Suppressing fever may increase the spread of infection because people can feel well enough to mix with others (Earn et al., 2014)
- Antipyretics do not affect the risk of death and serious adverse events in adults (Holgersson et al., 2022)

Prescription

- If antibiotics are indicated, prescribe in line with national guidelines or your local formulary (provided that it is up to date)
- For a flu-like illness, antiviral medicines (oseltamivir, zanamivir) may be recommended in primary care (UKHSA, 2021), but only when the Chief Medical Officer has announced that influenza is circulating in the community. However, they shorten the duration of the illness by <1 day and do not significantly reduce the risk of complications or hospital admission (Heneghan et al., 2016). For this reason, the World Health Organization (WHO) does not recommend their use in primary care (WHO, 2022)
- If people identified as being at high risk of adverse outcomes with COVID-19 test positive, they should contact 111 or their GP practice, who can then assess eligibility and refer for specific treatment (see Chapter 4)

 RED FLAGS

Feverish illness

- Severe illness, rigors, or prostration (unable to stand up) (*likely sepsis; admit very urgently under Medical/Paediatrics*)
- Urinary symptoms (*likely pyelonephritis or prostatitis; refer to experienced colleague*)
- Unexplained fever lasting ≥5 days (*unlikely to be viral; assess for urinary tract infection (UTI) or secondary bacterial infection. In a young child, check for signs of Kawasaki disease; see Box 2.3*)
- Pregnancy (*consider pyelonephritis and listeriosis; refer to experienced colleague. In the first trimester of pregnancy, there is concern that fever may increase the risk of neural tube defects such as spina bifida in the baby (Graham, 2020). However, there are also concerns that paracetamol in pregnancy increases the risk of neurodevelopmental disorders (Bauer et al., 2021). See Box 2.2*)
- Lactating (*mastitis may cause flu-like symptoms in a breastfeeding woman with only minimal signs in the breast; examine breasts and follow advice in Chapter 10*)
- Travel to tropical area in last 12 months (*malaria or other tropical disease; refer to experienced colleague*)
- Exposure to rats' urine (*risk of leptospirosis; arrange polymerase chain reaction (PCR) test and consider doxycycline*)
- Neutropenia or current chemotherapy (*high risk from infection; admit very urgently under Medical/Paediatrics*)
- High-risk for sepsis (*see Box 2.1 for potential risk factors; refer to experienced colleague*)
- Dehydration (*may need IV fluids; admit urgently under Medical/Paediatrics*)
- Photophobia, drowsiness, neck or back stiffness or non-blanching (purpuric) rash (*possible meningitis; give benzylpenicillin IV/IM (<1 year, 300 mg; 1–9 years, 600 mg; 10 years to adult, 1.2 g) and admit very urgently under Medical/Paediatrics*)

 RED FLAG CONDITION

BOX 2.3 KAWASAKI DISEASE

A form of vasculitis, thought to be due to an abnormal immune response to an infection, that affects children aged <5 years and may cause permanent damage to the heart (particularly the coronary arteries).

The key symptom is a prolonged fever lasting ≥5 days, and some of the following:
- Bilateral painless red conjunctivae
- Fissured lips, strawberry tongue
- Fingers and toes red or swollen, then peeling
- Polymorphous rash on trunk
- Cervical lymphadenopathy

If suspected, admit urgently under Paediatrics.

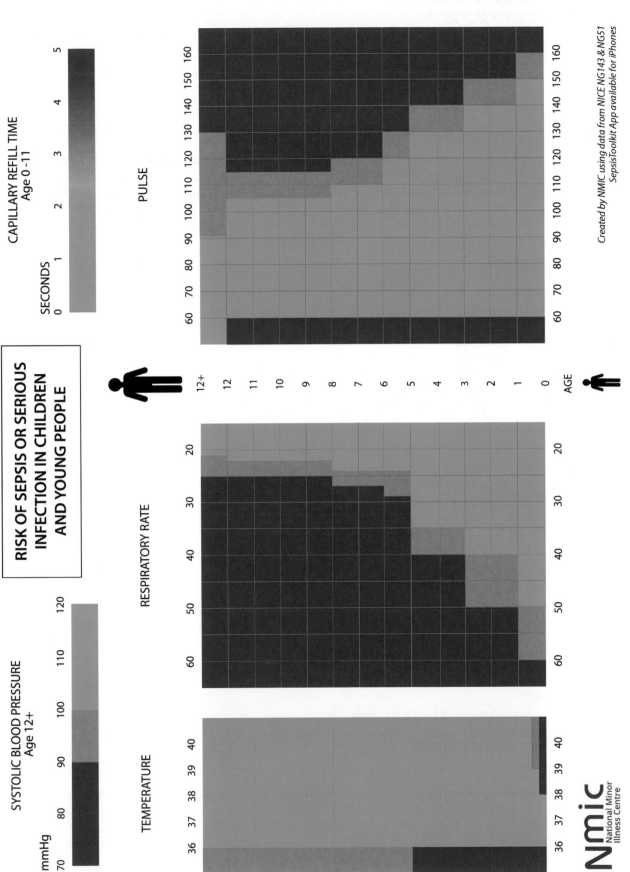

Figure 2.1 Risk of sepsis: the NMIC Sepsis Toolkit

Action for suspected sepsis

- Send urgently to hospital. If dialling 999 for an ambulance, use the word 'sepsis'
- Alert the hospital team
- Give high-flow oxygen in adults, if needed, to achieve saturations of ≥94%
- People with moderate-to-severe chronic obstructive pulmonary disease (COPD) should have oxygen saturation monitored to achieve 88%–92%
- Give oxygen to children if saturations are ≤90%
- If the journey to hospital is likely to take ≥1 hour:
    - If the cause is known, consider giving an appropriate **parenteral** antibiotic e.g., benzyl penicillin for meningococcal septicaemia or flucloxacillin for cellulitis
    - If (as is often the case) the cause is not apparent, give IM or IV ceftriaxone, 80 mg/kg, maximum dose 4 g (reduce dose to 50 mg/kg in baby aged <28 days)

FEVERISH ILLNESS IN CHILDREN UNDER FIVE: THE NICE 'TRAFFIC LIGHT' SYSTEM

We recommend that you study the summary of the National Institute for Health and Care Excellence (NICE) guideline NG143 (revised in 2021), which provides a framework for the assessment of feverish children. There are some differences in the reference ranges for pulse and respiratory rate between this guideline and NG51. We suggest that in this case you follow the advice from NG51, as in Figure 2.1, because it is more recent and more detailed. We would like to draw your attention to the following points.

The routine assessment of a feverish child should always include:

- Temperature (taken with an axillary thermometer in babies aged <4 weeks)
- Heart rate
- Respiratory rate
- Capillary refill time

A temperature of ≥38°C in a baby aged <3 months is an indication for hospital assessment. However, whether this should apply in the 48 hours after a meningitis B (Men B) vaccination is controversial (Vesikari et al., 2013; NICE, 2021). Our assessment is that most primary care clinicians would not routinely refer a feverish (but otherwise well) baby in the 48 hours following Men B vaccination. However, in the absence of clear advice from NICE, this decision should be taken after a face-to-face assessment by an experienced clinician.

A temperature of ≥39°C in a baby aged <6 months may be a sign of sepsis (amber – intermediate risk). Over the age of 6 months, a high fever alone is not a sign of sepsis, but a low temperature of ≤36°C in an unwell person of any age suggests sepsis. Antipyretic medicine is sometimes given to children by clinicians as part of an assessment, because of a misconception that a good response is thought to exclude serious illness. This is a dangerous assumption, and there is no evidence to support it (King, 2013; NICE, 2017; Gelernter et al., 2021).

Parents often worry that a rash with fever equals meningitis.

- Meningococcal infection is now very rare in the UK; the incidence has dropped by more than 70% since 2012 (UKHSA, 2023)
- It is an illness of rapid onset over a few hours and is more likely to affect children aged <5 years, with symptoms including fever, vomiting, headache, poor concentration and muscle pain. Apicella (2023) provides a useful summary
- Explore concerns and, provided that there is no evidence of meningitis, reassure them accordingly

The *Healthier Together* website (https://www.what0-18.nhs.uk/) has specific paediatric pathways for a range of common conditions (regional variations may not have a 'professionals' option). These pathways give extra red, amber and green symptoms which are specific to the condition. It also has the useful facility of sending a condition-specific self-care link (with Google Translate and Recite Me options) directly to the parent's phone.

Urgency of referral

If using remote assessment:

- A child with red features in Figure 2.1 or Table 2.1 should be seen as soon as possible (and certainly within 2 hours)

- A child with amber features should be seen urgently within a few hours

If using face-to-face assessment:

- A child with red features should be admitted for paediatric assessment (unless fever is the only sign in the 48 hours following Men B vaccination; see previous section)
- A child with amber features but no obvious diagnosis should be seen by an experienced clinician for assessment of the need for admission. If not admitted, appropriate treatment, careful safety-netting and follow-up should be arranged

Table 2.1 Traffic light system for identifying risk of serious illness in under 5s (NICE NG143)

	Green – low risk	Amber – intermediate risk	Red – high risk
Colour (of skin, lips or tongue)	• Normal colour	• Pallor reported by parent/carer	• Pale/mottled/ashen/blue
Activity	• Responds normally to social cues • Content/smiles • Stays awake or awakens quickly • Strong normal cry/not crying	• Not responding normally to social cues • No smile • Wakes only with prolonged stimulation • Decreased activity	• No response to social cues • Appears ill to a healthcare professional • Does not wake or if roused does not stay awake • Weak, high-pitched or continuous cry

Respiratory		• Nasal flaring
		• Tachypnoea:
		  – RR >50 breaths/minute, age 6–12 months
		  – RR >40 breaths/minute, age >12 months
		• Oxygen saturation ≤95% in air
		• Crackles in the chest
			• Grunting
			• Tachypnoea: RR >60 breaths/minute
			• Moderate or severe chest indrawing

Circulation and hydration	• Normal skin and eyes
	• Moist mucous membranes
		• Tachycardia:
		  – >160 beats/minute, age <12 months
		  – >150 beats/minute, age 12–24 months
		  – >140 beats/minute, age 2–5 years
		• CRT ≥3 seconds
		• Dry mucous membranes
		• Poor feeding in infants
		• Reduced urine output
			• Reduced skin turgor

Other	• None of the amber or red symptoms or signs	• Age 3–6 months, temperature ≥39°C • Fever for ≥5 days • Rigors • Swelling of a limb or joint • Non-weight bearing limb/not using an extremity	• Age <3 months, temperature ≥38°C* • Non-blanching rash • Bulging fontanelle • Neck stiffness • Status epilepticus • Focal neurological signs • Focal seizures
CRT, capillary refill time; RR, respiratory rate * Some vaccinations have been found to induce fever in children aged under 3 months			
This traffic light table should be used in conjunction with the recommendations in the NICE guideline on feverish illness in the under 5s			

REFERENCES

Andersen, A.M.N., Vastrup, P., Wohlfahrt, J., et al. 2002. Fever in pregnancy and risk of fetal death: a cohort study. *Lancet*; 360(9345):1552–6. https://doi.org/10.1016/S0140-6736(02)11518-2 *No increased risk of miscarriage or stillbirth.*

Apicella, M. 2023. Clinical manifestations of meningococcal infection. https://medilib.ir/uptodate/show/1300 *A useful review.*

Bauer, A.Z., Swan, S.H., Kriebel, D., et al. 2021. Paracetamol use during pregnancy — a call for precautionary action. *Nat Rev Endocrinol*; 17(12):757–66. https://doi.org/10.1038/s41574-021-00553-7 *Prenatal exposure to paracetamol could increase the risks of some neurodevelopmental, reproductive and urogenital disorders.*

Clark, A., Cannings-John, R., Blyth, M., et al. 2022. Accuracy of the NICE traffic light system in children presenting to general practice: a retrospective cohort study. *Br J Gen Pract*; 72(719), e398–e404. https://doi.org/10.3399/BJGP.2021.0633 *The traffic light categories of 6703 acutely unwell children aged under 5 years in primary care were linked with hospital admissions in the subsequent 7 days. Only 0.3% had serious illness, mostly pneumonia. The sensitivity and specificity of red and amber combined (versus green) was 100% and 5.7%, respectively.*

Corrard, F., Copin, C., Wollner, A., et al. 2017. Sickness behavior in feverish children is independent of the severity of fever. An observational, multicenter study. *PLOS One*; 12(3):e0171670. https://doi.org/10.1371/journal.pone.0171670 *The distress of an unwell child may be unrelated to their fever.*

Earn, D.J.D., Andrews, P.W., and Bolker, B.M. 2014. Population-level effects of suppressing fever. *Proc R Soc B*; 281(1778). https://doi.org/10.1098/rspb.2013.2570 *Suppressing fever is likely to increase the spread of infection, because people feel well enough to go out and mix with others.*

emc. 2023. SmPC for paracetamol 500mg tablets. https://www.medicines.org.uk/emc/product/9128/smpc#gref

Gelernter, R., Ophir, N., Goldman, M., et al. 2021. Fever response to ibuprofen in viral and bacterial childhood infections. *Am J Emerg Med*; 46:591–4. https://doi.org/10.1016/j.ajem.2020.11.036 *Failure of fever to respond to ibuprofen administration is not indicative of serious bacterial infections in children under 4 years of age.*

Graham Jr, J.M. 2020. Update on the gestational effects of maternal hyperthermia. *Birth Defects Res*; 112(12):943–52. https://doi.org/10.1002/bdr2.1696 *A review of epidemiological studies supports the causal nature of the relationship between maternal fever and specific birth defects.*

Hashimoto, R., Suto, M., Tsuji, M., et al. 2021. Use of antipyretics for preventing febrile seizure recurrence in children: a systematic review and meta-analysis. *Eur J Pediatr*; 180(4):987–97. https://doi.org/10.1007/s00431-020-03845-8 *There is clearly no role for antipyretic prophylaxis in preventing febrile seizures during distant fever episodes.*

Heneghan, C.J., Onakpoya, I., Jones, M.A., et al. 2016. Neuraminidase inhibitors for influenza: a systematic review and meta-analysis of regulatory and mortality data. *Health Technol Assess*; 20(42). https://doi.org/10.3310/hta20420 *No reduction in mortality.*

Holgersson, J., Ceric, A., Sethi, N., et al. 2022. Fever therapy in febrile adults: systematic review with meta-analyses and trial sequential analyses. *BMJ*; 378:e069620. https://doi.org/10.1136/bmj-2021-069620 *No evidence that antipyretics delay recovery in adults with fever.*

Jolliffe, D.A., Faustini, S.E., Holt, H., et al. 2022. Determinants of antibody responses to SARS-CoV-2 vaccines: population-based longitudinal study (COVIDENCE UK). *Vaccines*; 10(10):1601. https://doi.org/10.3390/vaccines10101601 *Fever indicates a good response to COVID vaccination; antipyretics do not affect this.*

King, D. 2013. Question 2: Does a failure to respond to antipyretics predict serious illness in children with a fever? *Arch Dis Child*; 98(8):644–6. http://dx.doi.org/10.1136/archdischild-2013-304497 Full text available at researchgate.net. *The majority of published evidence indicates that clinicians cannot rely on response to antipyretics to predict serious illness in febrile children.*

Kopczynska, M., Sharif, B., Cleaver, S., et al. 2018. Sepsis-related deaths in the at-risk population on the wards: attributable fraction of mortality in a large point-prevalence study. *BMC Res Notes*; 11(1):720. https://doi.org/10.1186/s13104-018-3819-2 *A large proportion of deaths from sepsis are in people with life-limiting conditions.*

Koufoglou, E., Kourlaba, G., and Michos, A. 2021. Effect of prophylactic administration of antipyretics on the immune response to pneumococcal conjugate vaccines in children: a systematic review. *Pneumonia*; 13(1):7. https://doi.org/10.1186/s41479-021-00085-8 *Up to 12% of children who were given paracetamol with their pneumococcal vaccine did not have protective levels of antibody.*

NICE. 2021. NG143. Fever in under 5s: assessment and initial management. https://www.nice.org.uk/guidance/ng143 *This guidance was revised in 2017 to acknowledge that 'Some vaccinations have been found to induce fever in children aged under 3 months'. Unfortunately no guidance is given about when such a baby with post-vaccination fever, but no other signs of serious illness, can safely be managed in primary care.*

NICE. 2024. NG51. Sepsis: recognition, diagnosis and early management. https://www.nice.org.uk/guidance/ng51

Nijman, R.G., Jorgensen, R., Levin, M., et al. 2020. Management of children with fever at risk for pediatric sepsis: a prospective study in pediatric emergency care. *Front Pediatr*; 8. https://www.frontiersin.org/articles/10.3389/fped.2020.548154 *The vast majority of children arriving in an emergency department with positive sepsis indicators do not have serious disease.*

RCGP (Royal College of General Practitioners). 2022. Sepsis Toolkit. https://elearning.rcgp.org.uk/mod/book/view.php?id=12896&chapterid=544

Rumbus, Z., Matics, R., Hegyi, P., et al. 2017. Fever is associated with reduced, hypothermia with increased mortality in septic patients: a meta-analysis of clinical trials. *PLOS One*; 12(1):e0170152. https://doi.org/10.1371/journal.pone.0170152 *Adults with sepsis who had a fever had a 50% lower mortality than those with normal temperatures.*

Saleh, E., Moody, M.A., and Walter, E.B. 2016. Effect of antipyretic analgesics on immune responses to vaccination. *Hum Vaccines Immunother*; 12(9):2391–402. https://doi.org/10.1080/21645515.2016.1183077 *A reduced immune response to vaccines has only been noted following prophylactic antipyretics before primary vaccination with novel antigens; it disappears following booster immunisation.*

Sass, L., Urhoj, S.K., Kjærgaard, J., et al. 2017. Fever in pregnancy and the risk of congenital malformations: a cohort study. *BMC Pregnancy Childbirth*; 17(1):413. https://doi.org/10.1186/s12884-017-1585-0 *No increased risk was found.*

Singer, M., Inada-Kim, M., and Shankar-Hari, M. 2019. Sepsis hysteria: excess hype and unrealistic expectations. *Lancet*; 394(10208):1513–514. https://doi.org/10.1016/S0140-6736(19)32483-3 *Age-specific data on sepsis cases and deaths.*

Sullivan, J.E., and Farrar, H.C. 2011. Fever and antipyretic use in children. *Pediatrics*; 127(3):580. https://doi.org/10.1542/peds.2010-3852 *The primary goal of treating the febrile child should be to improve the child's overall comfort rather than focus on the normalisation of body temperature.*

UKHSA (UK Health Security Agency). 2013. Vaccine safety and adverse events following immunisation: the green book, chapter 8. https://www.gov.uk/government/publications/vaccine-safety-and-adverse-events-following-immunisation-the-green-book-chapter-8 *See page 56 for advice on antipyretics and vaccination.*

UKHSA. 2021. Influenza: treatment and prophylaxis using anti-viral agents. https://www.gov.uk/government/publications/influenza-treatment-and-prophylaxis-using-anti-viral-agents *UKHSA are still recommending the use of antivirals in primary care, despite the lack of evidence. See WHO reference below.*

UKHSA. 2023. Invasive meningococcal disease in England: annual laboratory confirmed reports for epidemiological year 2021 to 2022. https://www.gov.uk/government/publications/meningococcal-disease-laboratory-confirmed-cases-in-england-in-2021-to-2022/invasive-meningococcal-disease-in-england-annual-laboratory-confirmed-reports-for-epidemiological-year-2021-to-2022

Vesikari, T., Esposito, S., Prymula, R., et al. 2013. Immunogenicity and safety of an investigational multicomponent, recombinant, meningococcal serogroup B vaccine (4CmenB) administered concomitantly with routine infant and child vaccinations: results of two randomised trials. *Lancet*; 381(9869):825–35. https://doi.org/10.1016/S0140-6736(12)61961-8 *Without prophylactic paracetamol, 77% of babies developed a fever after compound vaccination (including Men B), which would be sufficient to trigger admission to hospital under the guidance of NICE NG143. With paracetamol, this percentage dropped to 40%.*

Waterfield, T., Maney, J. A., Fairley, D., et al. 2020. Validating clinical practice guidelines for the management of children with non-blanching rashes in the UK (PiC): a prospective, multicentre cohort study. *Lancet Infect Dis*; 21(4):569–77. https://doi.org/10.1016/S1473-3099(20)30474-6 *Of 1329 children with fever and petechial rash, only 19 had meningococcal infection.*

WHO. 2022. WHO model list of essential medicines. https://www.who.int/publications/i/item/WHO-MHP-HPS-EML-2021.02 *Oseltamivir is recommended only for 'severe illness due to confirmed or suspected influenza virus infection in critically ill hospitalized patients'.*

Wise, J. 2022. Sixty seconds on . . . hydration. *BMJ*; 379. https://doi.org/10.1136/bmj.o2869 *Many conferences and articles urging us to drink more fluids have been sponsored by Hydration for Health, an organisation created by a company which produces bottled water.*

Wrotek, S., LeGrand, E.K., Dzialuk, A., et al. 2021. Let fever do its job: the meaning of fever in the pandemic era. *Evol Med Public Health*; 9(1):26–35. https://doi.org/10.1093/emph/eoaa044 *A review of the benefits of fever in infection.*

Yamamoto, S., Yamazaki, S., Shimizu, T., et al. 2016. Body temperature at the emergency department as a predictor of mortality in patients with bacterial infection. *Medicine*; 95(21). https://doi.org/doi: 10.1097/MD.0000000000003628 *Inverse relationship between fever and mortality.*

Zafeiri, A., Raja, E.A., Mitchell, R.T., et al. 2022. Maternal over-the-counter analgesics use during pregnancy and adverse perinatal outcomes: cohort study of 151,141 singleton pregnancies. *BMJ Open*; 12(5):e048092. https://doi.org/10.1136/bmjopen-2020-048092 *There is an increased risk of malformations with analgesic use in pregnancy.*

CHAPTER 3

Respiratory tract infections

Cough is a very common problem; other symptoms may accompany it and help to make a diagnosis. The person may seek help because the cough is persistent, interferes with sleep or because of anxiety that infection is 'going to the chest'. Quite often a friend or a relative has suggested that the person should seek medical help. Mothers may fear that their children may choke in the night.

ACUTE COUGH

History

- Duration
- Dry/productive/wheezy
- Hoarseness
- Colour of sputum, and if bloodstained (red or rusty) or frothy
- Fever
- Chest pain (and location)
- Breathlessness
- Previous similar episodes (how treated and what happened)
- Smoking (how much, duration)
- Immunosuppression
- Medication (e.g., angiotensin-converting enzyme [ACE] inhibitor, expectorant)

Examination

- Temperature
- Heart rate
- CRT in children aged <12 years/BP in adults and older children
- Respiratory rate
- Oxygen saturation
- Cyanosis (bluish tinge to fingers or lips, indicating poor oxygenation)
- Subcostal/intercostal recession (especially in babies)
- Use of accessory muscles
- Percussion
- Crackles or wheezing in chest (and where located)
- Asymmetrical breath sounds/bronchial breathing

Tests

- Peak expiratory flow rate (PEFR) if wheezing in adult or child aged >7 years (see later section on Asthma Exacerbation)
- C-reactive protein (CRP) point-of-care test if available and a diagnosis of pneumonia is uncertain
- Sputum culture is unhelpful except in special cases (e.g., cystic fibrosis, chronic obstructive pulmonary disease (COPD), bronchiectasis, or if tuberculosis (TB) is suspected)
- Consider chest x-ray (CXR) if any of the following:
  - Smoker aged >50
  - Cough duration >3 weeks
  - Sputum bloodstained
- Note that a normal CXR does not exclude lung cancer; further investigation is needed if there is clinical concern

SPECIFIC TYPES OF COUGH

Acute cough (<3 weeks' duration) may be due to:

- Upper respiratory tract infection (URTI; e.g., the common cold [viral]; see Chapter 5)
- COVID-19
- Acute bronchitis (usually viral)
- Acute laryngitis (viral), associated with hoarseness
- Pneumonia (bacterial or viral)
- Exacerbation of COPD or bronchiectasis (viral or bacterial)
- Exacerbation of asthma (viral)
- Bronchiolitis in children (viral)
- Croup in children (viral)
- Pulmonary embolism (unilateral pleuritic chest pain, dry cough, dyspnoea and sometimes haemoptysis, may follow lower limb deep vein thrombosis [DVT]; risk factors include previous DVT, cancer, recent surgery, immobility and pregnancy/within 6 weeks postpartum)
- Remember that the cough of more chronic causes will always seem acute if you see the person during the first 3 weeks

A persistent or relapsing cough may occur in:

- Post-viral cough (which may last for several weeks)
- Asthma (young children may present with cough without wheezing, often worse at night/early morning)
- Heavy smokers (but consider COPD or cancer)
- Lung cancer (a persistent cough in a smoker is suspicious, particularly if associated with chest pain, haemoptysis or weight loss)
- Allergic rhinitis (will often have typical 'hay fever' symptoms and seasonal timing if due to pollen)
- Acid reflux (may be accompanied by sore throat or heartburn symptoms; however, may be 'silent' with no indigestion pain or other typical symptoms)
- Upper-airway cough syndrome (previously called post-nasal drip)
- ACE inhibitor use – drug names ending in –pril, e.g., ramipril. (If the cough goes away immediately after stopping the drug, then you can be sure the drug was **not** responsible as it would typically take weeks to resolve. Remember the cough can occur in people who have been taking the drug for years)
- Heart failure (a typical history of being worse when lying down and producing frothy, pink or white, non-purulent sputum; may have fine crackles at both lung bases on examination. Usually a previous history of heart disease and/or hypertension)
- Pertussis (whooping cough; see later section)
- *Mycoplasma pneumoniae* (an unusual infection that occurs in cycles of 3–5 years and causes a cough that may last for 3 months. It is sensitive to clarithromycin or doxycycline but not amoxicillin; a 2-week course is necessary)
- TB; consider this in contacts of people with TB and people born (or who have spent time living) in Asia or Africa. It can be reactivated when immunosuppressed and may be accompanied by weight loss and night sweats
- Cough hypersensitivity syndrome (cough triggered by, e.g., cold air, tobacco smoke or perfume)
- Habit/tic

Self-care for coughs

- Most acute coughs are due to URTIs or acute bronchitis
- Advise that acute cough can persist for 3–4 weeks. People may expect proprietary cough medicines to cure the cough and come for something stronger because brand X 'hasn't worked'. They need gentle re-education on the likely effectiveness of these medicines
- The following may provide some symptomatic relief:
  - Simple linctus can be helpful and is unlikely to cause harm

- For people aged ≥12 years, NICE (2019) recommends over-the-counter cough medicines containing the expectorant guaifenesin (although expectorants can stimulate sputum production and contribute to a persistent cough)
- Pelargonium extract (e.g., Kaloba) has been shown to reduce sputum production in acute bronchitis in 11 manufacturer-sponsored trials (Timmer et al., 2013); there is some evidence to support using *Andrographis paniculate*, ivy, primrose or thyme herbal medicines (Wagner et al., 2015), but they may be difficult to obtain. The interactions of herbal medicines are not well understood, so they are best avoided if other regular medicines (particularly warfarin) are taken
- Menthol, either inhaled or in a linctus, appears to have a short-lived cough suppressant effect (Morice et al., 1994)
- Soothing drinks, e.g., honey and lemon (do not advise honey for child aged <1 year)
- Dark chocolate contains around 800 mg of theobromine per 100 g. A dose of 300 mg (nearly half a 100 g bar) twice daily has cough suppressant activity (Morice et al., 2017), although it comes with about 300 kcal!

- Adequate fluid intake
- Stop smoking (but warn that this may cause a transient increase in coughing); includes parents of coughing child
- Steam inhalations are no longer recommended due to the risk of scalding. However, this risk can be minimised by steaming up a bathroom by running a hot shower, or using one of the many humidified air devices available
- Remember to give safety-netting advice about 'second sickening'; bacterial secondary infection can occur after a viral respiratory tract infection

References

Abuelgasim, H., Albury, C., and Lee, J. 2021. Effectiveness of honey for symptomatic relief in upper respiratory tract infections: a systematic review and meta-analysis. *BMJ EBM*; 26(2):57. https://doi.org/10.1136/bmjebm-2020-111336

Dicpinigaitis, P. 2006. Angiotensin converting enzyme inhibitor-induced cough: ACCP evidence-based clinical practice guidelines. *Chest*; 129(1 Suppl): 169S–173S. https://doi.org/10.1378/chest.129.1_suppl.169S

Morice, A., Marshall, A., Higgins, K., et al. 1994. Effect of inhaled menthol on citric acid induced cough in normal subjects. *Thorax*; 49(10):1024. https://doi.org/10.1136/thx.49.10.1024

Morice, A., McGarvey, L., Pavord, I., et al. 2017. Theobromine for the treatment of persistent cough: a randomised, multicentre, double-blind, placebo-controlled clinical trial. *J Thorac Dis*; 9(7). https://doi.org/10.21037/jtd.2017.06.18

NICE. 2019. NG120. Cough (acute): antimicrobial prescribing. www.nice.org.uk/guidance/ng120

Scarborough, A., Scarborough, O., Abdi, H., et al. 2021. Steam inhalation: more harm than good? Perspective from a UK burns centre. *Burns*; 47(3):721–7. https://doi.org/10.1016/j.burns.2020.08.010

Timmer, A., Günther, J., Motschall, E., et al. 2013. *Pelargonium sidoides* extract for treating acute respiratory tract infections. *Cochrane Database Syst Rev*; 10:CD006323. https://doi.org/10.1002/14651858.CD006323.pub3

Usmani, O., Belvisi, M., Patel, H., et al. 2005. Theobromine inhibits sensory nerve activation and cough. *FASEB J*; 19:231-3. https://doi.org/10.1096/fj.04-1990fje

Wagner, L., Cramer, H., Klose, P., et al. 2015. Herbal medicine for cough: a systematic review and meta-analysis. *Forsch Komplementmed*; 22(6):359–68. https://doi.org/10.1159/000442111

ACUTE BRONCHITIS

- A lower respiratory tract infection of adults or children (90% viral) which affects the upper air passages
- This is the commonest diagnosis in acute cough, where the cough is the predominant symptom (i.e., without symptoms suggestive of an URTI [e.g., blocked/discharging nose, sore throat]). See Figure 3.1

History

- Cough, possibly with sputum
- Fever
- Wheeze or breathlessness

Examination

- Temperature (may be raised)
- Oxygen saturation (usually normal unless chronic lung disease)

- Heart rate and respiratory rate (usually normal)
- CRT in children aged <12 years/BP in adults and older children (usually normal)

Action

- See earlier section on Self-care for coughs
- An antibiotic is not usually indicated (Box 3.1)

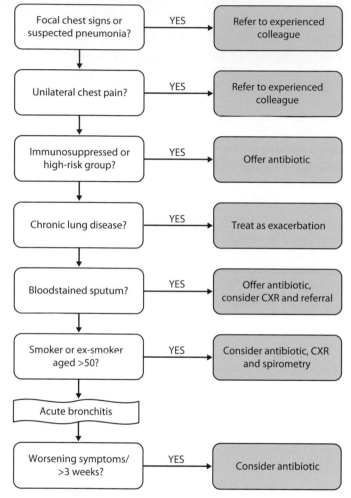

Figure 3.1 Adult with acute cough – is it acute bronchitis?

💊 BOX 3.1 ANTIBIOTICS FOR ACUTE BRONCHITIS

Prescribe an antibiotic if:

- Seriously ill
- High-risk group for severe infection, including immunosuppression (see Chapter 1)
- Bloodstained sputum

Consider an antibiotic if:

- Smoker aged >50 (may have undiagnosed COPD – consider CXR now, and then spirometry 6 weeks after recovery from acute infection)
- Prolonged (>3 weeks) or worsening symptoms
- Comorbidities such as diabetes or heart, lung, liver, kidney or neuromuscular disease
- Hospital admission for relevant cause in the last year

Antibiotic choice

- Doxycycline[PBC] for 5 days for adults (200 mg on first day then 100 mg daily for 4 more days)
- Amoxicillin for 5 days in children or pregnant women (500 mg three times daily for adults)
- Alternative: clarithromycin[PIQ] for 5 days (250–500 mg twice daily for adults)

RED FLAGS

- Persistent symptoms (*consider whooping cough, tuberculosis and lung cancer; consider CXR and refer to experienced colleague*)
- Cough with unexplained weight loss (*urgent CXR and refer to experienced colleague*)
- Previous asbestos exposure (*possible lung cancer or mesothelioma; urgent CXR*)
- Age >40 with unexplained haemoptysis (*suspected lung cancer; Urgent Suspected Cancer [USC] referral to Chest Clinic*)

References

Cornford, C., Morgan, M., and Ridsdale, L. 1993. Why do mothers consult when their children cough? *Fam Pract*; 10(2):193–6. https://doi.org/10.1093/fampra/10.2.193 *An old paper (but still the best) which gives fascinating insights into parents' concerns.*

Johnson, G., and Helman, C. 2004. Remedy or cure? Lay beliefs about over-the-counter medicines for coughs and colds. *BJGP*; 54:98–102. http://bjgp.org/content/54/499/98 *Common confusion between the ability of a medicine to relieve symptoms, and its ability to cure a disease or to hasten recovery.*

Little, P., Stuart, B., Smith, S., et al. 2017. Antibiotic prescription strategies and adverse outcome for uncomplicated lower respiratory tract infections: prospective cough complication cohort (3C) study. *BMJ*; 357:j2148. https://doi.org/10.1136/bmj.j2148

NICE. 2019. NG120. Cough (acute): antimicrobial prescribing. www.nice.org.uk/guidance/ng120

NICE. 2021. NG12. Suspected cancer: recognition and referral. www.nice.org.uk/guidance/ng12

NICE CKS. 2021. Chest infections – adult. https://cks.nice.org.uk/topics/chest-infections-adult

Smith, S., Fahey, T., Smucny, J., et al. 2017. Antibiotics for acute bronchitis. *Cochrane Database Syst Rev*; 6:CD000245. https://doi.org/10.1002/14651858.CD000245.pub4

LARYNGITIS

A viral infection of adults and children

History

- Hoarseness
- Sore throat (worse on swallowing)
- Fever
- Headache
- Dry irritating cough

Examination

- Usually normal apart from fever and hoarse voice

Self-care

- Rest the voice; speak as little as possible, don't whisper
- Advise that symptoms may last up to a week
- Avoid smoky environments
- Drink adequate fluids

- Try not to cough more than essential
- Take paracetamol or ibuprofen[P] if needed for headache or throat pain

 RED FLAGS

- Age ≥45 years with unexplained hoarseness for more than 3 weeks (*USC referral to Head and Neck Team*)
- Actual difficulty swallowing (not related to pain). This may be worse for solids than liquids (*USC referral to Gastroenterology*)

References

NICE. 2012. NG12. Suspected cancer: recognition and referral. www.nice.org.uk/guidance/ng12

Reveiz, L., and Cardona, A.F. 2015. Antibiotics for acute laryngitis in adults. *Cochrane Database Syst Rev*; 5:CD004783. https://doi.org/10.1002/14651858.CD004783.pub5

PNEUMONIA

- An infection of the lung tissue, usually bacterial
- High mortality
- Not a minor illness and should be managed by an experienced practitioner

History

- Fever
- Rigors
- Cough
- Breathlessness
- Bloodstained or rusty sputum (suggests *Streptococcus pneumoniae*)
- Unilateral chest pain
- Muscle or joint pains

Examination

- Temperature
- Heart rate (likely tachycardia)
- Respiratory rate (likely to be raised)
- Oxygen saturation
- CRT in children aged <12 years/BP in adults and older children
- There may be focal chest signs (e.g., dullness on percussion, bronchial breathing, coarse crackles)
- Elderly people may have non-specific symptoms and are less likely to have fever

Tests

- Consider CRP point-of-care test if available and there is diagnostic uncertainty (see Table 3.1)
- If smoker aged >50, arrange CXR now and then spirometry 6 weeks after recovery (if CXR suggests pneumonia, repeat after 6 weeks to confirm resolution and check for underlying cancer)

Table 3.1 Interpreting CRP blood test results in people with symptoms of lower respiratory tract infection

CRP result (mg/l)	Risk of mortality (%)	Action
<20	<1	No antibiotic
20–100	1	Offer delayed antibiotic
>100	10–19	Offer antibiotic and consider admission

Self-care

- Maintain adequate fluid intake
- Avoid physical exertion until the fever settles
- Paracetamol or ibuprofen[P] for pain relief
- Smoking cessation advice
- Advise on the likely progress, emphasising that the cough may persist for 6 weeks:
  - 1 week – fever should have resolved
  - 4 weeks – chest pain and sputum production should have substantially reduced
  - 6 weeks – cough and breathlessness should have substantially reduced
  - 3 months – most symptoms should have resolved, but fatigue might still be present
  - 6 months – symptoms should have fully resolved

Action

- If CRP point-of-care testing is available, action according to the result (Table 3.1). If not available, follow the approach below
- CRB-65 score for mortality risk (Table 3.2) – one point for each of the following:
  - Confusion (new disorientation in person, place or time)
  - Raised respiratory rate (≥30/min)
  - Low blood pressure (diastolic ≤60 mmHg or systolic <90 mmHg)
  - Age ≥65 years
- **Consider admission if CRB-65 score ≥1, especially if ≥2**
  - Use clinical judgement in addition to CRB-65 score to decide if admission is required
  - Other important factors include the person's preferences, comorbidities, pregnancy, and pulse oximetry
- If not admitting to hospital, offer an antibiotic (unless this is inappropriate, e.g., comfort care on an end-of-life pathway)
- Review within 3 days and again at 5 days
- Advise the person to seek help if symptoms worsen, or do not begin to improve within 3 days, as hospital admission may be needed

Table 3.2 Predictive value of CRB-65 score on mortality from pneumonia (based on data on people in hospital)

CRB-65 score	Risk of mortality (%)	Antibiotic choice
0	1	Single
1	5	Dual
2	12	Dual
3	18	Dual
4	33	Dual

Antibiotic choice

Note that all of the following regimens are adult doses for 5 days, with the expectation of a review taking place at 5 days and extension of antibiotic treatment to 10–15 days being considered at that time. Remember that sputum production is expected to continue for 4 weeks.

CRB-65 score 0:

- Amoxicillin 500 mg three times daily

If allergic to penicillin, use:

- Doxycycline[PBC] (200 mg on the first day, then 100 mg once daily) *or*
- Clarithromycin[PIQ] (500 mg twice daily) *or*
- Erythromycin[PIQ] (500 mg four times a day) if pregnant

CRB-65 score 1 or 2 (and clinical judgement):

- Amoxicillin 500 mg three times daily *and*
- Clarithromycin[PIQ] (500 mg twice daily) *or*
- Erythromycin[PIQ] (500 mg four times a day) if pregnant

If allergic to penicillin, use:

- Doxycycline[PBC] (200 mg on the first day, then 100 mg once daily) *or*
- Clarithromycin[PIQ] (500 mg twice daily)

If following flu-like illness, then use co-amoxiclav (500/125 mg three times daily) rather than amoxicillin (which does not cover *Staphylococcus*). If allergic to penicillin, then use doxycycline[PBC] for adults or clarithromycin[PIQ] for children

RED FLAGS

- Severe illness, breathlessness or confusion (*admit urgently under Medical/Paediatrics*)
- Worsening despite oral treatment (*needs IV antibiotics; admit urgently under Medical/Paediatrics*)
- Person with HIV (*possible Pneumocystis jiroveci pneumonia; admit urgently under Medical/Paediatrics*)
- Unilateral chest pain, worse on coughing or deep breathing (*suggests pleurisy, pulmonary embolism or pneumothorax; consider sending urgently to hospital*)
- Signs of sepsis (see Chapter 2) (*admit very urgently under Medical/Paediatrics*)
- Oxygen saturation <94% (*admit urgently under Medical/Paediatrics*)
- CRB-65 score of ≥1 (*especially if ≥2; consider admitting urgently under Medical/Paediatrics*)
- CRP >100 (*especially if very high; consider admitting urgently under Medical/Paediatrics*) (Travlos et al., 2022)
- Baby with abnormal chest examination, e.g., recession (*differential diagnosis includes bronchiolitis; refer to experienced colleague*)

References

Blackburn, R., Henderson, K., Lillie, M., et al. 2011. Empirical treatment of influenza-associated pneumonia in primary care: a descriptive study of the antimicrobial susceptibility of lower respiratory tract bacteria (England, Wales and Northern Ireland, January 2007–March 2010). *Thorax*; 66(5):389–95. https://doi.org/10.1136/thx.2010.134643

NICE. 2019. NG120. Cough (acute): antimicrobial prescribing. www.nice.org.uk/guidance/ng120

NICE. 2019. NG138. Pneumonia (community-acquired): antimicrobial prescribing. www.nice.org.uk/guidance/ng138

NICE CKS. 2021. Chest infections – adult: scenario: community-acquired pneumonia. https://cks.nice.org.uk/topics/chest-infections-adult/management/community-acquired-pneumonia/

NICE CKS. 2023. Cough – acute with chest signs in children: scenario: community-acquired pneumonia. https://cks.nice.org.uk/topics/cough-acute-with-chest-signs-in-children/management/community-acquired-pneumonia/#

Travlos, A., Bakakos, A., Vlachos, K., et al. 2022. C-reactive protein as a predictor of survival and length of hospital stay in community-acquired pneumonia. *J Pers Med*; 12(10). https://doi.org/10.3390/jpm12101710

Williams, D., Creech, C., Walter, E., et al. 2022. Short- vs standard-course outpatient antibiotic therapy for community-acquired pneumonia in children: the SCOUT-CAP randomized clinical trial. *JAMA Pediatr*; 176(3):253–61. https://doi.org/10.1001/jamapediatrics.2021.5547

COPD/BRONCHIECTASIS EXACERBATION

History

- Cough
- Wheeze
- Sputum quantity, colour and thickness
- Worsening breathlessness
- Fever
- Recent antibiotics
- Previous episodes and their treatment
- Any documented care plan

Rsp

Examination

- Temperature
- BP
- Respiratory rate
- Oxygen saturation (compare with their usual)
- Wheezing
- Pursed lip breathing
- Use of accessory muscles at rest
- ⚑ Cyanosis
- ⚑ Confusion/drowsiness
- ⚑ Peripheral oedema

Test

- NICE (2019) does not recommend routinely sending sputum for culture in people with exacerbations of COPD managed in primary care. However, it can be helpful if the infection turns out to respond poorly to initial treatment
- Sputum cultures should always be sent for exacerbations of bronchiectasis

Self-care

- In COPD, increase dose or frequency of short-acting bronchodilator to the maximum (salbutamol or ipratropium)
- Use a spacer (if the inhaler is a metered-dose inhaler [MDI])
- Smoking cessation advice and support; stopping smoking is the most effective intervention in avoiding progression of COPD and increasing survival
- Safety-netting advice

Prescription

- In COPD, if breathlessness has worsened, give prednisolone[PI] 30 mg/day for 5 days
- If sputum has increased and become purulent (green and thick), prescribe an antibiotic

Antibiotic choice

Be guided by the result of the most recent sputum culture or, if none, by what treatment proved helpful in the previous infective episode.

For adults for 5 days (COPD) or 7–14 days (bronchiectasis):

- Amoxicillin 500 mg three times daily
- If allergic to penicillin, use doxycycline[PBC] (200 mg on the first day, then 100 mg once daily) or clarithromycin[PIQ] (500 mg twice daily)
- If severe COPD with recurrent antibiotic use, consider co-amoxiclav (500/125 mg three times daily)
- If not responding to amoxicillin, add clarithromycin[PIQ] or change to doxycycline[PBC]

 RED FLAGS

Consider *admitting urgently under Medical* if any of the following:

- Living alone or limited support at home
- Severe breathlessness
- Cyanosis and/or oxygen sats <90%
- Significant comorbidities (e.g., heart disease), poor level of activity
- Worsening of peripheral oedema
- Impaired level of consciousness or acute confusion
- Already receiving long-term oxygen therapy
- Rapidly progressing symptoms

References

Grant, J., and Saux, N. 2021. Duration of antibiotic therapy for common infections. *J Assoc Med Microbiol Infect Dis Can*; 6(3):181–97. https://doi.org/10.3138/jammi-2021-04-29

NICE. 2018. NG114. Chronic obstructive pulmonary disease (acute exacerbation): antimicrobial prescribing. www.nice.org.uk/guidance/ng114

NICE. 2019. NG115. Chronic obstructive pulmonary disease in over 16s: diagnosis and management. www.nice.org.uk/guidance/ng115

Wedzicha, J., Miravitlles, M., Hurst, J., et al. 2017. Management of COPD exacerbations: a European Respiratory Society/American Thoracic Society guideline. *Eur Respir J*; 49(3). https://doi.org/10.1183/13993003.00791-2016 *Support for the use of oral corticosteroids and antibiotics for exacerbations.*

ASTHMA EXACERBATION

History

- Wheeze
- Breathlessness
- Cough
- Fever
- Sleep disturbance
- Current medication and concordance
- Any documented care plan; if so, has it been followed?
- Previous hospital admissions for asthma
- 🚩 Any previous intensive care admissions for asthma

Examination

- Temperature
- Heart rate
- Respiratory rate
- Oxygen saturation
- In severe episodes, CRT in children aged <12 years/BP in adults and older children
- PEFR (if they are able to comply)

  🚩 Moderate exacerbation: PEFR 50–75% of best or predicted

  🚩 Severe exacerbation: PEFR 33–50% of best or predicted

  🚩 Life threatening: PEFR <33% of best or predicted

🚩 Inability to complete sentences

🚩 Agitation

🚩 Cyanosis

🚩 Recession/use of accessory muscles

🚩 Exhaustion

Action

- Immediately use salbutamol inhaler; one puff at a time and inhale with 5 tidal breaths via spacer if available:
  - Adult: four puffs initially, followed by two puffs every 2 minutes according to response, up to 10 puffs
  - Child: a puff every 30-60 seconds (5 tidal breaths), up to 10 puffs
  - Repeat every 10–20 minutes according to response
- Afterwards (if symptoms improve), use inhaled salbutamol as required (if needing to use more frequently than every 4 hours, then seek help)
- Safety-netting advice: monitor PEFR and symptoms. If symptoms worsen or PEFR decreases, seek help

Prescription

- Do not give antibiotics unless there are signs of pneumonia
- Prescribe a short course of oral prednisolone[PI]:
  - Child aged <2 years: 10 mg daily for 3 days
  - Child aged 2–5 years: 20 mg daily for 3 days
  - Child aged 6–12 years: 30–40 mg daily for 3 days
  - Adult or child aged >12 years: 40–50 mg daily for 5 days
- Arrange follow-up in 24–48 hours. Once recovered, will need further review (after about a month) to adjust medication and potentially update asthma action plan

 RED FLAGS

Send very urgently to hospital (by ambulance, ideally with nebulised salbutamol driven with oxygen while waiting for transfer) if any of the following:

- A previous near-fatal asthma attack
- PEFR <33% of best or predicted
- Silent chest (severe airways constriction) or silent half of chest (pneumothorax)
- Cyanosis/oxygen saturation <92%
- Altered consciousness/confusion
- Exhaustion/poor respiratory effort
- Cardiac arrhythmia
- Low BP

Consider sending urgently to hospital if moderate exacerbation plus any of the following:

- Age <18
- No/limited improvement of symptoms with initial treatment with salbutamol
- Not adherent to treatment
- Living alone
- Psychological problems such as depression or substance misuse
- Physical or learning disability
- Previous severe asthma attack
- Current oral steroid use
- Presentation in afternoon or at night
- Recent symptoms at night
- Recent hospital admission
- Pregnancy

Note there is an important overlap between hay fever and asthma. Exposure to pollens can aggravate asthma and trigger worsening symptoms. The National Review of Asthma Deaths (2014) showed that 15% of asthma deaths had hay fever as the trigger for the exacerbation, and recommended that people with both asthma and hay fever should be encouraged to increase preventer medication prior to the hay fever season; it would also seem sensible for them to take a regular antihistamine. Asthma attacks have been tracked across countries following thunderstorms that split pollen particles which were then raised into the air by the electric field of the storm (Hajat et al., 1997; Venables et al., 1997; Douglass et al., 2022).

References

British Thoracic Society (BTS) and Scottish Intercollegiate Guidelines Network (SIGN). 2019. SIGN158: British guideline on the management of asthma. www.sign.ac.uk/media/1773/sign158-updated.pdf

Douglass, J.A., Lodge, C., Chan, S., et al. 2022. Thunderstorm asthma in seasonal allergic rhinitis: the TAISAR study. *J Allergy Clin Immunol*; 149(5):1607–16. https://doi.org/10.1016/j.jaci.2021.10.028

Hajat, S., Goubet, S.A., and Haines, A. 1997. Thunderstorm-associated asthma: the effect on GP consultations. *Br J Gen Pract*; 47(423):639. https://bjgp.org/content/bjgp/47/423/639.full.pdf

Kew, K., Flemyng, E., Quon, B., and Leung, C. 2022. Increased versus stable doses of inhaled corticosteroids for exacerbations of chronic asthma in adults and children. *Cochrane Database Syst Rev*; 9:CD007524. https://doi.org/10.1002/14651858. CD007524.pub5 *This Cochrane review concluded that increasing ICS dose at time of exacerbation was unlikely to have a clinically meaningful benefit.*

NICE. 2021. NG80. Asthma: diagnosis, monitoring and chronic asthma management. www.nice.org.uk/guidance/ng80

NICE CKS. 2022. Asthma. https://cks.nice.org.uk/topics/asthma/

Royal College of Physicians. 2014. Why asthma still kills: the National Review of Asthma Deaths (NRAD) Confidential Enquiry report. London. https://www.rcplondon.ac.uk/projects/outputs/why-asthma-still-kills

Venables, K.M., Allitt, U., Collier, C.G., et al. 1997. Thunderstorm-related asthma – the epidemic of 24/25 June 1994. *Clin Exp Allergy*; 27(7):725–36. https://doi.org/10.1046/j.1365-2222.1997.790893.x

VIRAL-INDUCED WHEEZE

Viral infections may cause wheezing and tightness in the chest in those who do not have asthma. Use salbutamol MDI via spacer, four times daily for 1 week. Affected children with a family history of atopy and exercise-induced wheeze are more likely to develop asthma later.

Reference

NICE CKS. 2022. Scenario: viral-induced wheeze/infective exacerbation of asthma. https://cks.nice.org.uk/topics/cough-acute-with-chest-signs-in-children/management/viral-induced-wheeze-possible-asthma/

BRONCHIOLITIS

- A viral infection of children aged <2 years, usually 3–6 months
- Mainly caused by respiratory syncytial virus (RSV)

History

- Persistent cough following an URTI (usually peaks at 3–5 days)
- May be breathless or have episodes of apnoea

Examination

- Temperature (usually <39°C)
- Heart rate
- Respiratory rate
- Oxygen saturation
- CRT
- Recession/use of accessory muscles
- Chest (often scattered crackles and wheezes)
- Percussion (no dullness)

Self-care

- Maintain adequate fluid intake
- There is no specific treatment. Steam inhalations are no longer recommended due to the risk of scalding. However, this risk can be minimised by steaming up a bathroom by running a hot shower, or using one of the many humidified air devices available
- This is a long illness: only 50% of children will be better by day 13
- Safety-netting advice, including to seek help if any of:
  - Faster breathing
  - Increasing difficulty in breathing
  - Episodes of apnoea
  - Recession (sucking in of the skin between the ribs)
  - Reduced feeding (<50% of normal)
  - Signs of dehydration
  - Fever ≥5 days

RED FLAGS

A child with suspected bronchiolitis should be reviewed by an experienced clinician in order to assess the need for hospital admission. It can be difficult to distinguish bronchiolitis from pneumonia.

- Episodes of apnoea (*admit urgently under Paediatrics*)
- Oxygen saturation <92% (*give oxygen and admit urgently under Paediatrics*)
- Recession or raised respiratory rate: 0–5 months, >60/min; 6–12 months, >50/min; >12 months, >40/min (*consider admitting urgently under Paediatrics*)
- Focal signs in chest (*possible pneumonia; consider admitting urgently under Paediatrics*)
- Baby aged <3 months of age or born prematurely, especially if born <32 weeks' gestation
- Feeding difficulties/signs of dehydration
- Background of lung or neuromuscular disease, or immunosuppressed
- Parents/carers lacking skill or confidence to look after the child at home and detect signs of deterioration

Rsp

References

NICE. 2021. NG9. Bronchiolitis in children: diagnosis and management. www.nice.org.uk/guidance/ng9

NICE CKS. 2023. Cough (acute) with chest signs in children. https://cks.nice.org.uk/topics/cough-acute-with-chest-signs-in-children/

Quinonez, R., Coon, E., Schroeder, A., et al. 2017. When technology creates uncertainty: pulse oximetry and overdiagnosis of hypoxaemia in bronchiolitis. *BMJ*; 358:j3850. https://doi.org/10.1136/bmj.j3850

Thompson, M., Vodicka, T., Blair, P., et al. 2013. Duration of symptoms of respiratory tract infections in children: systematic review. *BMJ*; 347:f7027. https://doi.org/10.1136/bmj.f7027

Umoren, R., Odey, F., and Meremikwu, M. 2011. Steam inhalation or humidified oxygen for acute bronchiolitis in children up to three years of age. *Cochrane Database Syst Rev*; 1:CD006435. https://doi.org/10.1002/14651858.CD006435.pub2

CROUP

A viral infection of children, most common between the ages of 6 months and 3 years.

History

- Cough (seal-like barking)
- Crowing noise on inspiration (stridor, worse at night)
- Fever
- May be breathless
- Prodromal URTI 12–72 hours beforehand
- ⚑ Immunosuppressed

Examination

- Temperature
- Heart rate
- Respiratory rate
- Oxygen saturation
- CRT
- Recession/use of accessory muscles
- Chest (usually normal)
- Throat

Self-care

- Croup can be categorised as mild, moderate or severe (Table 3.3). Mild croup can usually be managed at home
- Explain nature of illness – usually resolves within 48 hours, but can last up to 1 week
- Steam inhalations are no longer recommended due to the risk of scalding. However, this risk can be minimised by steaming up a bathroom by running a hot shower, or using one of the many humidified air devices available

- Safety-netting advice about symptoms of worsening severity according to Table 3.3

Table 3.3 Categorisation of croup

	Barking cough	Stridor at rest	Sternal recession	Agitation/lethargy
Mild	✔	✘	✘	✘
Moderate	✔	✔	✔	✘
Severe	✔	✔	✔	✔

Prescription

- Give all children with croup a single dose of oral dexamethasone[PI] (150 micrograms/kg). Tablets are available as 500 micrograms and 2 mg. Round the dose up to the nearest tablet available. We would caution against prescribing soluble tablets or liquid preparations because pharmacies may not stock them, and ordinary tablets dissolve in water adequately for young children
- If dexamethasone is unavailable, give a single dose of oral prednisolone[PI] (1–2 mg/kg) (Parker and Cooper, 2019). Soluble tablets are available but expensive; standard ones will dissolve in a little water if agitated for a few minutes

RED FLAGS

Consider admitting urgently under Paediatrics if:

- Abnormal airway (including Down's syndrome), heart or lung disease
- Immunosuppressed
- Parents not coping
- Moderate or severe croup (see Table 3.3)
- Mild croup and any of:
  - Age <3 months
  - Respiratory rate >60
  - High fever
  - Inadequate fluid intake

References

Moore, M., and Little, P. 2007. Humidified air inhalation for treating croup: a systematic review and meta-analysis. *Fam Pract*; 24(4):295–301. https://doi.org/10.1093/fampra/cmm022

NICE CKS. 2022. Croup. https://cks.nice.org.uk/topics/croup/

Parker, C., and Cooper, M. 2019. Prednisolone versus dexamethasone for croup: a randomized controlled trial. *Pediatrics*; 144(3):e20183772. https://doi.org/10.1542/peds.2018-3772

DIFFERENTIAL DIAGNOSIS OF ACUTE COUGH WITH CHEST SIGNS IN CHILDREN

Table 3.4 summarises the illnesses which may cause cough with chest signs in children: pneumonia, viral-induced wheeze, bronchiolitis and croup.

Table 3.4 Differential diagnosis of acute cough with chest signs in children

	Pneumonia	Viral-induced wheeze	Bronchiolitis	Croup
Age	Any age	1–5 years	<2 years	6 months–3 years
Fever	Yes	Maybe	Yes	Yes
Respiratory rate	Increased	Normal or increased	Increased	Increased
Recession	No	Maybe	Maybe	Maybe
Hyperinflation	No	Maybe	Often	No
Wheeze	No*	Present	Maybe	Stridor
Crackles	Coarse, localised	None	Fine, generalised	None

* Except with *Mycoplasma pneumoniae*.

WHOOPING COUGH

A bacterial infection caused by *Bordetella pertussis,* affecting all ages. Although most severe in babies aged <3 months (who are too young to be directly protected by routine immunisation), incidence in babies has reduced due to a vaccination programme in pregnant women. Whooping cough now mostly affects older children, particularly teenagers, as their immunity has waned. Recorded cases in England were markedly reduced in 2021 compared with previous years, although incidence tends to follow a cyclical pattern with surges every 3–4 years. It is a notifiable disease and probably underdiagnosed in adults.

History

- Consider in child if coughing for ≥2 weeks, especially if sputum is thick and vomiting occurs after coughing
- Median duration of cough is 112 days
- Three phases of symptoms:
  - Catarrhal phase – dry cough (usually 1 week)
  - Paroxysmal phase – coughing fit, whooping and post-tussive vomiting (may last a month). (Whoop: sharp inhalation of breath during bouts of paroxysmal cough)
  - Convalescent phase – gradual improvement in the frequency and severity of cough (may be an additional 2 months)

Examination

- Temperature
- Heart rate
- CRT in children aged <12 years/BP in adults and older children
- Respiratory rate
- Oxygen saturation
- Examination of chest is usually normal

Tests

- Contact the local Health Protection Team (HPT) – it will advise on the appropriate test (there are different possibilities including culture, serology, oral fluid testing and PCR)

Self-care

- Stay away from day care, school or work for 2 days after starting antibiotic, or 21 days after the onset of cough, whichever is sooner
- Expect recovery to take several weeks

Prescription

- Clarithromycin[PIQ] (500 mg twice daily for adults for 7 days); if given in the first 3 weeks of illness, it reduces transmission (but does not directly benefit the person treated)

Reference

UKHSA. 2022. Pertussis: guidance, data and analysis. www.gov.uk/government/collections/pertussis-guidance-data-and-analysis

CHAPTER 4

COVID-19 and pandemics

Much has changed since the last edition of *The Minor Illness Manual*. Perhaps most notable is the immense and far-reaching impact of the COVID-19 pandemic, which has extended across almost every aspect of our lives. The consequences on our working environments and health services have been particularly marked, with ongoing repercussions for elective care, long-term conditions and psychological wellbeing (to name a few) likely to continue for years to come.

Prior to early 2020, for most people the idea of a worldwide pandemic with lockdowns and personal restrictions would have seemed far-fetched. Now, having lived through this, the idea of further pandemics in our lifetimes feels all too real.

It can be difficult to look past the suffering, disruption and death of the past few years. Many of us have lost loved ones, either directly or indirectly due to the COVID-19 pandemic. These impacts cannot be understated. However, we can take some solace in the hope that, if we see a further pandemic in years to come, the world will likely be better prepared with coordinated, well-planned, international responses supported by rapidly generated, effective treatments.

Medical science and technology have progressed rapidly, with mRNA vaccines now having been deployed by the billions, and incredible advancements in the time taken from identification of pathogen to vaccine generation. Monoclonal antibodies and other targeted treatments can be produced in record time; processes that once took years now take just months and it is almost certain that the pace will further quicken.

With the COVID-19 pandemic having exposed weaknesses in some countries' early response and their approaches to avoiding disease transmission, lessons may be learned and investment may follow to ensure better pandemic preparedness. The ethos of 'it won't happen' has been quashed and if there's a 'next time round', we would expect to see the effect of such preparedness, investment, coordination and technological advancement in driving prompt, effective action to protect the population.

COVID-19

Entire books have been written about COVID-19 and its causative organism, SARS-CoV-2. It is likely that you will already know quite a lot about it, given its complete domination over our lives and daily activities for the better part of 2 years. You may have contracted COVID-19 yourself at some point, perhaps more than once, and you may be one of the many millions who have tragically lost friends and family to the disease.

Although COVID-19 seems to have largely fallen out of the headlines, it is still circulating and continuing to evolve; perhaps the key difference now compared with the early stages of the pandemic is that, for the vast majority, it tends to result in relatively minor illness (at least acutely). The reasons for this are likely to be multifactorial, but widespread vaccination and changes in the virus itself are perhaps the main contributors. For those with more severe symptoms (in hospital settings), or at high risk of adverse outcomes, we now have antivirals and monoclonal antibodies to treat COVID-19.

According to the WHO, the following are the symptoms of COVID-19:

- Most common symptoms:
  - Fever
  - Chills
  - Sore throat
- Less common symptoms:
  - Muscle aches
  - Severe fatigue or tiredness
  - Runny or blocked nose, or sneezing
  - Headache
  - Sore eyes

- Dizziness
- New and persistent cough
- Tight chest or chest pain
- Shortness of breath
- Hoarse voice
- Heavy arms/legs
- Numbness/tingling
- Nausea, vomiting, abdominal pain/bellyache, or diarrhoea
- Appetite loss
- Loss or change of sense of taste or smell
- Difficulty sleeping
- Serious symptoms:
  - Difficulty breathing, especially at rest, or unable to speak in sentences
  - Confusion
  - Drowsiness or loss of consciousness
  - Persistent pain or pressure in the chest
  - Skin being cold or clammy, or turning pale or a bluish colour
  - Loss of speech or movement

This list has changed markedly over the 12 months prior to publication of this book. The previously common symptoms of cough and loss of taste or smell are now less prominent, although the patterns of presentation may change again in the months and years to come. Particularly in older people, presentations may be with non-specific symptoms such as confusion, whereas children may have gastrointestinal symptoms.

Watching the COVID-19 pandemic unfold and its symptomatology and severity change over time has been unlike managing any other disease in the authors' experience. During the early stages of the pandemic, a healthcare professional could assess with some confidence that someone was likely to have COVID-19 (often due to the key indicator of anosmia); however, there tends to be little these days to differentiate acute infection with SARS-CoV-2 from infection with one of the multitude of rhinoviruses, influenza viruses, parainfluenza viruses, etc. The reduced access to testing (and disinclination of many to pay for such testing) further compounds diagnostic uncertainty.

Indeed, most people with suspected COVID-19 symptoms in the UK are no longer recommended to get tested unless they are at high risk of adverse outcomes. However, somewhat confusingly, COVID-19 remains a notifiable illness.

Except for those at highest risk of adverse outcomes with COVID-19, the key question therefore relates not to the identity of the specific causative virus, but, in keeping with the assessment of all illness (minor or otherwise), to the severity. Listen to the person and use your clinical examination skills to help guide you. As with any acute presentation, severe illness and/or hypoxia (oxygen saturation ≤92% and/or >4% lower than usual levels) will likely require hospital admission; see the Red Flags box for more detail.

Action

For those in the highest-risk groups (in England), there is a practical reason to establish if they have COVID-19, namely their eligibility for specific treatment including antivirals and monoclonal antibodies. Groups included in the definition of highest risk are those with immunosuppression – an up-to-date list can be found at https://www.nhs.uk/conditions/coronavirus-covid-19/self-care-and-treatments-for-coronavirus/treatments-for-coronavirus/. People within these groups should already know of this and are entitled to free COVID-19 tests.

If someone in the highest-risk groups suspects that they may have COVID-19, they should be advised to test using lateral flow tests; if the initial test is negative, then they should be advised to perform three tests over 3 days. If testing positive, they should contact 111 or their GP practice who can then assess eligibility and refer for specific treatment. The use of different treatments has changed over time as more evidence on effectiveness has become available (Amani and Amani, 2023; Tian et al., 2023) and NICE guidance/technology appraisals have been issued. At the time of writing, there is no facility or expectation for practitioners outside COVID-19 medicine delivery units to provide such treatments, although this may change in future.

RED FLAGS

Admit urgently under Medical if any of the following:

- Severe shortness of breath at rest or difficulty breathing
- Oxygen saturation ≤92% and/or >4% lower than usual levels
- Coughing up blood
- Blue lips or face
- Feeling cold and clammy with pale or mottled skin
- Collapse or fainting (syncope)
- New confusion
- Becoming difficult to rouse
- Reduced urine output

C19

REFERENCES

Amani, B., and Amani, B. 2023. Efficacy and safety of nirmatrelvir/ritonavir (Paxlovid) for COVID-19: a rapid review and meta-analysis. *J Med Virol*; 95(2):e28441. https://doi.org/10.1002/jmv.28441 *There was a significant difference between the Paxlovid and no-Paxlovid groups in terms of mortality rate (odds ratio [OR] = 0.25) and hospitalisation rate (OR = 0.40).*

NHS. 2023. Who can get a free NHS coronavirus (COVID-19) rapid lateral flow test. www.nhs.uk/conditions/coronavirus-covid-19/testing/get-tested-for-coronavirus/

NICE. 2022. NG191. COVID-19 rapid guideline: managing COVID-19. www.nice.org.uk/guidance/ng191/

Tian, F., Feng, Q., and Chen, Z. 2023. Efficacy and safety of molnupiravir treatment for COVID-19: a systematic review and meta-analysis of randomized controlled trials. *Int J Antimicrob Agents*; 62(2):106870. https://doi.org/10.1016/j.ijantimicag.2023.106870 *Molnupiravir can accelerate the rehabilitation of people with COVID-19, but it does not significantly reduce rates of mortality or hospitalisation.*

UK Health Security Agency. 2022. Guidance – notifiable diseases and causative organisms: how to report. www.gov.uk/guidance/notifiable-diseases-and-causative-organisms-how-to-report#list-of-notifiable-organisms-causative-agents

WHO (World Health Organization). Coronavirus disease (COVID-19). www.who.int/health-topics/coronavirus

CHAPTER 5

Ear, nose and throat

SORE THROAT

People with sore throats are often diagnosed as having either tonsillitis or pharyngitis. However, these are best considered as part of a spectrum of a single disease process, tonsillopharyngitis, which includes infection or inflammation of the pharynx and/or tonsils. Viral infection is the commonest cause of sore throat (75% for children and 90% for adults). Glandular fever is another diagnosis that needs to be considered. Far rarer, more serious problems such as quinsy and epiglottitis may also present with a history of sore throat and should be considered in the differential diagnosis.

History

- Reason for presenting – often pain relief
- Duration
- Fever
- Rash
- Treatment already tried
- Hydration in young children – fluid intake/wet nappies
- Other symptoms such as cough or blocked/discharging nose
- 🚩 Drooling/unable to swallow
- 🚩 Previous rheumatic fever (rare in the UK for decades, but prevalent in sub-Saharan Africa and South Asia)
- 🚩 Immunosuppressed
- 🚩 Medication that may affect the bone marrow (agranulocytosis), e.g., immunosuppressant (including corticosteroids), carbimazole, mirtazapine, sulfasalazine, clozapine and disease-modifying antirheumatic drugs (DMARDs)

Examination

- Temperature – consider any recent antipyretic (fever is common with sore throat and often >38°C)
- If systemically unwell, consider:
  - Heart rate
  - Respiratory rate
  - CRT in children aged <12 years/BP in adults and older children
- Examine throat to assess inflammation and check for tonsillar exudate – but do not examine if suspecting epiglottitis (suggested by fever, severe pain, difficulty swallowing and drooling; see Box 5.3). Table 5.1 summarises possible examination findings for differential diagnoses of sore throat
- When examining, asking the person to yawn, take a deep breath or pant may improve the view
- Consider using a tongue depressor on the sides of the tongue if tonsils are not visible
- If attempting examination is causing distress, consider the value of proceeding
- Check neck for enlarged lymph nodes (cervical lymphadenopathy)
- In a child, check for the rash of scarlet fever (small rough pinpricks)

Table 5.1 Specific examination findings in sore throat

Finding	Diagnosis
Petechiae on palate, tonsils or pharynx	GABHS (group A beta-haemolytic *Streptococcus*) infection or glandular fever
Swelling next to one tonsil only/ deviation of the uvula	Quinsy
Strawberry tongue	Scarlet fever or Kawasaki disease
Thick grey coating on the tonsils, larynx and/or pharynx	Diphtheria (very rare in the UK, but consider in migrant population)

Test

- Urgent FBC should be requested if taking medication which may affect bone marrow. The safe course of action is to stop the potentially causative drug until the FBC result is confirmed to be normal
- Rapid antigen throat swab tests designed to detect group A streptococcal infections are not recommended by NICE for routine care. They are unable to differentiate between carrier state and invasive infection

Self-care advice

- Reassure: symptoms resolve within 3 days in 40% of people and within 7 days in 85%, irrespective of whether the sore throat is viral or due to a streptococcal infection
- Warm saltwater mouthwash (half a teaspoon of salt in 250 ml of water) may help relieve symptoms
- Cold drinks and ice lollies may be soothing
- Benzydamine mouthwash, lozenges or spray (e.g., Difflam OTC) may relieve discomfort
- Lozenges containing local anaesthetic may help to reduce pain, but numbing the throat may result in accidental injury or superficial burns from food or drink that is too hot
- Paracetamol or ibuprofen[P] can relieve pain
- Flurbiprofen[PBC] lozenges (Strefen OTC) are an alternative (one 8.75 mg lozenge every 3–6 hours for maximum 3 days, allow lozenge to dissolve slowly in the mouth; maximum five lozenges per day). Adverse events occur in over a third of people using flurbiprofen lozenges, including taste disturbances, numbness, dry mouth and nausea (NICE, 2023)
- Oral corticosteroid may be prescribed if the pain is very severe, but carries risks including sepsis and venous thromboembolism (VTE)
- Safety-netting advice: seek help if they develop difficulty in breathing or are unable to swallow enough fluid to maintain hydration

When should we prescribe antibiotics for sore throat?

Antibiotics are typically of marginal benefit in sore throat and may only shorten the illness by 16 hours (remember that the immune system is designed to handle sore throats, both viral and bacterial in origin, and is usually highly competent in doing so). Against this must be weighed the cost to the person (prescription charge, burden of medicine-taking, risk of side effects) and to society (antibiotic resistance, medicalisation of self-limiting illness).

The late 2022 outbreak of GABHS and resultant child deaths understandably weighs on the minds of practitioners and parents of children presenting with sore throat, potentially influencing decisions about antibiotic prescribing. This persists despite the direction from NHS England to revert to normal NICE guidance for prescribing antibiotics for children with sore throats (interim guidance had temporarily lowered the threshold).

NICE recommends the use of two clinical prediction rules, FeverPAIN (Box 5.1) and Centor, to guide antibiotic decision-making. They may be better than nothing, but neither is very reliable (Seeley et al., 2021). The Centor criteria have been criticised for leading to overprescription of antibiotics and have been found to be of no value in children (Roggen et al., 2013). FeverPAIN is preferred because it has been validated for children aged ≥3 years.

BOX 5.1 FeverPAIN Score (Little et al., 2013)

One point for each of:

- Fever in last 24 hours
- Purulence
- Attends with symptoms rapidly (<3 days)
- Inflammation of tonsils (if severe)
- No cough or coryza

Score of 0–1: 13%–18% have *Streptococcus (close to background carriage); no antibiotic*
Score of 2–3: 34%–40% have *Streptococcus; consider delayed antibiotic*
Score of ≥4: 62%–65% have *Streptococcus; consider immediate antibiotic if severe symptoms or delayed antibiotic prescription*

Action

- Prescribe an antibiotic if:
  - Seriously ill
  - Prolonged and worsening symptoms
  - Immunosuppressed
  - Previous rheumatic fever (may be retriggered by streptococcal infection)
- Consider an antibiotic if:
  - FeverPAIN score ≥4
  - Preceding viral infection (including chickenpox)
  - Close contact of someone with scarlet fever/GABHS infection
- If antibiotic indicated:
  - Phenoxymethylpenicillin, 500 mg four times daily (or 1 g twice daily) for adults for 5–10 days (see NMIC Debates in the Members' section of the NMIC website for debate on duration)
  - If allergic to penicillin, use clarithromycin[PIQ] 250 mg twice daily for adults for 5 days
  - For children who are unable to swallow tablets or eat crushed tablets and refuse phenoxymethylpenicillin solution because of its bad taste, amoxicillin suspension may be used instead. It tastes much better than phenoxymethylpenicillin suspension but is broader spectrum and there is international concern about increasing resistance. Avoid amoxicillin if glandular fever is suspected (see next section)
- If not responding to antibiotic, then reassess. Viral causes are common and are the usual reason for poor response; consider glandular fever

 RED FLAGS

- Drooling, cannot swallow, respiratory distress (*possible epiglottitis [see Box 5.2]; do not examine throat; send very urgently to hospital with referral to Ear, Nose and Throat [ENT] Team*)
- Large swelling around one tonsil, feverish and unwell (*possible quinsy [see Box 5.3]; send urgently to hospital with referral to ENT*)
- Previous rheumatic fever (*risk of recurrence; prescribe antibiotic*)
- Taking medication that may be toxic to bone marrow (*urgent FBC and refer to experienced colleague*)

References

Aertgeerts, B., Agoritsas, T., Siemieniuk, R., et al. 2017. Corticosteroids for sore throat: a clinical practice guideline. *BMJ*; 358:j4090. https://doi.org/10.1136/bmj.j4090 *This controversial guideline recommends giving high-dose dexamethasone to reduce the symptoms of sore throat. However, in NMIC's opinion, the possible benefits do not outweigh the risks.*

Little, P., Hobbs, F., Moore, M., et al. 2013. Clinical score and rapid antigen detection test to guide antibiotic use for sore throats: randomised controlled trial of PRISM (primary care streptococcal management). *BMJ*; 347:f5806. https://doi.org/10.1136/bmj.f5806 *Evidence for the FeverPAIN score. Lack of evidence for the rapid antigen test.*

NHS England. 2023. Group A *Streptococcus*: reinstatement of NICE sore throat guidance for children and young people and withdrawal of NHS England interim guidance. www.england.nhs.uk/wp-content/uploads/2022/12/PRN00247_Group-A-Streptococcus-reinstatement-of-NICE-sore-throat-guidance-for-children-and-young-people-and-wi.pdf *This document provides some rationale for the change in recommended practice for sore throat that occurred in England between December 2022 and February 2023 due to an outbreak of group A Streptococcus.*

NICE. 2023. NG84. Sore throat (acute): antimicrobial prescribing. www.nice.org.uk/guidance/ng84

Roggen, I., van Berlaer, G., Gordts, F., et al. 2013. Centor criteria in children in a paediatric emergency department: for what it is worth. *BMJ Open*; 3(4):e002712. https://doi.org/10.1136/bmjopen-2013-002712 *The Centor score was of no value in identifying children with bacterial sore throats.*

Schachtel, B., Aspley, S., Shephard, A., et al. 2014. Utility of the sore throat pain model in a multiple-dose assessment of the acute analgesic flurbiprofen: a randomized controlled study. *Trials*; 15(1):263. https://doi.org/10.1186/1745-6215-15-263 *In this manufacturer-sponsored study, 34% of those taking flurbiprofen reported adverse events.*

Seeley, A., Fanshawe, T., Voysey, M., et al. 2021. Diagnostic accuracy of Fever-PAIN and Centor criteria for bacterial throat infection in adults with sore throat: a secondary analysis of a randomised controlled trial. *BJGP Open*; 5(6) https://doi.org/10.3399/BJGPO.2021.0122 *In those who do not require immediate antibiotics in primary care, neither clinical prediction rule provides a reliable way of diagnosing streptococcal throat infection.*

Shephard, A., Smith, G., Aspley, S., et al. 2015. Randomised, double-blind, placebo-controlled studies on flurbiprofen 8.75 mg lozenges in patients with/without group A or C streptococcal throat infection, with an assessment of clinicians' prediction of 'strep throat'. *Int J Clin Pract*; 69(1):59–71. https://doi.org/10.1111/ijcp.12536 *A single flurbiprofen lozenge provided better pain relief than placebo.*

Spinks, A., Glasziou, P., and DelMar, C. 2021. Antibiotics for treatment of sore throat in children and adults. *Cochrane Database Syst Rev*; 12:CD000023. https://doi.org/10.1002/14651858.CD000023.pub5

GLANDULAR FEVER (INFECTIOUS MONONUCLEOSIS)

- People aged 15–25 are most commonly affected
- Caused by Epstein–Barr virus (EBV)
- Long incubation period (1–2 months)
- Transmission by saliva

History

- Fever
- Neck pain due to enlarged lymph nodes
- Sore throat
- Malaise and fatigue

Examination

- Temperature
- Heart rate
- Respiratory rate
- CRT in children aged <12 years/BP in adults and older children
- Inflamed, enlarged tonsils with exudate
- Enlarged lymph nodes in both the anterior and posterior triangles of the neck (in bacterial sore throat, usually only the anterior nodes are enlarged). The lymph nodes of the axilla and groin may also be enlarged
- Other possible findings:
  - Oedema of the uvula or around the eyes
  - Petechial rash on the palate
  - Variable generalised skin rash
  - Jaundice may be visible

Tests

- Usually a clinical diagnosis – classic triad: fever, sore throat and posterior cervical lymphadenopathy
- FBC (glandular fever is likely if 20% of lymphocytes are atypical or reactive)
- Paul–Bunnell or Monospot blood test, after at least 7 days (slow to turn positive and high false-negative rate)
- EBV serology – useful when the previous tests leave the diagnosis in doubt and there is need to identify the virus, e.g., in pregnancy (EBV is not harmful in pregnancy, but cytomegalovirus, which may pose harm, can cause similar symptoms)

Self-care advice

- Paracetamol or ibuprofen[P] can relieve pain
- Symptoms can last for 2–4 weeks. Tiredness is common and can persist for months
- Avoid strenuous activity and contact/collision sport for 1 month (to reduce the risk of rupture of the spleen)
- Avoid spread of infection from saliva
- Safety-netting advice: seek help if they develop difficulty breathing, or are unable to swallow enough fluids to maintain hydration, or develop abdominal pain (may indicate rupture of the spleen)

Action

- Avoid amoxicillin, which causes a rash in about 30% of people with glandular fever (the rash is disease-specific, not due to an allergy)

References

Lennon, P., Crotty, M., and Fenton, J. 2015. Infectious mononucleosis. *BMJ*; 350:h1825. https://doi.org/10.1136/bmj.h1825

NICE CKS. 2021. Glandular fever (infectious mononucleosis). https://cks.nice.org.uk/topics/glandular-fever-infectious-mononucleosis/

Thompson, D.F., and Ramos, C.L. 2017. Antibiotic-induced rash in patients with infectious mononucleosis. *Annals of Pharmacotherapy*, 51(2), 154-62 doi: https://doi.org/10.1177/1060028016669525.

 RED FLAG CONDITION

BOX 5.2 EPIGLOTTITIS

This is very rare and is now seen more often in adults than in children due to the *Haemophilus influenzae* type b (Hib) vaccination. If suspecting epiglottitis, **do not examine the throat**, as this may trigger airway obstruction.

- Severe illness with acute onset
- High fever
- Severe sore throat
- Difficulty and pain when swallowing, may be drooling
- 'Hot potato' voice
- Check vaccination history, especially if not covered by UK childhood vaccination schedule
- Anterior neck tenderness
- Stridor may be present

Send very urgently to hospital with referral to ENT

Reference

Guerra, A.M., and Waseem, M. 2022. Epiglottitis. *StatPearls*. Treasure Island (FL): StatPearls Publishing. www.ncbi.nlm.nih.gov/books/NBK430960/

BOX 5.3 QUINSY (PERITONSILLAR ABSCESS)

Most common in young teenagers but may occur at any age (rare <5 years).

- Severe illness with high fever
- Unilateral sore throat
- May have earache on the affected side
- May have painful swallowing (can be so severe that they cannot swallow their own saliva, causing drooling)
- Offensive breath (as a result of poor oral hygiene due to the point above)
- 'Hot potato' voice as the abscess size progresses
- Trismus (unable to open mouth fully)
- The arch of the soft palate is red and swollen on the affected side
- Uvula is swollen and pushed to the opposite side

Send urgently to hospital with referral to ENT

Reference

Gupta, G., and McDowell, R.H. 2022. Peritonsillar abscess. *StatPearls*. Treasure Island (FL): StatPearls Publishing. www.ncbi.nlm.nih.gov/books/NBK519520/

MOUTH PROBLEMS

- Oral candidiasis (thrush)
- Aphthous ulcers
- Herpes simplex stomatitis
- (Hand, foot and mouth disease is covered in Chapter 8)

ORAL CANDIDIASIS (THRUSH)

Candida is a yeast-like fungus which is part of the normal commensal flora. In some cases these may multiply and lead to candidiasis. It is common in babies and rarely serious.

History

- Soreness in mouth and tongue
- Difficulty in eating/drinking
- Foul taste in the mouth/loss of taste
- Explore risk factors:
  - Immunosuppressed
  - Use of a steroid inhaler
  - Wearing dentures
  - Recent antibiotics
  - Smoker
  - Condition or medication that can cause a dry mouth
  - Low iron

Examination

- White patches on tongue and oral mucosa that can be removed with some effort
- Redness of tongue or denture contact areas

Tests

- Swabs are unhelpful because *Candida* is a common commensal

- In adults consider arranging FBC, haematinics (B12, folate, ferritin), fasting plasma glucose (FPG) or HbA1c, and HIV serology to investigate possible underlying cause

Self-care

- Smoking cessation advice if appropriate
- Good dental/denture hygiene in adults
- For those using inhaled steroids, recommend rinsing out mouth with water after use. If the steroid inhaler is an MDI then use with a spacer (e.g., AeroChamber)
- Miconazole[I] oral gel (OTC if aged >4 months or >6 months if born pre-term) is the most effective treatment. Recommend use for at least 14 days, with treatment continued for 7 days after symptoms have resolved
- Avoid reinfection to baby from teats/nipples/dummies. Consider miconazole[I] cream for the breastfeeding mother's nipples (remove the cream from the breast before breastfeeding)

Prescription

- Miconazole[I] oral gel – a prescription will be required for babies aged <4 months or <6 months if born preterm (*unlicensed indication*). For babies, parents should be advised to take care that the gel does not obstruct the throat; avoid application to the back of the throat and subdivide doses. In adults, avoid using with warfarin, statin or sulphonylurea (e.g., gliclazide) due to interactions
- Nystatin suspension is an alternative but is 50% less effective. It is not licensed for babies aged <1 month
- Fluconazole[PCIQ] (50 mg daily for 14 days) may be used in people aged ≥16 who have severe or resistant cases or who are significantly immunosuppressed

RED FLAG

- Oral candidiasis is unusual in a healthy adult. If there is no obvious trigger (e.g., inhaled corticosteroids, dentures or recent broad-spectrum antibiotic) offer screening for immunosuppression including HIV

References

Ainsworth, S., and Jones, W. 2009. It sticks in our throats too. *BMJ*; 338:a3178. https://doi.org/10.1136/bmj.a3178 *Explains why the licence for miconazole was revoked for babies under 4 months.*

Medicines and Healthcare products Regulatory Agency (MHRA). 2016. Topical miconazole, including oral gel: reminder of potential for serious interactions with warfarin. www.gov.uk/drug-safety-update/topical-miconazole-including-oral-gel-reminder-of-potential-for-serious-interactions-with-warfarin

NICE CKS. 2022. *Candida* – oral. https://cks.nice.org.uk/topics/candida-oral/

Specialist Pharmacy Service. 2021. Using miconazole oral gel to treat oral thrush in adults taking a statin. www.sps.nhs.uk/articles/using-miconazole-oral-gel-to-treat-oral-thrush-in-adults-taking-a-statin/

Xiao, Y., Yuan, P., Sun, Y., et al. 2022. Comparison of topical antifungal agents for oral candidiasis treatment: a systematic review and meta-analysis. *Oral Surg Oral Med Oral Pathol Oral Radiol*; 133(3):282–91. https://doi.org/10.1016/j.oooo.2021.10.023

APHTHOUS ULCERS

These are painful mouth ulcers affecting 20% of the population, often presenting in childhood or adolescence, and not associated with systemic disease. The causes are not well understood. They are often recurrent, with spontaneous resolution with age.

History

- Duration (usually <3 weeks for aphthous ulcers)
- Any family history of recurrent ulcers? (Present in around 50%)
- Fever (if so, consider hand, foot and mouth disease; see Chapter 8)
- Any history of ulcers elsewhere (suggests possible systemic disorder)
- Systemic symptoms such as fatigue, gastrointestinal issues (possible systemic disorder such as inflammatory bowel disease [IBD], coeliac disease, Behçet's disease or immunosuppression)

ENT

Examination

- Red, round lesions, sometimes with white crater
- Look for evidence of trauma, e.g., poorly fitting dentures

Tests

There is no specific laboratory test; diagnosis is based on the history and examination with exclusion of a systemic cause. The following tests may be considered, depending on the history:

- Immunoglobulin A-tissue transglutaminase (IgA-TTG) (for coeliac disease)
- Faecal calprotectin test if available (for IBD)
- HIV serology
- Erythrocyte sedimentation rate (ESR) and CRP (may be raised in systemic inflammatory disease such as Behçet's disease and inflammatory bowel disease)

Self-care

- Advise that most will heal within 10–14 days
- Reduce oral trauma (e.g., softer toothbrush)
- Encourage maintaining/improving mouth hygiene (to reduce risk of exacerbating ulcer and secondary infection)
- Benzydamine spray (e.g., Difflam OTC) to reduce pain (for adults, four to eight sprays onto affected area every 1.5–3 hours)
- Topical anaesthetic gels may be helpful. However, care must be taken not to use any products containing salicylates in children due to the risk of Reye's syndrome.
  - In adults: e.g., Bonjela^C adult gel OTC, apply half an inch with gentle massage, not more often than every 3 hours
  - In children: e.g., Bonjela junior gel OTC, apply half an inch with gentle massage, not more often than every 3 hours
- Chlorhexidine mouthwash (OTC) to prevent secondary bacterial infection. Rinse or gargle 10 ml twice daily (for about 1 minute)
- Applying probiotic lozenges (e.g., Luvbiotics) may help reduce pain in recurrent aphthous ulcers (Cheng et al., 2020)

Prescription

- Hydrocortisone^P mucoadhesive buccal tablets, used at the first sign (one 2.5 mg tablet four times a day, allowed to dissolve slowly in the mouth in contact with the ulcer)
- For severe recurrent aphthous ulcers, a short course of prednisolone may be prescribed

RED FLAGS

- Persisting ≥3 weeks (in an adult, *USC referral to Oral Surgery*)
- Ulceration affects other parts of body, or presence of gastrointestinal symptoms or systemic symptoms such as fatigue (*consider alternative diagnoses, e.g., [IBD], coeliac disease, Behçet's disease or immunosuppression; refer to experienced colleague*)

References

Cheng, B., Zeng, X., Liu, S., et al., 2020. The efficacy of probiotics in management of recurrent aphthous stomatitis: a systematic review and meta-analysis. *Scientific Reports*; 10(1):21181. https://doi.org/10.1038/s41598-020-78281-7

Johnston, L., Warrilow, L., Fullwood, I., et al. 2022. Fifteen-minute consultation: oral ulceration in children. *Arch Dis Child Educ Pract Ed*; 107(4):257–64. https://doi.org/10.1136/archdischild-2021-321597

Ledford, D. 2019. Aphthous ulcers from food allergy. www.aaaai.org/allergist-resources/ask-the-expert/answers/old-ask-the-experts/aphthous *Experts believe there is no evidence of food allergy being related to aphthous ulcers.*

NICE CKS. 2022. Aphthous ulcer. https://cks.nice.org.uk/topics/aphthous-ulcer/

HERPES SIMPLEX STOMATITIS

As well as the familiar cold sore (see section on Other Localised Rashes in Chapter 8), the herpes simplex virus (HSV-1) may cause a systemic illness with extensive mouth ulceration when first encountered. It is spread by direct contact or via droplets of secretions (from someone who may be asymptomatic). Once infected with the virus, it can recur as a cold sore with intermittent re-activation occurring throughout life.

History

- Usually a child aged <5 years
- Painful ulcers inside the mouth/blisters in and around the mouth
- Short history of fever and malaise
- May be refusing to eat or drink
- Immunosuppressed

Examination

- Temperature
- Heart rate
- Respiratory rate
- Capillary refill time
- Check for evidence of dehydration
- Enlarged cervical lymph nodes (especially submandibular)
- Multiple small ulcers on tongue, palate and buccal mucosa (cheek lining)
- Gums may be inflamed

Self-care

- Advise that it is self-limiting and should resolve in 7–10 days
- Ensure adequate fluid intake (a straw or very cold drinks may help)
- Paracetamol may be used for pain relief
- Benzydamine spray (e.g., Difflam OTC) may be helpful
- Take precautions to reduce infection spread
- Avoid contact with babies aged <4 weeks

Prescription

- If onset within the last 3 days, offer a 5-day course of oral aciclovir (longer course may be needed if new lesions appear during treatment or if healing is incomplete):
  - If aged between 1 month and 2 years, dose is 100 mg five times a day
  - If aged ≥2 years, dose is 200 mg five times a day
  - Double the dose if immunosuppressed

RED FLAGS

Consider *admitting urgently under Paediatrics* if:

- Unable to maintain adequate hydration (*for IV fluids*)
- Immunosuppressed (*may need IV aciclovir*)
- Complication of infection (e.g., severe pain)
- Confused, very drowsy, significant behaviour change (*possible herpes simplex encephalitis*)

References

Goldman, R. 2016. Acyclovir for herpetic gingivostomatitis in children. *Can Fam Physician*; 62(5),403–4.

Johnston, L., Warrilow, L., Fullwood, I., et al. 2022. Fifteen-minute consultation: oral ulceration in children. *Arch Dis Child Educ Pract Ed*; 107(4):257–64. https://doi.org/10.1136/archdischild-2021-321597

NICE CKS. 2023. Scenario: herpes labialis (cold sores) and gingivostomatitis. https://cks.nice.org.uk/topics/herpes-simplex-oral/management/herpes-labialis-gingivostomatitis/

'SWOLLEN GLANDS' (ENLARGED CERVICAL LYMPH NODES)

History

- Duration of swelling
- Any sore throat, earache or rashes
- Fever
- 🏴 Night sweats
- 🏴 Weight loss
- 🏴 Recurrent infections
- 🏴 Unexplained bruising
- 🏴 Progressive enlargement over time (if present >3 weeks)

Examination

- Temperature
- Location, number and size of enlarged nodes
- Local tenderness or heat
- Any enlargement of lymph nodes of the axilla or groin
- Throat – any inflammation or exudate

Tests (if symptoms last >3 weeks)

- FBC
- CRP
- Paul–Bunnell/Monospot test for glandular fever (especially if aged 15–25)
- Consider HIV test

Self-care advice

- Explain that the 'glands' are the body's defence against infection
- Can use paracetamol or ibuprofen[P] if pain is severe
- Safety-netting advice: seek help if not settling within 3 weeks

 RED FLAGS

Refer to experienced colleague if:

- Node >2 cm in size (*unlikely to be a normal reaction to infection*)
- Single very large painful node or one enlarging rapidly (*may contain an abscess*)
- Supraclavicular node (*possible sign of abdominal cancer*)
- Nodes are hard, fixed or enlarging progressively over 3–6 weeks (*possible sign of HIV, lymphoma, leukaemia, sarcoidosis or TB*)
- Night sweats or weight loss (*possible serious systemic infection or cancer*)
- Recurrent infections (*may be a sign of HIV or leukaemia*) or unexplained bruising (*may be a sign of leukaemia*)

Reference

Willacy, H. 2019. Generalised lymphadenopathy. Patient professional article. https://patient.info/doctor/generalised-lymphadenopathy

MUMPS

History

- Swelling/pain of parotid glands, worse on chewing
- Dry mouth, making it harder to swallow
- Fever
- Malaise
- Headache
- Earache
- Contact with mumps (up to 28 days before)
- Vaccination history
- 🚩 Drowsiness/photophobia/vomiting/severe headache
- 🚩 Abdominal pain
- 🚩 Testicular pain

Examination

- Temperature
- Parotid glands (swelling may be unilateral or bilateral)
- Earlobe may be pushed upward and outward
- 🚩 Neck stiffness, confusion/drowsiness, photophobia
- 🚩 Abdominal tenderness
- 🚩 Swollen/tender testicle(s)

Tests

- Confirmation of the diagnosis (using a special salivary sample kit) may be requested by the HPT; note that mumps is a notifiable disease and the HPT must be informed

Self-care

- Advise that it is a self-limiting viral condition which usually resolves in 1–2 weeks
- Paracetamol or ibuprofen[P] may ease the discomfort
- Maintain fluid intake
- Acidic fruit juices may intensify the pain and should be avoided
- Infectious from 2 days before to 5 days after the onset of swelling
- To stay off school or work for 5 days after the initial development of parotid swelling
- Vulnerable contacts (who have not previously received two doses of mumps vaccine) should be vaccinated. Unfortunately, vaccination will not give immediate protection
- Safety-netting advice: seek help if severe headache, vomiting, neck stiffness, photophobia, confusion, drowsiness or abdominal or testicular pain

RED FLAGS

- Symptoms of meningitis or encephalitis due to mumps (*e.g., severe headache, vomiting, neck stiffness, photophobia, confusion, drowsiness; admit urgently under Medical/Paediatrics*)
- Abdominal tenderness (*may have pancreatitis; admit urgently Medical*)
- Testicular symptoms (*may have orchitis; refer to experienced colleague*)

EARACHE

History

- Duration and type of pain/discomfort
- Hearing impairment
- Discharge from ear
- Fever
- Previous ear problems/perforation
- Any previous treatment
- ⚑ Immunosuppressed
- ⚑ Cochlear implant

Examination

- Temperature
- If feverish, view ear from behind to look for outward and downward displacement of pinna (due to mastoiditis) and check mastoid area for tenderness and swelling
- Use an otoscope to check:
  - Ear canal for inflammation, foreign body, discharge or swelling (generalised or local, e.g., boil); pain on insertion of the otoscope suggests that inflammation is present
  - Tympanic membrane to assess colour, dullness, perforation, bulging/retraction and fluid level

Differential diagnosis

The most likely causes of acute earache are otitis media, otitis externa, a boil in the ear canal, impacted wax or Eustachian tube dysfunction.

OTITIS MEDIA

- Inflammation of the middle ear
- Can be caused by viruses and/or bacteria. It is difficult to distinguish between them
- Most commonly affects children from birth to 4 years; less common in adults

History

- Younger children may present with fever, crying, poor feeding, holding/rubbing of ear, cough, runny nose, or vomiting
- Older children and adults present more specifically with earache
- Other possible symptoms: vertigo, hearing loss, sudden discharge from the ear

Examination

- Tympanic membrane is pink/red, yellow or cloudy and may be bulging (note that other causes of bilateral pink/red tympanic membrane include an URTI, fever, and a distressed crying baby)
- If the tympanic membrane cannot be visualised, but the history is suggestive, assume that otitis media is present

Self-care

- Advise that symptoms usually last for around 3 days, but can last up to 1 week
- Reassure that ear infections in the UK today very rarely cause complications
- Recommend paracetamol or ibuprofen[P] given regularly at maximum dose for age to treat the pain
- Explain that antibiotics are not helpful for most people with otitis media. 60% will be pain-free within 24 hours, whether or not they take antibiotics, and the chance of experiencing a side effect from the antibiotic is greater than the chance of benefiting
- Flying or diving may cause severe pain and even perforation, and should be avoided while pain is present
- Severe infections may cause temporary deafness by perforation of the eardrum, which will usually heal within 3 weeks

- If perforation is present, avoid getting water in the ear
- Safety-netting advice: seek help if symptoms worsen significantly or there is no improvement within 3 days

Prescription

- Prescribe an antibiotic if:
  - Seriously ill
  - Immunosuppressed
  - Symptoms for ≥3 days and not improving
- Consider an antibiotic if:
  - Discharge and perforation
  - Grommet in place (the only indication for a topical antibiotic in otitis media; NICE 2023)
- If an oral antibiotic is indicated (see BNFC for children's doses):
  - Amoxicillin for 5–7 days (500 mg three times daily for adults)
  - If allergic to penicillin, give clarithromycin[PIQ] (500 mg twice daily for adults)
  - If not responding to amoxicillin within 3 days, change to co-amoxiclav (500/125 mg three times daily for adults)
- If a topical antibiotic is indicated:
  - Ciprofloxacin with dexamethasone. Apply four drops twice daily for 7 days (*unlicensed indication*)
- Topical ciprofloxacin drops are safe and more effective than oral antibiotics in children with grommets (NICE, 2023; Mather et al., 2022; Steele et al., 2017). Note that other types of antibiotic ear drops (aminoglycoside) can cause hearing damage if they are allowed past the eardrum. Topical antibiotics will be ineffective in otitis media when the tympanic membrane is intact
- Note that there is limited evidence on the role of antibiotics in adults with otitis media
- If an immediate antibiotic is not prescribed and there is no perforation or discharge, consider topical anti-inflammatory and anaesthetic ear drops for pain (Hay et al., 2019; NICE, 2022); phenazone and lidocaine (Otigo), four drops two or three times a day for up to 7 days

RED FLAGS

- Cochlear implant (*will need IV antibiotics; send urgently to hospital with referral to ENT*)
- Suspected mastoiditis (*send urgently to hospital with referral to ENT*)
- Immunosuppressed person with hearing loss, pain and discharge (*if not responding to treatment within 72 hours, send urgently to hospital with referral to ENT*)
- Persistent foul-smelling discharge and hearing loss (*possible cholesteatoma; refer urgently to ENT*)
- If hearing does not return to normal within 21 days (*may need ENT referral for monitoring of perforation*)

References

Antonelli, P.J., and Durand, M.L. 2022. Cochlear implant infections. UpToDate. Waltham, MA: UpToDate. https://medilib.ir/uptodate/show/5534

Cushen, R., and Francis, N. 2020. Antibiotic use and serious complications following acute otitis media and acute sinusitis: a retrospective cohort study. *Br J Gen Pract*; 70(693):e255. https://doi.org/10.3399/bjgp20X708821

Hay, A., Downing, H., Francis, N., et al. 2019. Anaesthetic–analgesic ear drops to reduce antibiotic consumption in children with acute otitis media: the CEDAR RCT. *Health Technol Assess*; 23(34). https://doi.org/10.3310/hta23340

Mather, M.W., Talks, B., Dawe, N., et al. 2022. Ototopical therapies for post tympanostomy tube otorrhoea in children. *Translational Pediatrics*; 11(10):1739–42. https://doi.org/10.21037/tp-22-387

NICE. 2018. NG98. Hearing loss in adults: assessment and management. www.nice.org.uk/guidance/ng98

NICE CKS. 2022. Otitis media – acute. https://cks.nice.org.uk/topics/otitis-media-acute/

NICE. 2022. NG91. Otitis media (acute): antimicrobial prescribing. www.nice.org.uk/guidance/ng91

NICE. 2023. NG233. Otitis media with effusion in under 12s. https://www.nice.org.uk/guidance/ng233 *Consider non-ototoxic topical antibiotic ear drops (such as ciprofloxacin) for 5 to 7 days for otorrhoea after grommet insertion.*

Steele, D., Adam, G., Di, M., et al. 2017. Prevention and treatment of tympanostomy tube otorrhea: a meta-analysis. *Pediatrics*; 139(6):e20170667. https://doi.org/10.1542/peds.2017-0667

Venekamp, R., Sanders, S., Glasziou, P., et al. 2015. Antibiotics for acute otitis media in children. *Cochrane Database Syst Rev*; 6:CD000219. https://doi.org/10.1002/14651858.CD000219.pub4

OTITIS EXTERNA

- Inflammation of the outer ear
- More commonly affects adults; less common in children
- Typically caused by *Pseudomonas aeruginosa* or *Staphylococcus aureus*
- Risk factors include underlying skin conditions such as eczema, acute otitis media, trauma to the ear canal (including hearing aids), foreign body and water exposure (swimming)
- The treatment may vary depending on the presence of perforation of the tympanic membrane or grommets (see Box 5.4)

History

- Itch, discomfort or discharge
- Hearing loss (due to occlusion of the ear canal)
- Current perforation
- Grommet in place
- ⚑ Immunosuppressed

Examination

- Temperature (a high-grade fever is uncommon in otitis externa; if present, reconsider the diagnosis)
- Tenderness of the tragus and/or pinna
- Pain/discomfort on inserting otoscope
- Red and swollen ear canal
- Sometimes the tympanic membrane may also appear red
- Discharge (scant white mucus suggests bacterial infection and fluffy white/off-white or black/grey small balls suggests fungal infection)

Test

- Consider taking a swab if there is copious discharge or resistant/recurrent infection, but results may be misleading – remember that the antibiotic sensitivity data relate to oral antibiotics whereas topical treatment gives higher concentrations

Self-care

- Avoid putting anything into the ear canal (remember the old adage 'put nothing in your ear smaller than your elbow'!)
- Use cotton wool and Vaseline to keep shampoo and shower gel out of inflamed ears while showering or washing hair
- Dry inside ears with hairdryer on lowest heat setting
- Use ear plugs when swimming. Avoid swimming while ear is inflamed
- People aged ≥12 can use acetic acid spray (EarCalm^C OTC) twice daily and after swimming or showering, for a maximum of 7 days. Maximum dosage frequency is one spray every 2–3 hours

---

BOX 5.4 IS THE TYMPANIC MEMBRANE PERFORATED?

If the tympanic membrane cannot be seen (e.g., due to wax in canal), then suspect perforation if:

- Medication placed in the ear can be tasted, *or*
- Air can be blown out of the ear when the nose is pinched, *or*
- Grommet inserted in the past year (and not known to have fallen out)

Prescription

- If very inflamed, offer ear drops containing an antibiotic and a corticosteroid for 7–14 days. These should be warmed to room temperature before use

- **If there is a grommet/perforation (see Box 5.4), all antibiotic ear drops except ciprofloxacin are contraindicated**, as they contain aminoglycoside antibiotics, which could potentially cause long-term hearing damage. Instead, use ciprofloxacin with dexamethasone[PC]; apply four drops twice daily for 7 days

- In other situations there is little evidence to inform the choice; be guided by price and availability. Options include:
  - Otomize[PC] spray (containing neomycin); one spray three times a day for adults and children aged ≥2 years
  - Sofradex[P] (containing framycetin and gramicidin); apply two or three drops, three to four times a day (note that this is listed by the BNF as 'less suitable for prescribing')

- Oral antibiotics may be indicated in some situations – see Box 5.5

- If swab shows a fungal cause (around 10% of otitis externa cases), then first try clotrimazole 1% solution two or three times a day, continued for 2 weeks after the infection appears to have cleared. Treatment may be needed for up to a few months. Occasionally, oral antifungal treatment is needed

> **BOX 5.5 ORAL ANTIBIOTICS FOR OTITIS EXTERNA**
>
> Topical antibiotic treatment is usually preferable. *Prescribe an oral antibiotic (with or without topical treatment)* only if:
>
> - Canal completely blocked with debris and suction not available
> - Signs of systemic infection
> - Cellulitis
> - Immunosuppressed
>
> Seek advice from an experienced colleague on the choice of antibiotic. Flucloxacillin will not cover *Pseudomonas*; dual therapy with topical antibiotic and oral ciprofloxacin[PCIQ] (500 mg twice daily for adults) may be recommended, particularly if suspicion of *Pseudomonas* due to history of swimming or blue-green discharge. Note that fluoroquinolone antibiotics, such as ciprofloxacin, should only be prescribed for systemic use when other commonly recommended antibiotics are inappropriate

> **RED FLAGS**
>
> - Severe infection in person with immunosuppression which has not responded to treatment within 72 hours (*possible 'malignant' otitis externa extending into bone; send to hospital urgently with referral to ENT*)
> - Facial palsy (*possible Ramsay Hunt syndrome; send to hospital urgently with referral to ENT*)
> - Canal completely occluded or persistent/recurrent symptoms (*referral for microsuction according to local pathway*)
> - Bloodstained discharge (*possible cancer; refer to experienced colleague*)

References

Al Aaraj, M., and Kelley, C. 2020. Malignant otitis externa. *StatPearls*. www.ncbi.nlm.nih.gov/books/NBK556138/

NICE CKS. 2022. Otitis externa. https://cks.nice.org.uk/topics/otitis-externa/

Rosenfeld, R., Schwartz, S., Cannon, C., et al. 2014. Clinical practice guideline: acute otitis externa. *Otolaryngol Head Neck Surg*; 150(S1):S1–S24. https://doi.org/10.1177/0194599813517083

Willacy, H. 2022. Otomycosis; fungal ear infection. Patient professional article. https://patient.info/doctor/fungal-ear-infection-otomycosis

BOIL IN EAR CANAL

This staphylococcal infection is very painful and causes a localised red swelling in the canal, often with unilateral deafness. Introduce the otoscope gradually and gently, looking through it as you do this because impacting the earpiece directly on to a boil can cause severe pain.

ENT

Self-care

- Take paracetamol or ibuprofen[P] to relieve the pain
- The ear may discharge

Prescription

- Prescribe an antibiotic if:
  - Cellulitis spreading to pinna
  - Fever
  - Immunosuppressed/diabetes
- If antibiotic is indicated, first line would be flucloxacillin, 250–500 mg four times daily for adults for 7 days
- If allergic to penicillin, give clarithromycin[PIQ], 250 mg twice daily for adults (use erythromycin[PIQ] if pregnant)

Reference

NICE CKS. 2022. Boils, carbuncles, and staphylococcal carriage: scenario: boils and carbuncles. https://cks.nice.org.uk/topics/boils-carbuncles-staphylococcal-carriage/management/boils-carbuncles/

EUSTACHIAN TUBE DYSFUNCTION

The Eustachian tube is responsible for drainage of middle ear secretions, equalising pressure differences between the environment and the body, and protection from potentially deafening sounds. Dysfunction is common in children and may follow an episode of otitis media, URTI, sinus infection or hay fever, causing the Eustachian tube to become blocked (a different mechanism of the loss of fatty tissue supporting the tube can cause similar symptoms after rapid weight loss).

History

- Reduced/muffled hearing (as if underwater)
- Feeling of fullness in the ear
- Ear intermittently 'popping'
- Discomfort/pain
- Tinnitus

Examination

- The tympanic membrane may appear retracted or bulging, indicating a pressure difference between the inner and outer ear; a normal appearance neither supports nor refutes the diagnosis
- A fluid level may be seen behind the drum, which is not inflamed

Self-care

- Explain that the eardrum is a sensitive structure that hurts when pressure changes. When catarrh blocks the Eustachian tube, changes in atmospheric pressure cause earache that comes and goes
- Paracetamol or ibuprofen[P] may ease the discomfort
- Nasal decongestant drops or sprays may help unblock the tube (e.g., Otrivine[PC] OTC, for no more than 3 days [two or three drops or one spray up to three times a day]). Otrivine[PC] is licensed for 7 days' use, but see Dykewicz et al., 2020
- Carefully 'pop' the ears by trying to breathe out with mouth closed and nostrils shut (pinching the nose). Yawning and swallowing can also help
- If these manoeuvres fail, an Otovent balloon (OTC) can help open the Eustachian tube
- Nasal douching with saline can help flush out excess mucus and debris from the nose and sinuses
- Antihistamines or nasal corticosteroids may reduce nasal congestion and/or inflammation of the lining of the Eustachian tube

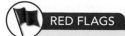

RED FLAGS

- Sudden onset (taking ≤3 days) of unexplained hearing loss which occurred within the last 30 days (*possible autoimmune disease, infection, tumour or stroke; send urgently to hospital with referral to ENT*)
- Sudden onset (taking ≤3 days) of unexplained hearing loss which occurred more than 30 days ago (*refer urgently to ENT*)
- Hearing loss which is unexplained and rapidly worsening over a period of 4–90 days (*refer urgently to ENT*)
- Persistent asymmetric, unexplained hearing loss (*refer to ENT*)

ENT

References

Dykewicz, M., Wallace, D., Amrol, D., et al. 2020. Rhinitis 2020: A practice parameter update. *J Allergy Clin Immunol*; 146(4):721–67. https://doi.org/10.1016/j.jaci.2020.07.007 *Rebound congestion may develop within 5 days of use of topical decongestants.*

Llewellyn, A., Norman, G., Harden, M., et al. 2014. Interventions for adult Eustachian tube dysfunction: a systematic review. *Health Technol Assess*; 18(46). https://doi.org/10.3310/hta18460

NICE CKS. 2019. Hearing loss in adults. https://cks.nice.org.uk/topics/hearing-loss-in-adults/

EAR WAX

Wax is a mixture of several substances including dead skin cells, cerumen (produced by special glands in the ear canal) and sebum from sebaceous glands. It is mildly acidic and antibacterial. The gradual migration of cells in the ear canal causes wax to travel, assisted by jaw movement, towards the outside of the ear over a few weeks, so it cleans and protects the delicate surfaces.

History

- Hearing loss
- Ear discomfort/blockage
- Tinnitus
- Itching
- Use of cotton buds
- Ask about any previous perforation of tympanic membrane

Examination

- Note extent of wax and whether it is impacted against tympanic membrane
- Check for perforation if the tympanic membrane is visible
- Check for inflammation of any visible parts of the ear canal skin

Self-care

- Do not insert cotton buds inside the ear canal
- There is no evidence to prefer one type of wax-softening ear drop over another. The BNF counsels that sodium bicarbonate drops may cause dryness. Use olive oil or sodium bicarbonate ear drops, at body temperature, three times daily for at least 7 days. Warn that they may cause discomfort, dizziness and irritation of the skin and can make hearing and symptoms worse before getting better. DO NOT recommend if there is a suspected perforated tympanic membrane, active dermatitis or active infection of the ear canal
- The use of ear candles is not supported by evidence

Action

- If self-care is ineffective, consider microsuction (preferred) or irrigation. Check local availability of these services
- Pre-softening of wax is not required for microsuction; contraindications are severe dizziness and inability to keep the head still
- Contraindications to irrigation include:
  - Perforation of the tympanic membrane (some ENT specialists may permit irrigation if there is an old, healed perforation, but this should be agreed in advance)
  - Active inflammation or infection of the ear canal

- Grommets
- Previous ear surgery
- Discharge from ear in the previous 12 months
- Otitis media in the previous 6 weeks
- Cleft palate, even after surgical correction
- Foreign body in the ear
- Previous problem with irrigation
- 'Precious ear' (i.e., only one hearing ear)

References

Meyer, F., Preuß, R., Angelow, A., et al. 2020. Cerumen impaction removal in general practices: a comparison of approved standard products. *J Prim Care Community Health*; 11:2150132720973829. https://doi.org/10.1177/2150132720973829
NICE CKS. 2021. Earwax. https://cks.nice.org.uk/topics/earwax/

COMMON COLD (CORYZA)

A mild, self-limiting URTI caused by a wide range of different viruses. Though usually associated with a dry cough, even a productive cough with green phlegm is most likely viral in origin (in people without COPD).

History

- Duration
- Fever
- Sore throat
- Blocked or discharging nose, sneezing
- Hoarse voice
- Cough
- Joint and muscle pain

Examination

- Temperature
- Throat (usually appears normal)
- Cervical lymph nodes
- Ears
- Chest

Self-care

- Consider a COVID-19 test if in a high-risk group (see Chapter 4)
- Reassure that, although unpleasant, the symptoms of a cold are self-limiting; usually peaking at day 2–3 and resolving after 7 days in adults and 14 days in younger children. A mild cough may persist for 3 weeks
- For symptomatic relief:
  - Paracetamol or ibuprofen[P] if needed for sore throat/headache/body pains
  - Gargling with salt water (half a teaspoon of salt in 250 ml of water)
  - Honey (if aged ≥1 year) and lemon (Paul et al., 2007)
  - Sodium chloride nasal drops (for babies) or spray (e.g., Sterimar Hypertonic) (Cabaillot et al., 2020)
  - Nasal decongestant drops or sprays, e.g. Otrivine[PC], for no more than 3 days (two or three drops or one spray up to three times a day)
  - Although steam inhalation has been recommended as a home remedy for many years, there is no evidence of benefit, and children are at risk of serious burns (Scarborough et al., 2021). However, this risk can be minimised by steaming up a bathroom by running a hot shower, or using one of the many humidified air devices available
- Some evidence suggests that high-dose zinc (15 mg/day) and vitamin C (at least 1000 mg/day) may shorten the duration of colds (Abioye et al., 2021)

- Frequent handwashing and avoiding sharing towels and toys may reduce the spread of infection
- Prophylaxis – taking a probiotic for 3 months in the winter reduced:
  - The chance of having at least one URTI by 24%
  - The chance of having three or more URTIs by 41%
  - The mean duration of a URTI by 1.2 days (Zhao et al., 2022)

References

Abioye, A., Bromage, S., and Fawzi, W. 2021. Effect of micronutrient supplements on influenza and other respiratory tract infections among adults: a systematic review and meta-analysis. *BMJ Global Health*; 6(1):e003176. https://doi.org/10.1136/bmjgh-2020-003176

Al Himdani, S., Javed, M., Hughes, J., et al. 2016. Home remedy or hazard? Management and costs of paediatric steam inhalation therapy burn injuries. *Br J Gen Pract*; 66(644):e193. https://doi.org/10.3399/bjgp16X684289

Cabaillot, A., Vorilhon, P., Roca, M., et al. 2020. Saline nasal irrigation for acute upper respiratory tract infections in infants and children: a systematic review and meta-analysis. *Paediat Respir Rev*; 36:151–8. https://doi.org/10.1016/j.prrv.2019.11.003

Deckx, L., DeSutter, A., Guo, L., et al. 2016. Nasal decongestants in monotherapy for the common cold. *Cochrane Database Syst Rev*; 10:CD009612. https://doi.org/10.1002/14651858.CD009612.pub2

DeSutter, A., Eriksson, L., and vanDriel, M. 2022. Oral antihistamine-decongestant-analgesic combinations for the common cold. *Cochrane Database Syst Rev*; 1:CD004976. https://doi.org/10.1002/14651858.CD004976.pub4

Dykewicz, M., Wallace, D., Amrol, D., et al. 2020. Rhinitis 2020: a practice parameter update. *J Allergy Clin Immunol*; 146(4):721–67. https://doi.org/10.1016/j.jaci.2020.07.007 *Rebound congestion may develop within 5 days of use of topical decongestants.*

Karsch-Völk, M., Barrett, B., Kiefer, D., et al. 2014. Echinacea for preventing and treating the common cold. *Cochrane Database Syst Rev*; 2:CD000530. https://doi.org/10.1002/14651858.CD000530.pub3

Paul, I., Beiler, J., McMonagle, A., et al. 2007. Effect of honey, dextromethorphan, and no treatment on nocturnal cough and sleep quality for coughing children and their parents *Arch Pediatr Adolesc Med*; 161(12):1140–6. https://doi.org/10.1001/archpedi.161.12.1140

Paul, I., Beiler, J., King, T., et al. 2010. Vapor rub, petrolatum, and no treatment for children with nocturnal cough and cold symptoms. *Pediatrics*; 126(6):1092–9. https://doi.org/10.1542/peds.2010-1601

Public Health England. 2013. Green phlegm and snot 'not always a sign of an infection needing antibiotics'. www.gov.uk/government/news/green-phlegm-and-snot-not-always-a-sign-of-an-infection-needing-antibiotics

Scarborough, A., Scarborough, O., Abdi, H., et al. 2021. Steam inhalation: more harm than good? Perspective from a UK burns centre. *Burns*; 47(3):721–7. https://doi.org/10.1016/j.burns.2020.08.010

Timmer, A., Günther, J., Motschall, E., et al. 2013. Pelargonium sidoides extract for treating acute respiratory tract infections. *Cochrane Database Syst Rev*; 10:CD006323. https://doi.org/10.1002/14651858.CD006323.pub3

Zhao, Y., Dong, B.R., and Hao, Q. 2022. Probiotics for preventing acute upper respiratory tract infections. *Cochrane Database Syst Rev*; 8:CD006895. https://doi.org/10.1002/14651858.CD006895.pub4

SINUSITIS

This is usually viral in origin and can be difficult to diagnose because the traditional symptoms and signs are unreliable. It is defined as symptomatic inflammation of the paranasal sinuses, worsening after 5 days or persisting beyond 10 days, and often follows a common cold. It is much less common in children because their sinuses are not fully developed.

History

- Duration (average 18–20 days)
- Diagnostic features in adults:
  - Nasal blockage/purulent nasal discharge (may be anterior and/or posterior) *with*
  - Facial pain/headache (typically worse on bending forward) and/or reduction in sense of smell
- Other associated symptoms may include:
  - Fever
  - Cough
  - Toothache
- 🚩 Bloody nasal discharge
- 🚩 Eye/visual symptoms (e.g., periorbital oedema, double vision, reduced acuity)

ENT

Examination

- Temperature
- Heart rate
- Respiratory rate
- BP in adults
- Throat (look for post-nasal discharge)
- Ears
- 🚩 Localised swelling or redness anywhere on the face (consider cellulitis)

Self-care

- If appropriate, reassure that sinusitis is most often caused by a viral infection and is only complicated by a bacterial infection in 2% of cases (NICE, 2017). It can take 2–3 weeks to resolve
- Avoid smoky atmospheres
- Using a sinus rinse kit available OTC (e.g., NeilMed Sinus Rinse) may help, or irrigate the nose with sodium chloride solution (e.g., Sterimar Hypertonic)
- Analgesia with paracetamol or ibuprofen[P] if needed
- Decongestant nasal drops or spray, e.g., Otrivine[PC] (for no more than 3 days) may also provide symptomatic relief

Prescription

- Consider high-dose nasal corticosteroid, e.g., mometasone 200 micrograms twice daily or fluticasone 100 micrograms twice daily (*unlicensed indication*)
- Prescribe an antibiotic if any of the following:
  - Seriously ill
  - Immunosuppressed
  - Symptoms not improving within 10 days
  - Purulent discharge and severe local pain (particularly if unilateral)
- If prescribing an antibiotic in adults:
  - First choice: phenoxymethylpenicillin, 500 mg four times daily for adults for 5 days
  - If allergic to penicillin, use doxycycline[PBC] (200 mg on the first day then 100 mg once daily for adults for 5 days in total) or clarithromycin[PIQ] (250 mg twice daily for adults for 5 days)
  - If systemically unwell, at a high risk of complications, or symptoms are worsening despite 2–3 days of the first-line antibiotic, use co-amoxiclav (500/125 mg three times daily for adults for 5 days) or azithromycin[PQ] (500 mg once daily for adults for 3 days)
- If prescribing an antibiotic in children:
  - First choice: phenoxymethylpenicillin for 5 days. An alternative if the child cannot tolerate the taste of phenoxymethylpenicillin suspension is amoxicillin
  - If allergic to penicillin, use clarithromycin[PIQ] for 5 days
  - If systemically unwell, at high risk of complications or symptoms are worsening despite 2–3 days of the first-line antibiotic, use co-amoxiclav for 5 days or azithromycin[PQ] for 3 days

RED FLAGS

- Eye symptoms, e.g., periorbital oedema, double vision, reduced visual acuity (*intraorbital complications; send urgently to hospital with referral to ENT*)
- Severe frontal headache or swelling over frontal bone (*intracranial complications; send urgently to hospital with referral to ENT*)
- Persistent unilateral nasal obstruction with bloody discharge (*USC referral to ENT*)
- Inflammation of the face, especially near eyes/nose (*facial cellulitis; consider urgent admission under Medical/Paediatrics*)

References

Cushen, R., and Francis, N. 2020. Antibiotic use and serious complications following acute otitis media and acute sinusitis: a retrospective cohort study. *Br J Gen Pract*; 70(693):e255. https://doi.org/10.3399/bjgp20X708821

Foden, N., Burgess, C., Shepherd, K., et al. 2013. A guide to the management of acute rhinosinusitis in primary care management strategy based on best evidence and recent European guidelines. *Br J Gen Pract*; 63(616):611. https://doi.org/10.3399/bjgp13X674620

Lemiengre, M., vanDriel, M., Merenstein, D., et al. 2018. Antibiotics for acute rhinosinusitis in adults. *Cochrane Database Syst Rev*; 9:CD006089. https://doi.org/10.1002/14651858.CD006089.pub5

Little, P., Stuart, B., Mullee, M., et al. 2016. Effectiveness of steam inhalation and nasal irrigation for chronic or recurrent sinus symptoms in primary care: a pragmatic randomized controlled trial. *CMAJ*; 188(13):940. https://doi.org/10.1503/cmaj.160362 *Steam inhalations were not effective, but nasal irrigation provided some symptom relief*

NICE. 2017. NG79. Sinusitis (acute): antimicrobial prescribing. www.nice.org.uk/guidance/ng79

Zalmanovici Trestioreanu, A., and Yaphe, J. 2013. Intranasal steroids for acute sinusitis. *Cochrane Database Syst Rev*; 12:CD005149. https://doi.org/10.1002/14651858.CD005149.pub4

ENT

HAY FEVER (SEASONAL ALLERGIC RHINITIS)

Seasonal (usually April to September) reaction to tree, grass or weed pollen (listed in their annual sequence of release). Many people assume they are allergic to a particular plant, such as oilseed rape that appears in bright yellow crops each year, but it is usually no more than a coincidence of timing. Plants with obvious flowers use them to attract insects as pollinators, whereas those with insignificant flowers may rely on the wind, so are more likely to trigger an allergic response (Smith, 2011). Note that allergy to mould spores can cause very similar symptoms to hay fever and tends to reach a peak in the Autumn.

History

- Frequent sneezing
- Blocked nose
- Nasal itching
- Red, itchy, watery eyes
- Dry, sore throat
- Wheeze, chest tightness, cough (hay fever may trigger/worsen asthma and has been implicated in ~15% of asthma deaths; controlling hay fever should also improve the asthma)
- Any treatment tried already? If so, with what effect?

Examination

- Check eyes for discharge (suggests infection)
- Check nose for polyps

Action

Non-pharmacological approaches

Pollen grains are very, very small, so avoidance is impossible. Advice can aim only to reduce the exposure to high concentrations. Some form of treatment for residual symptoms is necessary for most people.

- Nasal irrigation with saline
- Check pollen forecasts and try to avoid going outdoors, if possible, when counts are high, particularly during early mornings, early evenings and thunderstorms
- Avoid long grass and newly mowed lawns
- Avoid drying clothes outdoors when the pollen count is high
- When choosing a car, consider one with a pollen filter
- Consider investing in an 'air purifier' with a high-efficiency particulate air (HEPA) filter at home
- There is no evidence to support the standard advice to sleep with windows closed, except during thunderstorms
- Useful information about hay fever and other allergic conditions can be found at www.itchysneezywheezy.co.uk
- Advice is available from AllergyUK – www.allergyuk.org/types-of-allergies/hay fever

Pharmacological treatments (summarised in Table 5.2 and Figure 5.2)

- **Intranasal antihistamine spray (azelastine hydrochloride[PBC])**
  - Recommended as an initial treatment option, particularly if symptoms are intermittent
  - Available only on prescription and is licensed for adults and children aged ≥5 years
  - At least as effective as oral anthistamines but works much faster (15-30 min vs. 150 min)
  - Particularly good for nasal symptoms and provides the same relief for eye symptoms as intranasal corticosteroids
  - Side effects include drowsiness and a bitter taste
- **Intranasal steroid sprays** are recommended as an initial treatment for moderate/severe and persistent hay fever in people aged ≥15
  - Help with nasal and eye symptoms
  - More effective if started a few days (ideally 2 weeks) before symptoms are expected to begin. Their benefits will be reduced if they are not used correctly; see Figure 5.1
  - May be used in children and during pregnancy and breastfeeding, but a prescription will be required. There is concern that beclomethasone[PC] or fluticasone[C] may slow growth in children (Lee et al., 2014; Passali et al., 2016); instead use mometasone[C] for children aged ≥3 years
- **Intranasal anticholinergic sprays** can dry up nasal secretions and help manage runny nose in hay fever
  - Contain ipratropium, are prescription-only and only licensed for people aged ≥12 years
  - There is only one preparation available in the UK (Rinaspray[PC]: two sprays in each nostril, two or three times a day)
- **Intranasal saline sprays** (e.g., Sterimar isotonic) provide some improvement in symptoms with few side effects and may be a useful choice in pregnancy
- **Intranasal decongestants** are suggested only for short-term and intermittent treatment of nasal congestion (e.g., Otrivine[PC], OTC, two or three drops or one spray up to three times a day for adults)
  - Can provide quick relief for adults
  - Should not be used for more than 3 days as they can cause rebound symptoms
- **Oral antihistamines** are recommended for mild or intermittent symptoms
  - Second-generation antihistamines (e.g., cetirizine[PB], loratadine[PB] and fexofenadine[PBC]) are preferred to first-generation antihistamines (e.g., chlorphenamine[PBI]), as they have less potential side effects including sedation, performance impairment and anticholinergic-mediated symptoms (e.g., dry eyes, dry mouth, constipation, urinary hesitancy and urinary retention)
  - First-generation antihistamines are widely used by the public, but have a long half-life and are associated with poor performance in exams (Walker et al., 2007)
  - Be aware that even second-generation antihistamines may not be permitted for people in safety-critical occupations
  - No evidence that one antihistamine is more effective than others overall, but people may differ in their individual response
  - There is rarely a need to prescribe oral antihistamines, as they are available OTC for much less than a prescription charge
  - Loratadine[PB] is available OTC for children aged ≥2 years. However, a prescription would be required in pregnancy and breastfeeding
  - Despite a large body of evidence on loratadine[PB] showing no detrimental effects (Gilboa et al., 2014; emc, 2023), the manufacturers advise its avoidance in pregnancy; this appears in most patient information leaflets. Similar advice to avoid taking antihistamines in pregnancy appears for other antihistamines. Generally it is best to avoid medication in the first trimester when possible, but, given the evidence, the risk is low
  - When given to a breastfeeding mother, antihistamines may reduce the milk supply and cetirizine[PB] may sedate the baby (loratadine[PB] is preferred)
- **Eye drops** are recommended for symptomatic eyes
  - Sodium cromoglicate eye drops (OTC, four times daily) can be bought as an additional treatment (although a prescription will be needed if pregnant or breastfeeding), but they are slow to take effect. These may sting, especially if the eyes are already inflamed, and should be started at least 2 weeks before the season

- Otrivine Antistin[PBC] drops (OTC, two or three times daily) are faster acting but should not be used for more than 3 days because of their vasoconstrictor effect (Table 5.2)
- Topical antihistamine eye drops containing azelastine[PBC] (apply twice daily, increase if necessary to four times a day) are quicker acting but less effective than sodium cromoglicate eye drops and are available only with a prescription

Table 5.2 Choice of medication for hay fever

Medication	Over the counter	Prescription
Intranasal antihistamine	Not available	Azelastine hydrochloride[PBC]
Steroid nasal spray	Whichever is best value	Beclometasone[PC] (adult) Mometasone[C] (≥3 years)
Antihistamine – oral	Whichever second-generation drug is best value	Loratadine[PB] Cetirizine[PB] Fexofenadine[PBC]
Decongestant nasal spray	Whichever is best value	Otrivine[PC]
Intranasal anticholinergic (to 'dry up' runny nose)	Not available	Ipratropium[PC] (≥12 years)
Antihistamine – eye (for short-term symptom relief)	Otrivine Antistin[PBC] for no more than 3 days (≥12 years)	Azelastine[PBC] (≥4 years)
Long-term eye drop	Sodium cromoglicate	Sodium cromoglicate

- If usual treatment ineffective, consider prescribing:
  - Fluticasone/azelastine[PBC] nasal spray (Dymista[PBC], one spray twice daily into each nostril). This is a combination of intranasal antihistamine and steroid
  - Montelukast[PB] (as effective as antihistamines in children). A shared decision-making conversation is helpful to alert people to the rare (1 in 10,000) risk of neuropsychiatric events, including suicidal thoughts or behaviour (MHRA, 2019)
  - Famotidine[PBCQ] (*unlicensed indication*) 150 mg twice daily for adults (for more information, see the drug's entry in Prescribing Insights in the Members' section of the NMIC website)
  - In severe cases, prednisolone[PI] for 7 days (15–20 mg daily for adults, 5–10 mg daily for children)

(A)

1. Shake bottle well
2. Look down
3. Using right hand for left nostril put nozzle just inside nose aiming towards outside wall
4. Squirt once or twice (2 different directions)
5. Change hands and repeat for other side
6. Breathe in gently through the nose
7. Do not sniff

(B)

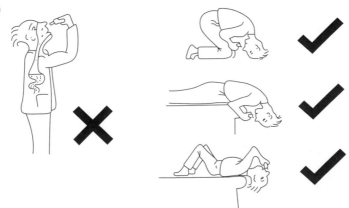

Figure 5.1 The correct use of nasal drops and sprays. (Scadding et al., 2017.)

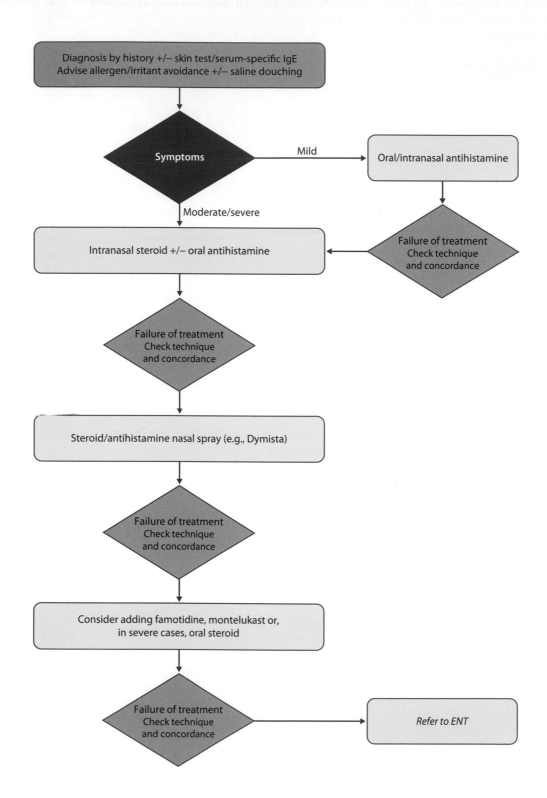

Figure 5.2 Management of allergic rhinitis in adults. (Derived from Lipworth et al., 2017.)

References

Dykewicz, M., Wallace, D., Amrol, D., et al. 2020. Rhinitis 2020: a practice parameter update. *J Allergy Clin Immunol*; 146(4):721–67. https://doi.org/10.1016/j.jaci.2020.07.007 *Rebound congestion may develop within 5 days of use of topical decongestants.*

emc. 2023. Loratadine 10 mg tablets. www.medicines.org.uk/emc/product/8911/smpc/print#PREGNANCY

Gilboa, S., Ailes, E., Rai, R., et al. 2014. Antihistamines and birth defects: a systematic review of the literature. *Expert Opin Drug Saf*; 13(12):1667–98. https://doi.org/10.1517/14740338.2014.970164

King, D. 2019. What role for saline nasal irrigation? *Drug Ther Bull*; 57(4):56. https://doi.org/10.1136/dtb.2018.000023 *In allergic rhinitis, symptom scores were improved with a decrease of 2 points on a 0–10 point visual analogue scale for nasal symptoms.*

Krishnamoorthy, M., Mohd Noor, N., MatLazim, N., et al. 2020. Efficacy of montelukast in allergic rhinitis treatment: a systematic review and meta-analysis. *Drugs*; 80(17):1831–51. https://doi.org/10.1007/s40265-020-01406-9

Lee, L., Sterling, R., Máspero, J., et al. 2014. Growth velocity reduced with once-daily fluticasone furoate nasal spray in prepubescent children with perennial allergic rhinitis. *J Allergy Clin Immunol Pract*; 2(4):421–7. https://doi.org/10.1016/j.jaip.2014.04.008

Lipworth, B., Newton, J., Ram, B., et al. 2017. An algorithm recommendation for the pharmacological management of allergic rhinitis in the UK: a consensus statement from an expert panel. *NPJ Prim Care Respir Med*; 27(1):3. https://doi.org/10.1038/s41533-016-0001-y *Suggested order of trying different treatments.*

Meltzer, E.O., Tripathy, I., Máspero, J.F., et al. 2009. Safety and tolerability of fluticasone furoate nasal spray once daily in paediatric patients aged 6–11 years with allergic rhinitis. *Clin Drug Investig*; 29(2):79–86. https://doi.org/10.2165/0044011-200929020-00002

MHRA. 2019. Montelukast (Singulair): reminder of the risk of neuropsychiatric reactions. www.gov.uk/drug-safety-update/montelukast-singulair-reminder-of-the-risk-of-neuropsychiatric-reactions

Royal College of Physicians. 2014. Why asthma still kills: the National Review of Asthma Deaths (NRAD). www.rcplondon.ac.uk/projects/outputs/why-asthma-still-kills

Passali, D., Spinosi, M., Crisanti, A., et al. 2016. Mometasone furoate nasal spray: a systematic review. *Multidiscip Respir Med*; 11(1):18. https://doi.org/10.1186/s40248-016-0054-3

Scadding, G., Kariyawasam, H., Scadding, G., et al. 2017. BSACI guideline for the diagnosis and management of allergic and non-allergic rhinitis (Revised edition 2017; first edition 2007). *Clin Exp Allergy*; 47(7):856–89. https://doi.org/10.1111/cea.12953

Skoner, D., Rachelefsky, G., Meltzer, E., et al. 2000. Detection of growth suppression in children during treatment with intranasal beclomethasone dipropionate. *Pediatrics*; 105(2):E23. https://doi.org/10.1542/peds.105.2.e23

Smith, H. 2011. Hay fever and allergic rhinitis. *InnovAiT*; 5(4):220–5. https://doi.org/10.1093/innovait/inr082

Wang, D., Clement, P., and Smitz, J. 1996. Effect of H1 and H2 antagonists on nasal symptoms and mediator release in atopic patients after nasal allergen challenge during the pollen season. *Acta Oto-Laryngologica*; 116(1):91–6. https://doi.org/10.3109/00016489609137720

Walker, S., Khan-Wasti, S., Fletcher, M., et al. 2007. Seasonal allergic rhinitis is associated with a detrimental effect on examination performance in United Kingdom teenagers: case–control study. *J Allergy Clin Immunol*; 120(2):381–7. https://doi.org/10.1016/j.jaci.2007.03.034

EPISTAXIS (NOSEBLEEDS)

Bleeding from the nose is usually self-limiting and often caused by damage to the blood vessels of the nasal mucosa. Most cases are anterior bleeds (80%–95%). Posterior bleeds are much less common but may occur in the elderly; they cause more profuse bleeding from both nostrils and the bleeding site will not be visible on examination. People with hypertension are 50% more likely to have epistaxis requiring hospital assessment (Byun et al., 2021).

History

- Which nostril, or both?
- Duration
- Blood loss – quantify, if possible, to identify if heavy or light bleeding
- Any previous episodes and, if so, how they were treated
- Has anything been inserted into the nose, e.g., cotton wool? (To reduce the risk of it being pushed in any further during examination/insertion of formal nasal packing)

ENT

- Questions to determine possible cause:
  - A history of nasal surgery or trauma such as nose picking, rubbing, sneezing
  - Other nasal symptoms of hay fever or bacterial sinusitis, or nasal polyps
  - Current medications (e.g., aspirin, anticoagulants or nasally administered drugs)
  - Recreational drug use (cocaine in particular)
  - Conditions predisposing to bleeding (e.g., haemophilia or leukaemia)
  - Family history of bleeding disorders
  - Environmental factors such as cold, dry weather, low humidity
- ⚑ Child aged <2 years (epistaxis is unusual in this age group and the possibility of non-accidental injury should be considered; it has been associated with intentional and non-intentional asphyxia)
- ⚑ Feeling faint (may have significant blood loss)
- ⚑ Symptoms of leukaemia – fever, fatigue, frequent infections, weight loss, swollen lymph nodes, easy bleeding or bruising (*refer to experienced colleague*)
- ⚑ Symptoms of nasal/paranasal cancer – blockage of one side of nose that does not go away, decreased sense of smell (*USC referral to ENT*)

Examination

- Heart rate
- CRT in children aged <12 years/BP in adults and older children (to assess severity of the blood loss/check for hypertension in adults)

Action

- Educate regarding nasal first aid. The person should be advised to be upright and leaning forward, and firmly pinch the **soft** part of the nose, compressing both nostrils for at least 10 minutes. Encourage them to spit out blood and advise to suck on an ice cube or apply ice pack to the nose
- Advise avoiding the following for the next 24 hours: blowing or picking the nose, heavy lifting, strenuous activity, lying flat, drinking alcohol or hot drinks
- Consider prescribing Naseptin (chlorhexidine and neomycin) cream to be applied to the nostrils four times daily for 10 days. If concordance is an issue, advise that it can instead be used twice daily for up to 2 weeks
  - If there is a history of allergy to peanut or soya, do not prescribe Naseptin; it has been reformulated to remove peanut products (available 2023), but there may be previous formulations still in the supply chain until November 2025
  - If Naseptin is not appropriate, consider prescribing mupirocin^P nasal ointment to be applied to the nostril two or three times a day for 5–7 days
- Safety-netting advice: seek help if there is further bleeding that does not respond to first aid measures

RED FLAGS

Consider *sending urgently to A&E* if:

- Nasal first aid fails
- On anticoagulant medications (will need international normalised ratio [INR] blood test if on warfarin)
- Concern that there may have been significant blood loss
- Significant comorbidity such as bleeding disorder, severe hypertension, ischaemic heart disease, severe anaemia
- Child aged <2 years (safeguarding concern)
- Elderly

References

Byun, H., Chung, J.H., Lee, S.H., et al. 2021. Association of hypertension with the risk and severity of epistaxis. *Jama Otolaryngol Head Neck Surg*; 147(1):34–40. https://doi.org/10.1001/jamaoto.2020.2906

Knott, L. 2021. Nosebleed: epistaxis. Patient info. https://patient.info/doctor/nosebleed-epistaxis-pro

McIntosh, N., Mok, J., and Margerison, A. 2007. Epidemiology of oronasal hemorrhage in the first 2 years of life: implications for child protection. *Pediatrics*; 120(5):1074–8. https://doi.org/10.1542/peds.2007-2097

NICE CKS. 2022. Epistaxis (nosebleeds). https://cks.nice.org.uk/topics/epistaxis-nosebleeds/

ENT

CHAPTER 6

Eyes

Your local Integrated Care Board (ICB) may have commissioned a Minor Eye Conditions Service (MECS), where people with acute eye problems can self-refer to an optometrist for NHS treatment. Check your postcode at primaryeyecare.co.uk. Eye injury requires urgent referral to Ophthalmology directly or via A&E, unless very minor and not affecting vision (such as a suspected scratch or small foreign body on the surface), when it can be managed by MECS.

SORE OR RED EYES

Red eye is a sign of inflammation of the eye. It is usually benign, with conjunctivitis being the most common cause. Other common causes include, a foreign body and subconjunctival haemorrhage. The cause of red eye can be diagnosed from a detailed history and examination of the eye; treatment is then based on the cause. Recognising when an urgent Ophthalmology assessment is needed is important. There are alternative, rarer diagnoses that threaten sight unless treated promptly, such as corneal ulcer (see Box 6.1), iritis (see Box 6.2) or acute glaucoma. Common, more benign causes usually do not affect visual acuity, so be suspicious of anyone presenting with what they think is conjunctivitis when their vision has deteriorated. A Snellen chart to check visual acuity (with distance glasses if worn, and after blinking away secretions) is an essential tool for managing eye complaints in primary care.

A sore eye or eyelid may or may not always be associated with a red eye. For example, dry eyes, blepharitis, stye and meibomian cyst may cause discomfort but no redness.

History

- Duration
- Associated upper respiratory tract infection (URTI) or rhinitis (suggests viral conjunctivitis)
- Bilateral or unilateral
- Discharge – watery (allergy) or purulent (infection)
- Pattern of symptoms (worse outdoors suggests allergic conjunctivitis, worse after computer work suggests dry eyes)
- Treatment already tried

🚩 Any problem with vision that does not resolve with blinking, for example vision loss or double vision

🚩 Pain or photophobia

🚩 History of trauma/foreign body/drilling or grinding, especially metal

🚩 Contact lens use

🚩 Previous eye problems, such as iritis

🚩 Background of autoimmune conditions, such as inflammatory bowel disease or ankylosing spondylitis

Examination

A magnifying glass and a light are helpful, but an ophthalmoscope examination is not needed. In uncomplicated conjunctivitis, examination may be unnecessary.

- Normal visual acuity is the most helpful sign in excluding a serious eye condition. If the person is not sure that there has been no change in the affected eye/s, check with a Snellen chart (with distance glasses if worn, and after blinking away secretions)
- Check eyelids (stye, meibomian cyst, cellulitis)
- Examine roots of eyelashes for scales (blepharitis)
- Look for vesicles on the surrounding skin (shingles)
- Discharge
- Redness – diffuse or localised

- Pupil shape and responsiveness to light
- Look for foreign body (evert eyelid), especially if symptoms unilateral

Test

- Stain the conjunctiva with fluorescein if unilateral symptoms or history of superficial trauma. Ensure any contact lens is removed first. Ask the person to hold a tissue to their cheek to catch any drops to prevent staining their clothing. If using a fluorescein strip as opposed to drops, moisten the orange tip (ideally with one drop of sterile normal saline) and touch it on the inner aspect of the lower eyelid. Ask the person to blink. Examine the conjunctival surface, ideally using a blue light, but, if unavailable, the green setting on an ophthalmoscope or any bright light may suffice. Areas of damage to the surface are highlighted and may appear a different colour from the light being used (Allen, 2016)

Action

The action to take will vary depending on the cause; see the next relevant section.

RED FLAGS

Send urgently to hospital with referral to Eye Clinic/A&E if any red flags identified. Example causes are given in brackets.

- Reduced visual acuity (*corneal ulcer, iritis, acute glaucoma*)
- Pain, not gritty discomfort (*corneal ulcer, iritis, acute glaucoma*)
- Photophobia (*corneal ulcer, iritis*)
- Previous serious eye disease or background of autoimmune disease (*iritis*)
- Baby aged <4 weeks with red eye/s (*chlamydia, gonorrhoea*)
- Possible metallic or glass foreign body, or high-speed injury (*intraocular foreign body, eye trauma – refer even if no external abnormality*)
- Contact lens wearer (*keratitis – ask them to take lenses and cleaning solution to appointment*)
- Severe inflammation, especially around cornea (*corneal ulcer or iritis*)
- Any abnormality seen using fluorescein (*corneal ulcer or trauma*)
- Irregular pupil or non-reactive (*iritis, acute glaucoma*)
- Facial shingles (*ophthalmic herpes zoster, corneal ulcer; if referral delayed, start aciclovir [both oral and eye ointment]*)
- Cellulitis of eyelid (*risk of affecting the brain*)

INFECTIVE CONJUNCTIVITIS

This presents with sore eyes and red conjunctival membranes, usually with discharge. It may be unilateral, especially in early stages. Check for scales on roots of eyelashes; if present, see next section on Blepharitis. Most cases of infective conjunctivitis in adults are viral. In children, the majority are caused by bacteria (Johnson et al., 2022). Despite this, routine use of topical antibiotics gives little benefit over placebo drops, which do provide lubrication that can be helpful to symptoms if needed.

Avoid the temptation to recommend a topical antibiotic 'just in case'. There has been concern about the boric acid content of chloramphenicol eye drops and its potential harm to future fertility. Reassurance has come from the fact that the eye can retain only a small volume of fluid, so for doses high enough to cause harm, much of what is administered will simply fall out from the eyelids, leaving little to pass down the nasolacrimal duct and be absorbed systemically.

The debate becomes irrelevant when you accept that most children and adults presenting with acute infective conjunctivitis in primary care will get better by themselves and do not need treatment with any antibiotic. At best, topical antibiotic may shorten the illness by 0.3 days (NNT 13; Jefferis et al., 2011); while up to 10% of people treated with chloramphenicol[PB] suffer an adverse reaction. And children often resist: 'Giving your child eye drops is one of the most annoying and unpleasant tasks in parenthood, because children are never cooperative when they're being given eye drops for the first time. I would probably have better luck taking our cat's temperature using a rectal thermometer' (Mendes, 2017).

Self-care

- Should settle without treatment in 1–2 weeks
- Clean discharge away with cotton wool soaked in cooled boiled water
- Remove contact lenses, if worn, until problem has completely settled
- Lubricant eye drops such as hypromellose 0.3% or Viscotears may reduce discomfort
- Viral conjunctivitis is very likely if there is an associated URTI
- Chloramphenicol[PB] makes little difference to comfort or speed of recovery and should not be used unless symptoms are severe, for example the eyelids stuck together with thick discharge. If used, one drop of chloramphenicol[PB] should be applied to the affected eye/s three or four times daily. If severe, also apply ointment at night (treat only the infected eye/s). On the rare occasions when chloramphenicol is needed, it should be obtained OTC (unless for a child aged <2 years)
- Wash hands after touching eyes, use own facecloth, make-up, pillowcase and towel. If used, mascara and eyeliner may carry bacteria
- Schools and nurseries often prefer that children with conjunctivitis do not attend until the discharge has gone. The UK Health Security Agency does not recommend exclusion, and topical antibiotics do not reduce the infective period. The Royal College of GPs (RCGP) wrote to Ofsted about this issue in 2016
- Complications are rare, but urgently seek advice if:
  - Severe eye pain or photophobia
  - Visual problems
  - Eye redness becomes severe

Action

- None for most
- Chloramphenicol[PB] is not available OTC for children aged <2 years; if it is indicated, then a prescription should be issued. Ointment may be easier to apply to babies
- Avoid chloramphenicol if:
  - History of bone marrow problem, for example aplastic anaemia (use ofloxacin eye drops[PBQ] instead)
  - Pregnant or breastfeeding (use fusidic acid eye drops, but narrow spectrum and currently very expensive)

References

Allen, R.C. 2016. Fluorescein staining of the cornea. https://webeye.ophth.uiowa.edu/eyeforum/atlas-video/fluorescein-staining.htm

Chen, Y.Y., Liu, A.H.S., Nurmatov, U., et al. 2023. Antibiotics versus placebo for acute bacterial conjunctivitis. *Cochrane Database Syst Rev*; 3:CD001211. https://doi.org/10.1002/14651858.CD001211.pub4 *Modest benefit from antibiotics but two-thirds of the studies were pharma-sponsored and few were based in primary care.*

Finnikin, S., and Jolly, K. 2016. Nursery sickness policies and their influence on prescribing for conjunctivitis: audit and questionnaire survey. *Br J Gen Pract*; 66(650):e674–9. https://doi.org/10.3399/bjgp16X686125

Jefferis, J., Perera, R., Everitt, H., et al. 2011. Acute infective conjunctivitis in primary care: who needs antibiotics? An individual patient data meta-analysis. *Br J Gen Pract*; 61(590):e542. https://doi.org/10.3399/bjgp11X593811

Johnson, D., Liu, D., and Simel, D. 2022. Does this patient with acute infectious conjunctivitis have a bacterial infection? The Rational Clinical Examination Systematic Review. *JAMA*; 327(22):2231–7. https://doi.org/10.1001/jama.2022.7687 *No single symptom or sign differentiated viral from bacterial conjunctivitis.*

Mendes, I. 2017. 5 tips for giving your kid eye drops. *Today's Parent*. www.todaysparent.com/family/parenting/5-steps-for-giving-your-child-eye-drops/

MHRA. 2021. Chloramphenicol eye drops containing borax or boric acid buffers: use in children younger than 2 years. www.gov.uk/drug-safety-update/chloramphenicol-eye-drops-containing-borax-or-boric-acid-buffers-use-in-children-younger-than-2-years

Rose, P.W., Harnden, A., Brueggemann, A.B., et al. 2005. Chloramphenicol treatment for acute infective conjunctivitis in children in primary care: a randomised double-blind placebo-controlled trial. *Lancet*; 366(9479):37–43. https://doi.org/10.1016/S0140-6736(05)66709-8 *The NNT in this Oxford primary care trial was 24.*

UK Health Security Agency. 2023. Children and young people settings: tools and resources. Exclusion table. www.gov.uk/government/publications/health-protection-in-schools-and-other-childcare-facilities/children-and-young-people-settings-tools-and-resources#exclusion-table

Eye

BLEPHARITIS

This common condition causes inflammation of the eyelids with stickiness and characteristic yellow scales at roots of eyelashes. It often presents as recurrent episodes separated by periods with no symptoms. The cause is not known but may be a reaction to the commensal bacteria that live naturally on the eyelid. Thus it is not possible to catch blepharitis from someone else. Seborrhoeic dermatitis may co-exist. The eyes become sore and the eyelids itchy, and blockage of the ducts of the meibomian glands reduces the oil content of the tear film.

- Remove scales by applying warm compresses, then wiping lids twice daily for 2 weeks with cotton wool dipped in a cleaning solution. This can be made at home with either a teaspoon of 'no tears' baby shampoo or a pinch of bicarbonate of soda in a cup of cooled, boiled water. Long-term lid hygiene should be recommended
- Treat dry eyes with lubricant drops (e.g., hypromellose 0.3% or Viscotears)
- Chloramphenicol[PB] eye ointment rubbed into the lid margin once or twice a day may be added if lid hygiene alone is ineffective
- Severe and persistent symptoms may require oral antibiotics

References

Lindsley, K., Matsumura, S., Hatef, E., et al. 2012. Interventions for chronic blepharitis. *Cochrane Database Syst Rev*; 5:CD005556. https://doi.org/10.1002/14651858.CD005556.pub2

NICE CKS. 2023. Scenario: management of blepharitis. https://cks.nice.org.uk/topics/blepharitis/management/management-of-blepharitis/

ALLERGIC CONJUNCTIVITIS

- Bilateral itchy eyes
- Generalised conjunctival inflammation
- Recurrent symptoms
- Sneezing, itchy throat
- History of triggers, for example animal fur, hay fever
- Watering rather than discharge

Self-care

- Avoid triggers, if possible
- Oral antihistamine (e.g., loratadine[PB], cetirizine[PB], fexofenadine[PBC])
- An antihistamine eye drop is available OTC (Otrivine Antistin[PBC]), but this also contains a vasoconstrictor. To avoid the risk of rebound effects on withdrawal, aim to limit use to 3 days (well within the BNF recommended maximum of 7 days). By this time, alternative, slower-acting topical eye treatments will have had time to start working
- Sodium cromoglicate eye drops are an alternative but are slower acting, with a delay of a few days before a benefit may be noticed and regular dosing needed for a few weeks for the full benefit to be seen. They may sting

Action

- If self-care is ineffective, prescribe azelastine[PBC] eye drops (or sodium cromoglicate eye drops if pregnant, breastfeeding or aged <6 years). Azelastine is a topical antihistamine which, when taken twice daily, tends to be more effective than oral antihistamines at managing allergic conjunctivitis. However, oral antihistamines may be preferred if there are also other allergy symptoms and a single treatment is desired

References

Bielory, L., Lien, K.W., and Bigelsen, S. 2005. Efficacy and tolerability of newer antihistamines in the treatment of allergic conjunctivitis. *Drugs*; 65(2):215–28. https://doi.org/10.2165/00003495-200565020-00004

Castillo, M., Scott, N.W., Mustafa, M.Z., et al. 2015. Topical antihistamines and mast cell stabilisers for treating seasonal and perennial allergic conjunctivitis. *Cochrane Database Syst Rev*; 6:CD009566. https://doi.org/10.1002/14651858.CD009566.pub2

Subconjunctival haemorrhage

This may sometimes be confused with conjunctivitis. It causes a sudden uniform red area in the eye with a clearly defined edge. You should be able to see the posterior margin. There is no discharge or deterioration in vision, and only mild discomfort. It is usually caused by minor trauma, coughing, straining or vomiting, but sometimes may be the first presenting symptom of hypertension. Lubricant drops such as hypromellose 0.3% or Viscotears may help to ease any discomfort.

- Since it is asymptomatic, it may have been detected by looking in a mirror or by someone else noticing it

- Reassurance is usually all that is needed. It will clear within 1–2 weeks

- Check BP and examine the margins of the red area

- 🏴 After trauma, if the posterior margin of the haemorrhage is not visible, this should raise suspicion of a fracture of the orbital bone or an intracranial haemorrhage

- 🏴 If taking warfarin, check international normalised ratio (INR)

- 🏴 If any unexplained bleeding or bruises elsewhere, check the FBC and clotting screen and consider safeguarding issues

Reference

Shah, S. 2022. Subconjunctival haemorrhage. https://patient.info/doctor/subconjunctival-haemorrhage-pro

Eye

DRY EYES

This common condition occurs when not enough tears are secreted, or they dry up quickly. Women and older people are more often affected (up to a third of people aged ≥65 may have it), as well as people who use computer screens for long periods of time without a break, wear contact lenses or take certain medications. Clinical features do not always correlate with severity. The history may include a 'gritty' sensation of the eye, transient blurring or photosensitivity. On examination there may be redness of the eyelids or conjunctiva.

Self-care

- Advise that, paradoxically, dry eyes can cause people to experience symptoms of watery eyes – the excess tears, however, are not oily enough to be effective

- Reduce the use of contact lenses

- If possible, stop or switch medication that may exacerbate dry eyes, for example antihistamines, antidepressants, aspirin, ibuprofen. Whilst many such drugs can be predicted from pharmacodynamics, such as anticholinergic agents impairing the signal to produce tears, the list is long and includes some unexpected medications; see the corrected version of table 3 developed from the National Registry of Drug-Induced Ocular Side Effects in America (Nakhla and Killeen, 2018)

- Avoid long periods without blinking (e.g., staring at a computer or gaming screen)

- Artificial tears help, but must be used frequently (hypromellose 0.3% or Viscotears, available OTC)

- Omega-3 oral supplements may be helpful, but there is low-certainty evidence that olive oil used as a placebo comparator may be just as beneficial

References

American Academy of Ophthalmology. 2018. Dry eye syndrome PPP. www.aao.org/preferred-practice-pattern/dry-eye-syndrome-ppp-2018

Downie, L.E., Ng, S.M., Lindsley, K.B., et al. 2019. Omega-3 and omega-6 polyunsaturated fatty acids for dry eye disease. *Cochrane Database Syst Rev*; 12:CD011016. https://doi.org/10.1002/14651858.CD011016.pub2

Epitropoulos, A.T., Donnenfeld, E.D., Shah, Z.A., et al. 2016. Effect of oral re-esterified omega-3 nutritional supplementation on dry eyes. *Cornea*; 35(9): 1185–91. https://doi.org/10.1097/ICO.0000000000000940

Nakhla, N., and Killeen, R. 2018. Comment on 'The role of medications in causing dry eye'. *J Ophthalmol*; 2018:7396982. https://doi.org/10.1155/2018/7396982

The Dry Eye Assessment and Management Study Research Group. 2018. N–3 fatty acid supplementation for the treatment of dry eye disease. *N Engl J Med*; 378:1681–90. https://doi.org/10.1056/NEJMoa1709691

STYE

This is a staphylococcal infection of one eyelash root causing an acute painful swelling on the lash margin, sometimes with a small area of pus at the tip. A swelling deeper in the lid would indicate a chalazion (see next section).

Self-care

- Should resolve within a few weeks. Warm compresses three or four times daily can help
- Advise about the risk of infecting others; use own facecloth and towel
- Avoid using make-up and contact lenses
- Advise the person not to puncture the stye themselves
- Topical antibiotics are not recommended

Reference

NICE CKS. 2019. Styes (hordeola). https://cks.nice.org.uk/topics/styes-hordeola/

CHALAZION (MEIBOMIAN CYST)

This is a firm, localised swelling in one eyelid, not on the lash margin, usually developing over several weeks. It is initially uncomfortable and is caused by blockage in drainage of an eyelid gland, not an infection.

Self-care

- Clean eyelid margin with cotton bud dipped in baby shampoo diluted 1:10 with warm water
- Warm compresses three or four times daily to liquefy cyst contents (eyebags are available which can be warmed in the microwave; these tend to retain heat better than a damp cloth)
- Massage cyst in direction of eyelashes twice daily using clean fingers or cotton buds
- Usually resolve within 6–8 weeks

Action

- Antibiotic therapy is not recommended unless cellulitis is suspected (see Table 6.1)
- If not resolving, then Ophthalmology referral for surgery may be needed, particularly if swelling is pulling eyelid away from the eye or causing excessive watering
- Although it is possible that a large chalazion can interfere with vision (the pressure on the eye can deform the cornea, temporarily leading to blurred vision), any visual disturbance would usually warrant urgent assessment in an Eye Clinic (or send to A&E if direct referral to Ophthalmology is not possible)

Table 6.1 Take care to distinguish a chalazion from cellulitis of the eyelid

	Chalazion	🏴 Cellulitis
Shape of swelling	Localised, like a marble	Diffuse
Speed of onset	Usually slow	Rapid
Fever	Absent	May be present
Eyelid temperature	Normal	Hot
Action required	Self-care	If mild and low risk, *refer urgently to experienced colleague*; otherwise, *admit urgently under Ophthalmology*

References

Carlisle, R.T., and Digiovanni, J. 2015. Differential diagnosis of the swollen red eyelid. *Am Fam Physician*; 92(2):106–12. www.aafp.org/pubs/afp/issues/2015/0715/p106.html

NICE CKS. 2015. Meibomian cyst (chalazion). https://cks.nice.org.uk/topics/meibomian-cyst-chalazion/

RED FLAG CONDITION

BOX 6.1 CORNEAL ULCER

It is important not to miss this condition, which may cause permanent damage to the cornea if not treated promptly. It is usually caused by a viral infection, for example herpes simplex or varicella zoster, but contact lens users may suffer from a range of different infections.

- History: unilateral pain, photophobia, no purulent discharge, reduced visual acuity
- Examination: unilateral red eye. Cornea may be hazy with red edge. Check visual acuity
- Test: stain with fluorescein and observe with light (ideally blue light) and magnification. Ulcer stains green
- Action: *send urgently to hospital with referral to Eye Clinic/A&E* (slit lamp examination is needed to confirm the diagnosis)

Reference

NICE CKS. 2021. Red eye. https://cks.nice.org.uk/topics/red-eye/

Eye

RED FLAG CONDITION

BOX 6.2 IRITIS (ANTERIOR UVEITIS)

Inflammation of the uveal tract most often affects the anterior compartment of the eye that includes the iris. In about half of cases, it is associated with the gene variant known as HLA-B27, which is linked to ankylosing spondylitis, inflammatory bowel disease and other autoimmune conditions.

- History: pain, photophobia, blurred vision, watering of the eye
- Examination: red eye, constricted or irregular pupil or not reactive to light
- Action: *send urgently to hospital with referral to Eye Clinic/A&E*

Reference

NICE CKS. 2021. Uveitis. https://cks.nice.org.uk/topics/uveitis/

CHAPTER 7

Neurology

HEADACHE

Headache is common, but people often fear that they have an underlying brain tumour. Fortunately, this is rare, being the cause in only 1 in 500 people presenting in primary care with new onset of headaches, or 1 in 300 of those aged >50 years. Severe headaches are not necessarily the ones of greater concern. Typical features that are either reassuring or suspicious are given in Table 7.1.

Many common infections cause headache (leading to concerns about meningitis), but overall, the commonest cause of headache is psychosocial stress. Beware of routinely suggesting simple analgesics as a solution. By the time a person seeks professional advice about a headache, they have often tried at least one OTC analgesic already and are understandably unimpressed by being advised to try it again or to try something similar, unless this is accompanied by a clear explanation of the nature of the headaches and why an alternative analgesic might be better. Furthermore, frequent use of analgesics risks leading to a repetitive cycle of medication-overuse headaches.

If you can identify a cause for headaches, then the prime aim is to remove or ameliorate it. When no cause can be found but there are no concerning features to the headache, reassurance may be all that is needed. Reducing anxiety about the headaches may, in turn, lead to their disappearance. Balance this with a recognition that even without suspicious features, recurring headaches can be disabling, and so may benefit from more specialist assessment.

Table 7.1 Features of headache

Reassuring	Suspicious
On the top of my head/like a tight band around my head	Localised/asymmetrical
It can come on at any time	There when I wake up/wakes me up
Gradual onset during the day	Sudden onset
Not exacerbated by coughing or position	Hurts more when I cough or bend over
I have had it for years on and off	Unusual for me to have headaches
Headaches feel much the same every time	Getting worse over the past few weeks
Apart from the headaches I feel well	Associated with neurological or visual symptoms
Family history of similar headaches	No family history of similar headaches

History

- We all get headaches – what is different about this one?
- What is worrying you? (Often a brain tumour)
- Duration: episodic/unremitting
- If recurrent, are they getting worse?
- Onset: sudden/gradual
- Aura? (Visual or other, e.g., sensory disturbance)
- Timing: waking from sleep/later in the day/related to menstrual cycle
- Severity of pain
- Quality: sharp/like a pressure or band/throbbing
- Site
- Any known triggers?
- Exacerbating factors, e.g., coughing or change in posture
- Relieving factors, e.g., rest, sleep or darkness

- Impact on daily life
- Treatments tried and how often
- Previous recurrent headaches
- Family history of similar headaches
- Depression/anxiety/stress/insomnia
- Sleep pattern/shift work/using a screen for long periods
- Fluid, alcohol and caffeine intake
- Medication
  - Analgesics (if headache keeps recurring consider medication-overuse headache)
  - Recent new medication (e.g., nitrates, calcium-channel blockers and, in children, loratadine[PB])
  - Long-term medication (e.g., oestrogen-containing contraceptives, doxazosin, statins, antidepressants)
  - Many other drugs can cause headache (for further information, see Ferrari et al., 2009 and Monteiro et al., 2021; Table 14.1)
- Associated symptoms (ask whether simultaneous or before headache):
  - Visual disturbance/eye pain
  - Nausea/vomiting
  - Any feverish illness and its symptoms
  - Sinus problems
  - Neck pain
  - ⚑ Sudden onset with maximum intensity within 5 minutes
  - ⚑ Confusion
  - ⚑ Neurological symptoms (e.g., sensory disturbance, double vision, incoordination)
  - ⚑ Rash
  - ⚑ Scalp or temple tenderness
- ⚑ Recent head injury (within the past 3 months)
- ⚑ Cancer (including past history) or human immunodeficiency virus (HIV)
- ⚑ Carbon monoxide exposure; symptoms may be related to one building and others may be affected
- ⚑ Pregnancy (see Box 7.2)

Examination

- Temperature (if infection suspected)
- BP (this must be really high – usually above 180/120 mmHg – to cause headache, but also it is important to check because migraine is associated with hypertension)
- Heart rate (while infection would drive tachycardia, brain tumours or intracranial hypertension may cause a reflex slowing of the heart rate)
- Palpate temporal arteries for tenderness if person aged ≥50 years
- If meningitis or cerebral haemorrhage is suspected, check for neck or back stiffness or a stiff gait

Tests

- CRP and ESR if giant cell (temporal) arteritis suspected (Box 7.1)

Self-care

- Reassure (if appropriate) that headache without neurological or visual symptoms is very unlikely to indicate brain tumour
- Regular meals, adequate fluids, avoid sudden changes in caffeine consumption
- Stress reduction or management (e.g., exercise, meditation, relaxation techniques. Apps such as Breathe2Relax or Headspace: Mindful Meditation may be helpful)
- Paracetamol or ibuprofen[P] *for occasional use*, if not tried or taken in inadequate dose

- Analgesics for headache should not be taken on more than 10 days per month (this is an average – people vary in their susceptibility to medication-overuse headache)

- Avoid codeine (high risk of medication-overuse headache, dependency and exacerbation of nausea) and caffeine (withdrawal effects may compound the problem)

- Adequate, but not excessive, time for sleep

- A headache diary may be useful (template available at migrainetrust.org)

- Frontal, muscular-tension headaches may happen when someone needs glasses or their job involves fine detail or using a screen for a long time, as their eyes are straining to try to get clear vision. An assessment by an optometrist may solve the problem

- If headaches are persistent, arrange assessment by experienced colleague and consider acupuncture

 RED FLAG CONDITION

BOX 7.1 GIANT CELL (TEMPORAL) ARTERITIS

This autoimmune condition causes inflammation in small- to medium-sized arteries, including those on the temples. It occurs in people aged ≥50, but occasionally it may affect younger people. It is twice as common in women as it is in men.

The headache is severe, usually unilateral and often associated with tenderness of the scalp and temples, aching of the jaw muscles on eating and sometimes visual disturbance. There may be fever and fatigue; 40% also have associated weakness of other muscles with morning stiffness, aches and weight loss (polymyalgia rheumatica). It is a 'red flag' because it may cause sudden occlusion of important blood vessels, resulting in blindness, stroke or myocardial infarction, so people in whom it is suspected should be *referred urgently to an experienced colleague.*

A raised CRP or ESR will help in confirming the diagnosis (British guideline recommends testing both; Mackie et al., 2020) but normal results do not rule out the condition. The person should start prednisolone[1] (without waiting for test results) (40–60 mg once daily); however, if there are any symptoms of cranial ischaemia, including visual disturbance, hospital assessment is required and intravenous methylprednisolone will be needed. Symptoms typically respond quickly to steroids; a lack of response within a week is highly suggestive of a diagnosis other than giant cell arteritis.

Referral is needed for specialist colour Doppler ultrasound or temporal artery biopsy, ideally performed within a week of starting prednisolone. Once the diagnosis is confirmed, tapering treatment is needed for 6–24 months with prednisolone, with steroid-sparing drugs used to reduce the risks from long-term, high-dose prednisolone.

References

Mackie, S.L., Dejaco, C., Appenzeller, S., et al. 2020. British Society for Rheumatology guideline on diagnosis and treatment of giant cell arteritis. *Rheumatology*; 59(3):e1–e23. https://doi.org/10.1093/rheumatology/kez672

Piccus, R., Hansen, M.S., Hamann, S., et al. 2022. An update on the clinical approach to giant cell arteritis. *Clin Med*; 22(2):107. https://doi.org/10.7861/clinmed.2022-0041

RED FLAGS

- History of cancer (*possible cerebral metastases; refer to experienced colleague or discuss with Oncology*)
- Pregnant and BP >140/90 (*pre-eclampsia [see Box 7.2]; send urgently to hospital with referral to Obstetrics*)
- New-onset headaches and age ≥50 (*needs investigation; refer to experienced colleague*)
- First episode of migraine and age ≥40 (*needs investigation; refer to experienced colleague*)
- First migraine or migraine with aura or localised symptoms in woman taking oestrogen-containing contraceptive (*risk of stroke; change contraceptive method to non-hormonal or progesterone-only*)
- Sudden 'thunderclap' headache (*possible subarachnoid haemorrhage; send very urgently to hospital*)
- Recent head injury (*possible subdural haemorrhage; admit urgently under Surgical*)
- Symptoms suggesting meningitis (*give benzylpenicillin [ideally administer IV, but if this would cause delay or be difficult, administer IM] and admit very urgently under Medical/Paediatrics*)
- Suspected carbon monoxide poisoning (*send urgently to A&E if currently symptomatic; otherwise check appliances. Gas Emergency Helpline: 0800 111 999*)
- Acute eye pain/red eye/visual disturbance (*consider acute glaucoma; if suspected, send urgently to hospital with referral to Eye Clinic*)
- Headache waking from sleep (*possible cerebral tumour or cluster headache; refer to experienced colleague*)
- Neurological symptoms (*possible cerebral haemorrhage/tumour; refer to experienced colleague*)
- Temporal artery tenderness (*possible giant cell arteritis; measure ESR and CRP, give prednisolone[l] [40–60 mg], refer urgently to Rheumatology [and Ophthalmology if any new visual loss or double vision]*)
- Worsening/persistent headaches (*need investigation; refer to experienced colleague*)

RED FLAG CONDITION

BOX 7.2 PRE-ECLAMPSIA

- Defined as new hypertension (BP >140/90) after 20 weeks' gestation with proteinuria (≥1+ on dipstick) or maternal organ dysfunction (renal, liver, neurological, blood, uterine or placental)
- More common in the second half of first pregnancy, first pregnancy with a new partner, or in subsequent pregnancies after previous episodes
- Symptoms may include:
    - Severe increasing headaches
    - Visual problems, for example blurred vision, flashing lights, double vision
    - Pain in epigastrium or right upper quadrant
    - Vomiting
    - Breathlessness
    - Sudden swelling of face, hands or feet

Send to hospital urgently with referral to Obstetrics if pre-eclampsia is suspected.

Reference

NICE CKS. 2022. Hypertension in pregnancy. https://cks.nice.org.uk/topics/hypertension-in-pregnancy/

References

Ahmed, F., Anish, B., Alok, T., et al. 2019. *National Headache Management System for Adults.* https://headache.org.uk/landing-page/bash-guideline/

Ferrari, A., Spaccapelo, L., Gallesi, D., et al. 2009. Focus on headache as an adverse reaction to drugs. *J Headache Pain*; 10(4):235–9. https://doi.org/10.1007/s10194-009-0127-1

Kernick, D., Stapley, S., Goadsby, P.J., et al. 2008. What happens to new-onset headache presented to primary care? A case–cohort study using electronic primary care records. *Cephalalgia*; 28(11):1188–95. https://doi.org/10.1111/j.1468-2982.2008.01674.x

Monteiro, C., Dias, B., and Vaz-Patto, M. 2021. Headache as an adverse reaction to the use of medication in the elderly: a pharmacovigilance study. *Int J Environ Res Public Health*; 18(5):2674. https://doi.org/10.3390/ijerph18052674

NICE. 2021. CG150. Headaches in over 12s: diagnosis and management. www.nice.org.uk/guidance/cg150

NICE CKS. 2022. Headache – assessment. https://cks.nice.org.uk/topics/headache-assessment/

The Migraine Trust. Keeping a headache diary. https://migrainetrust.org/live-with-migraine/self-management/ keeping-a-migraine-diary/

MIGRAINE

Migraine affects 12% of adults and 10% of children and is commoner in females. At least 90% of people with migraine experience their first attack before the age of 40. Symptoms of the aura do not last more than 60 minutes (typically 20–30 minutes) and usually resolve before the pain begins. Early symptoms such as emotional or personality changes, muddled thinking, excessive tiredness, yawning, pallor, visual disturbances and restlessness may start 1–48 hours before the headache. A partner or a friend may notice these changes before the patient does. In children, visual symptoms are less common and may be simultaneous with the headache, or they may have abdominal pain, vomiting or dizziness without headache.

Migraine causes instability in the size of the blood vessels in the head and the neck, although the initial event that starts an attack occurs in the brainstem. It is helpful for people to be informed that the reason they are susceptible to migraine, resulting from triggers that do not cause headache in other people, may be down to an inherited predisposition, so it is worth enquiring about a family history of migraine.

A wide variety of factors are known to trigger migraine:

- Change in stress level
- Excessive sensory stimuli, for example bright light, noise
- Menstruation – migraine is most likely to develop in either the 2 days leading up to a period or the first 3 days during a period, but may also occur at other times of the cycle
- Missing meals
- Overexertion
- Sleep disturbance – too much or too little
- Change in climate
- Hypoxia

Dietary factors are often suspected but rarely found; searching too hard may divert attention away from more likely factors, such as those mentioned previously. The widespread belief that chocolate is a trigger lacks evidence (Lippi et al., 2014; Nowaczewska et al., 2020). It is more likely to be a food craving in the prodromal phase. Alcohol does not cause migraine initially, but can trigger an attack as its effects wear off. For most people, the attacks seem to be multifactorial, and it is often not possible to identify any one trigger that will always cause attacks when encountered, and eliminate attacks when avoided. Often there is a build-up of different triggers, with a 'last straw' tipping the sufferer over the threshold and resulting in a migraine. Whatever the cause, the final part of the sequence of events leading to symptoms involves the neurotransmitter 5-hydroxytryptamine (serotonin, 5-HT).

The headache usually gradually subsides. Sleep can help to end an episode; for children, a sleep of a few minutes can be enough. This is followed by a recovery phase, which can take hours or days, where the person may feel drained by fatigue, feel weak, have difficulty concentrating and suffer generalised aches and pains.

Diagnostic history of migraine

- Episodes lasting 4–72 hours (occasionally longer – 'status migrainosus')
- Often unilateral (though not always)
- Pulsating/throbbing
- Moderate or severe pain
- Exacerbated by physical activity
- Nausea and/or vomiting
- Photophobia or phonophobia (sensitivity to noise)
- Focal migraine may also cause one of the following types of aura:
  - Visual symptoms (e.g., flickering lights and/or partial visual loss)
  - Sensory symptoms (pins and needles and/or numbness)
  - Dysphasia (speech disturbance)

- Medication history (oestrogen-containing contraceptives, hormone replacement therapy [HRT], nasal decongestants, proton pump inhibitors [PPIs] may contribute)

Self-care

- Being able to recognise the early features of their migraine can help the person decide when to take treatment or adapt activities
- Regular meals, exercise, sleep routines and keeping hydrated all help to reduce the frequency of attacks
- Simple analgesics (paracetamol, aspirin[PBCI] or ibuprofen[P]) work for many people, but to be most effective are best taken early, when the headache is mild. Ask what has been tried already and at what dose, as there is little point in suggesting something that has been found ineffective
- If there is associated nausea, it is important to treat this as well with an antiemetic such as buccal prochlorperazine[PBCQ] (OTC – see the following section for further information), ideally taken at the first sign of symptoms
- If simple analgesics are ineffective, consider sumatriptan[CQ] (adult dose: 50 mg. If the migraine improves but recurs, a second dose of 50 mg can be taken after at least 2 hours if required. Packs of two 50 mg tablets OTC). If they have aura, triptans should be taken at the start of the headache and not at the start of the aura (unless the aura and headache start simultaneously)
- The Migraine Trust is a research charity providing helpful information (https://migrainetrust.org)

Action

- Review medications that may be contributing and consider stopping. If taking an oestrogen-containing contraceptive and it is the first episode of migraine, or a migraine with aura or localised symptoms, advise stopping it immediately and discuss alternative contraceptive methods
- Migraine associated with difficulty reading, particularly in children or young people, may respond to colour tinting of spectacles. Referral to an optometrist for an intuitive colorimeter test may both help the migraine and (importantly) improve educational potential (Evans and Allen, 2016)
- Adults with frequent dyspepsia or heartburn as well as migraine should be tested for *Helicobacter pylori* – if the presence of *Helicobacter* is confirmed, eradication therapy may abolish the migraine as well as the gut symptoms (Su et al., 2014).

Prescription

- For migraine in adults, NICE recommends a combination of a triptan and a non-steroidal anti-inflammatory drug (NSAID), although monotherapy with a triptan is nearly as effective
- Naratriptan[PBCQ] is our first-choice triptan because of its low side-effect profile and low rate of migraine recurrence. If it is effective, it can continue to be used without a high burden of side effects; if it is not effective, other triptans are available that have greater efficacy. People vary in their response, so if the initial treatment is not working well, it is worth trying an alternative triptan or NSAID (Belvis et al., 2009; Saper, 2001)
- Note that triptans are contraindicated in uncontrolled hypertension and symptomatic cardiovascular or cerebrovascular disease
- Avoid enteric-coated NSAIDs (e.g., diclofenac sodium e/c) as they are too slow in onset to be effective
- An antiemetic can increase the effectiveness of the analgesic as well as reducing nausea; prochlorperazine[PBCQ] is available in a buccal tablet and, therefore, does not require the person to 'keep it down'
- If nausea and vomiting are prominent, then an alternative route of analgesia may be needed, for example diclofenac[PC] suppositories or zolmitriptan[PBCQ] nasal spray

Doses for adults

- Naratriptan[PBCQ], 2.5 mg. If the migraine improves but recurs, a second dose of 2.5 mg can be taken after at least 4 hours if required. Maximum 5 mg/24 hours
- Buccal prochlorperazine[PBCQ] (OTC), 3–6 mg up to twice daily; tablets to be placed high between upper lip and gum and left to dissolve
- Diclofenac[PC], 100 mg suppository once in 24 hours

- Zolmitriptan[PBCQ] nasal spray, 5 mg as soon as possible after onset of pain, into one nostril only. If the migraine improves but recurs, a second dose of 5 mg can be taken after at least 2 hours if required. Maximum 10 mg/24 hours

RED FLAGS

- Migraine lasting more than 72 hours and not responding to usual care (*status migrainosus; admit urgently under Medical for parenteral treatment*)
- First episode of migraine if age >40 (*needs investigation; refer to experienced colleague*)
- First migraine, migraine with aura or localised symptoms in woman taking oestrogen-containing contraceptive (*risk of stroke; change contraceptive method to non-hormonal or progesterone-only*)

References

Belvis, R., Pagonabarraga, J., and Kulisevsky, J. 2009. Individual triptan selection in migraine attack therapy. *Recent Pat CNS Drug Discov*; 4(1):70–81. https://doi.org/10.2174/157488909787002555

Evans, B.J., and Allen, P.M. 2016. A systematic review of controlled trials on visual stress using Intuitive Overlays or the Intuitive Colorimeter. [Review]. *J Optom*; 9(4):205–18. https://doi.org/10.1016/j.optom.2016.04.002

Evans, E.W., and Lorber, K.C. 2008. Use of 5-HT1 agonists in pregnancy. *Ann Pharmacother*; 42(4):543–9. https://doi.org/10.1345/aph.1K176 *Sumatriptan is the preferred triptan during pregnancy and breastfeeding.*

Law, S., Derry, S., and Moore, R.A. 2016. Sumatriptan plus naproxen for the treatment of acute migraine attacks in adults. *Cochrane Database Syst Rev*; 4:CD008541. https://doi.org/10.1002/14651858.CD008541.pub3

Linde, K., Allais, G., Brinkhaus, B., et al. 2016. Acupuncture for the prevention of episodic migraine. *Cochrane Database Syst Rev*; 6:CD001218. https://doi.org/10.1002/14651858.CD001218.pub3

Lippi, G., Mattiuzzi, C., and Cervellin, G. 2014. Chocolate and migraine: the history of an ambiguous association. *Acta Biomedica*; 85(3):216–21. www.mattioli1885journals.com/index.php/actabiomedica/article/view/3449 *Double-blind studies demonstrate that the risk of developing a headache attack after ingestion of chocolate is as likely as administering placebo in people with migraine.*

National Migraine Centre. 2017. Migraine triggers. www.nationalmigrainecentre.org.uk/migraine-and-headaches/migraine-and-headache-factsheets/migraine-triggers/

NICE CKS. 2022. Migraine. https://cks.nice.org.uk/topics/migraine/

Nowaczewska, M., Wiciński, M.Ł., Kaźmierczak, W., et al. 2020. To eat or not to eat: a review of the relationship between chocolate and migraines. *Nutrients*; 12(3):608. https://doi.org/10.3390/nu12030608 *This review found insufficient evidence for a link between eating chocolate and having migraine.*

Pringsheim, T., and Becker, W.J. 2014. Triptans for symptomatic treatment of migraine headache. *BMJ*; 348:g2285. https://doi.org/10.1136/bmj.g2285

Saper, J.R. 2001. What matters is not the differences between triptans, but the differences between patients. *Arch Neurol*; 58(9):1481–2. https://doi.org/10.1001/archneur.58.9.1481

Su, J., Zhou, X., and Zhang, G. 2014. Association between *Helicobacter pylori* infection and migraine: a meta-analysis. *World J Gastroenterol*; 20(40):14965–72. https://doi.org/10.3748/wjg.v20.i40.14965

Xu, S., Yu, L., Luo, X., et al. 2020. Manual acupuncture versus sham acupuncture and usual care for prophylaxis of episodic migraine without aura: multicentre, randomised clinical trial. *BMJ*; 368:m697. https://doi.org/10.1136/bmj.m697

DIZZINESS

There are fundamentally two types of dizziness: vertigo (caused by a disturbance of the balance system) and fainting/near-fainting (caused by a lack of oxygen in the brain).

History

- What is worrying you? (Often a stroke)
- Duration
- Circumstances:
  - If triggered or exacerbated by head movement, suggests vertigo
  - If occurring at rest or sitting/lying still, suggests neurological cause

Neu

- - If triggered by exercise, suggests a cardiac cause
  - If triggered by heat, emotion or toileting, suggests a vasovagal cause (simple faint)
- If loss of consciousness, try to obtain an eyewitness account. Was there any injury or incontinence?
- Description of experience (when you have dizzy spells, do you feel the world spin around you as if you had just got off a playground roundabout?)
  - Spinning or movement (vertigo – see Box 7.3 and Table 7.2)
  - Faint feeling (as if about to black out) (see Table 7.3)
- Previous episodes
- Ear surgery
- Recent head injury
- Recent blood loss
- Pregnancy
- Heart disease
- Diabetes
- Medication (especially if newly started or increased, for example antihypertensives, glucose-lowering medicines, tramadol, gabapentin, antidepressants)
- Associated symptoms:
  - Nausea
  - Earache
  - Cough/coryza (*viral infection*)
  - 🚩 New deafness/tinnitus (*sudden – cochlear disease; gradual – acoustic neuroma*)
  - 🚩 Headache/photophobia/visual loss/clumsiness/other neurological symptoms (*headache is not usually a feature of benign vertigo*)
  - 🚩 Palpitations (*arrhythmia*)
  - 🚩 Chest pain (*ischaemic heart disease*)
- 🚩 **Family history of sudden arrhythmic death** (*high risk of fatal arrhythmia*)

Examination

- If vertigo, check ears for signs of infection and look for nystagmus on lateral gaze. If nystagmus fits with the features in column 2 of Table 7.2, this suggests vestibular neuronitis as a common cause, but if not then refer to experienced colleague for further assessment as there are more serious causes to consider
- Measure BP after the person is lying for 5 minutes (if impractical take the first measurement sitting), then recheck after a minute of standing. If the history is of dizziness delayed by a few minutes after standing, check again after 3–5 minutes of standing (Schwenk, 2017). A positive result for postural hypotension is a drop in systolic BP of ≥20 mmHg and/or a drop to <90 mmHg on standing, and/or a drop in diastolic BP of ≥10 mmHg with symptoms
- Heart rate and rhythm
- Pallor/anaemia
- Gait (are they at risk of falls?)

Tests

- FBC if anaemia is suspected
- Oxygen saturation if hypoxia is suspected
- Capillary blood glucose if hypoglycaemia is suspected
- ECG if cardiac cause is suspected (but a normal ECG does not exclude a cardiac cause)

Self-care for vertigo

- Dizziness is common, and nausea often accompanies it
- Symptoms usually settle but may sometimes take several weeks
- Encourage activity, even if it worsens the vertigo, as it can speed recovery

- If the person is at risk of falls, advise them to stand up slowly and take practical measures to minimise the risk of injury. Consider referral to a falls prevention clinic
- Driving or other critical tasks may be affected (see DVLA form DIZ1)
- For BPPV (see below), simple exercises also may be helpful (e.g., Brandt–Daroff, Epley; search for one of the many videos available online)

BOX 7.3 VERTIGO

Vestibular neuronitis, labyrinthitis, benign paroxysmal positional vertigo (BPPV), and vestibular migraine are common causes of vertigo in primary care. Other diagnoses are possible, for example Ménière's disease and cerebral ischaemia.

Although the diagnoses of vestibular neuronitis and labyrinthitis are often used interchangeably, strictly they are different conditions; labyrinthitis tends to have hearing loss associated with vertigo whereas vestibular neuronitis does not. However, they both can be managed in the same way and, irrespective of treatment, should improve with time.

Table 7.2 Vertigo: common differential diagnoses

	Vestibular neuronitis	BPPV	Vestibular migraine	Cerebral ischaemia
Background	Recent URTI	Spontaneous, or after head trauma	Migraine history, or family history	History of cardiovascular disease
Characteristic signs/ symptoms	Nystagmus	Brought on by movement	Other migraine symptoms, maybe no headache	Other neurological symptoms
Associated features	Nausea and vomiting	Vertigo lasts less than a minute	Vertigo lasts 5 minutes to 72 hours	Maybe visual disturbance, drowsiness or headache
Timing	One episode may give symptoms over 18 months	Recurrent	Recurrent	Usually single event

Prescribing

- Offer buccal prochlorperazine[PBCQ] or cinnarizine[PBC] for vertigo for up to 7 days. These are for symptomatic relief, not a cure; they cause sedation and may delay recovery if taken for more than a week (Smith et al., 2023)
- Although these medications are available OTC, they are not licensed to be sold for conditions other than nausea/ vomiting in previously diagnosed migraine or travel sickness, so a prescription will be needed
- Doses for adults:
  - Buccal prochlorperazine[PBCQ], 3–6 mg up to twice daily; tablets to be placed high between upper lip and gum to dissolve
  - Cinnarizine[PBC], 30 mg three times daily
- Oral corticosteroids are not recommended because there is too little evidence of effectiveness

RED FLAGS

- Neurological symptoms or signs (*suspect stroke; send very urgently to hospital*)
- Headache/photophobia (*could be vestibular migraine, but stroke, tumour or infection all need considering; refer urgently to experienced colleague or admit urgently under Medical*)
- Sudden unilateral hearing loss or tinnitus (*possible vascular or immune disease of cochlea; refer urgently to ENT*)
- Head injury in previous 3 weeks, especially if on anticoagulant (*possible subdural haemorrhage; admit urgently under Surgical*)
- Previous ear surgery (*refer urgently to ENT*)
- Vertigo not improving after 1 week or not resolved after 6 weeks (*possible acoustic neuroma or cerebrovascular disease; refer urgently to ENT*)
- Palpitations (*arrhythmia; arrange immediate ECG if possible and admit urgently under Medical*)
- Chest pain (*ischaemic heart disease; if new then admit urgently under Medical*)
- Family history of sudden arrhythmic death (*high risk of fatal arrhythmia; arrange ECG and refer urgently to Cardiology even if the ECG appears normal*)

References

Harding, M. 2019. Dizziness, giddiness, and feeling faint. https://patient.info/doctor/dizziness-giddiness-and-feeling-faint

International Headache Society. 2016. Vestibular migraine. www.ichd-3.org/appendix/a1-migraine/a1-6-episodic-syndromes-that-may-be-associated-with-migraine/a1-6-6-vestibular-migraine/

Juraschek, S.P., Daya, N., Rawlings, A.M., et al. 2017. Association of history of dizziness and long-term adverse outcomes with early vs later orthostatic hypotension assessment times in middle-aged adults. *JAMA Intern Med*; 177(9):1316–23. https://doi.org/10.1001/jamainternmed.2017.2937

NICE CKS . 2023. Vestibular neuronitis. https://cks.nice.org.uk/topics/vestibular-neuronitis/

Oliveira J. e Silva L., Khoujah, D., Naples, J.G., et al. 2023. Corticosteroids for patients with vestibular neuritis: an evidence synthesis for guidelines for reasonable and appropriate care in the emergency department. *Acad Emerg Med*; 30(5):531–40. https://doi.org/10.1111/acem.14583

Royal College of Physicians. 2017. Measurement of lying and standing blood pressure: a brief guide for clinical staff. www.rcplondon.ac.uk/projects/outputs/measurement-lying-and-standing-blood-pressure-brief-guide-clinical-staff

Schwenk, T.L. 2017. No need to wait 3 minutes after standing to assess orthostatic hypotension [comment]. *NEMJ Journal Watch*. www.jwatch.org/na44690/2017/08/03/no-need-wait-3-minutes-after-standing-assess-orthostatic

Smith, T., Rider, J., Cen, S., et al. 2023. Vestibular neuronitis. *StatPearls*. StatPearls Publishing. www.ncbi.nlm.nih.gov/books/NBK549866/#article-31140.s8

FAINTING

Fainting occurs when there is not enough oxygen available to the brain. Vasovagal syncope, hypotension, hypovolaemia, anaemia, arrhythmias, cardiac failure, epilepsy and postural orthostatic tachycardia syndrome (POTS) are among the many causes of feeling faint (see Table 7.3 and Box 7.4).

Table 7.3 Feeling faint: common differential diagnoses (N.B. many other causes are possible, including anaemia and hypoglycaemia)

	Vasovagal	Hypotensive	Cardiac	Epileptic
Background	Any age, but first episode usually <40 years	History of blood loss, dehydration (including diarrhoea/vomiting)	Commoner in elderly	Any age
Typical trigger	Situational trigger, for example blood test, prolonged standing, micturition	Symptoms exacerbated by standing	Can occur in any position, even lying down	May occur in a situation unusual for other causes – like sitting at rest
Features/associations	Loss of consciousness not usually >20 seconds	May be low fluid intake	Preceding nausea or sweating	Aura before, or drowsiness/amnesia after
Features/associations	Pallor and sweating	On antihypertensive medicines	Palpitation, dyspnoea or chest pain	Twitching, jerking or abnormal movements
Features/associations	Most common cause – often preceded by feeling faint and vision narrowing	BP low or drops by >20/10 mmHg within 3 minutes of standing	Known cardiac disease or abnormal ECG	Injury or tongue biting

Self-care for fainting

- Avoid hot baths and prolonged standing, especially in the heat
- Drink adequate fluids; have two large glasses of water before situations that are likely to make you faint
- When getting out of bed, roll to sit on the edge of the bed for a few minutes before standing
- Avoid your own triggers and be aware of your warning signs
- At the first sign of feeling faint, lie down flat with your legs up on a chair or against a wall or sit down with your head between your knees
- If this is not possible, squat down on your heels. Both positions move blood from the legs back into the circulation
- When you feel better, get up slowly, but return to the position if symptoms return

> ### BOX 7.4 POSTURAL ORTHOSTATIC TACHYCARDIA SYNDROME (POTS)
>
> Feeling faint on becoming upright may result from a defect in the normal adjustment of BP to suit the change in position. A normal response to standing up is peripheral vasoconstriction and an increase in heart rate ≤20. Without the vasoconstriction, the heart rate may increase more in an effort to compensate.
>
> - Most common in young people aged 14–50
> - Five times more common in women than men
> - Often starts abruptly after an apparent trigger such as pregnancy, surgery, infection or immunisation, but the teenage form may come on gradually
> - Can be secondary to autonomic neuropathy due to a wide range of conditions, including diabetes, long COVID, glandular fever
> - There is an association with chronic fatigue syndrome
> - Examination findings to support the diagnosis are a sustained increase in heart rate of ≥30 (≥40 for teenagers) within 10 minutes of standing, standing heart rate >120, and acrocyanosis (purplish discolouration of the lower legs on standing and the feet are cold)
>
> If suspected, *refer to experienced colleague* to investigate possible causes.

RED FLAGS

- Family history of sudden arrhythmic death (*high risk of fatal arrhythmia; arrange ECG and refer urgently to Cardiology even if the ECG appears normal*)
- Systolic BP <90 mmHg, or drops by >20 mmHg on standing (*suspect medication or other causes of postural hypotension; refer to experienced colleague or admit under Medical*)
- Sustained increase in heart rate ≥30 within 10 min of standing (*suspect postural orthostatic tachycardia syndrome; refer to experienced colleague or admit under Medical*)
- Heart disease, known or suspected because of palpitations or chest pain (*refer to experienced colleague or admit urgently under Medical*)
- Injury or tongue biting during episode (*suggests epilepsy; refer urgently to Neurology*)

References

Saccilotto, R.T., Nickel, C.H., Bucher, H.C., et al. 2011. San Francisco Syncope Rule to predict short-term serious outcomes: a systematic review. *CMAJ*; 183(15):E1116. https://doi.org/10.1503/cmaj.101326

Tidy, C. 2021. Postural orthostatic tachycardia syndrome. Professional article. https://patient.info/doctor/postural-tachycardia-syndrome-pots-pro

Willacy, H. 2020. Syncope. https://patient.info/doctor/syncope

CHAPTER 8

Skin

ASSESSMENT

Healthcare professionals often find skin problems daunting initially. Remember two important principles, which apply equally to all types of minor illness: take a good history first and find out the person's agenda. Here is how to apply these principles to the diagnosis of skin conditions.

1. **Take a good history first**. This is where to find the diagnosis – your examination is for confirmation. The brain is a pattern-matching organ; if you don't know what you are looking for, you are unlikely to find it. The four most useful questions are about:

- Distribution (unilateral suggests an external trigger [or shingles])
- Itch or pain
- Systemic features, for example fever, malaise
- Duration

Other questions, depending on the answers so far, include the following:

- Any previous episodes?
- Have any suspected triggers been identified?
- Are there any associated symptoms?
- Are the spots of different ages? Are they spreading?
- Anyone else affected?

2. **Find out and address the person's/parent's agenda**. This is commonly:

- (For a rash) is it meningitis?
- Is it contagious?
- (For an isolated lesion) is it cancer?

The UK Primary Care Dermatology Society (PCDS) has a useful website with diagnostic algorithms as well as management advice. If you have made a working diagnosis, then it may be helpful to compare the rash with images; DermNet has good online resources, or use one of the many books available. Rashes look very different on darkly pigmented skin; check out the resources at Skin Deep and Black and Brown Skin.

Don't be surprised if you are unable to make a definite diagnosis. If you have addressed the person's concerns and ruled out serious illness, knowing the exact diagnosis may not matter. If the problem does not resolve, you could offer them an appointment with a more experienced clinician.

Websites

- Black and Brown Skin: www.blackandbrownskin.co.uk
- DermNet: https://dermnetnz.org
- PCDS: www.pcds.org.uk
- Skin Deep: https://dftbskindeep.com/

Reference

Ashton, R., Leppard, B., and Cooper, H., 2021. *Differential Diagnosis in Dermatology*, 5th edition. CRC Press, London. ISBN-13: 978-0367085971 *This book has very useful algorithms that explain the likely diagnoses for a particular presentation and their distinguishing features.*

RASHES

History

- Duration
- Unwell with fever/malaise?
- Distribution
- Itch or pain
- Did all spots appear at same time, or sequentially?
- Is rash constant, spreading or coming and going?
- Previous episodes
- Any contacts who are itching
- Any new medication
- Any identified triggers
- Recent travel
- What has been tried already and what was the response?

Examination

- Distribution/symmetry either side of the midline
- Discrete (separate 'spots') or confluent (merging 'rash')
- Colour, but beware: in darkly pigmented skin it is difficult to assess the degree of inflammation
- Does the rash blanch on pressure?
- Surface – feel with ungloved fingertips. Is it hot?
- Are the areas:
  - Wheal-like (irregular, raised, blotchy)?
  - Flat (macules) or raised (papules)?
  - Containing fluid (vesicles or pustules)?
- For itchy rashes, are burrows visible? Look at sides of fingers, finger webs, edges of hands, wrists and feet
- If person is unwell, check:
  - Temperature
  - Heart rate
  - Respiratory rate
  - CRT in children aged <12 years/BP in adults and older children

Tests

- If exudate is present, a swab for bacterial culture may be helpful. But swabbing intact skin will yield only normal skin flora
- If fungal infection is suspected, skin scrapings or 'dust' from around the edges of the nail may be sent for culture – the results may take around 3 weeks. Do not refrigerate the sample

RASH IN A SERIOUSLY ILL PERSON

🚩 Anaphylaxis

🚩 Measles

🚩 Meningococcal septicaemia (now extremely rare in the UK)

Remember to ask about the travel history of these people. If recently returned from a tropical area, seek advice from a microbiologist or the University College London (UCL) Tropical Medicine Registrar on 020 3456 7890 (24-hour service).

⚑ ANAPHYLAXIS

Anaphylaxis is a severe, potentially life-threatening allergic reaction that may develop rapidly. Features of anaphylaxis include:

- Feeling unwell, confusion, acting strangely
- Feeling lightheaded or faint
- Swollen eyes, lips, hands and feet
- Swelling of the mouth, throat or tongue, which can cause breathing and swallowing difficulties
- Wheezing
- Abdominal pain, nausea and vomiting
- Collapse and unconsciousness

If suspecting anaphylaxis, **call for an ambulance and get help from colleagues without delay**. Regular basic life support and anaphylaxis training will help you to be prepared; make sure you know where the emergency adrenaline is kept.

Reference

Resuscitation Council UK. 2021. *Emergency Treatment of Anaphylactic Reactions: Guidelines for healthcare providers*. www.resus. org.uk/library/additional-guidance/guidance-anaphylaxis/emergency-treatment

⚑ MEASLES

Measles is uncommon but outbreaks still occur, especially in groups with low vaccination rates (e.g., Travellers and migrants).. The number of annual UK cases varied between 2 and 2032 in the 10 years prior to 2022. It is 'the most infectious pathogen known to humankind' (Munro, 2023), but a rash is unlikely to be measles if the person has had two measles, mumps and rubella (MMR) vaccinations. Since 2020, all reported measles deaths in England and Wales have been in unvaccinated people; vaccination rates in London have dropped to the point where the UKHSA has warned that there is a risk of a major outbreak (UKHSA, 2023). At the time of writing, Birmingham Children's Hospital was seeing 6 cases of measles per day.

History

- Vaccination history
- Incubation period of 1–3 weeks
- 1–4 days of malaise, loss of appetite, nasal discharge, cough and conjunctivitis
- Rash starts on face on the hairline or behind the ears and then spreads down the body
- High fever >39°C, starting at onset of rash
- ⚑ Immunosuppressed
- ⚑ Pregnant
- ⚑ Baby aged <12 months

Examination

- Koplik's spots may appear just before the rash; blue-grey specks (like grains of salt) on a red base on the lining of the cheek or gums
- Bright red maculopapular (flat and raised) areas appear, coalesce and then peel after 5–7 days. They usually start on the face and spread down the body, affecting palms and soles
- Check ears and chest if secondary infection suspected (*may need urgent admission if evidence of pneumonia*)
- Check for signs of dehydration (*consider urgent admission if dehydrated*)

Self-care

- Infectious from 4 days before, to 4 days after, the onset of the rash – stay off work/school and avoid contact with high-risk groups (see Box 8.1)
- Recovery may take 10 days

- Take paracetamol if needed for muscular pains
- Drink adequate fluids
- Wash hands frequently. Avoid sharing cutlery, cups and towels; dispose of used tissues immediately

Action

- Exclude from school or work for 4 days after onset of rash
- Notify Health Protection Team
- Saliva tests will be requested to confirm the diagnosis. Most people who are suspected of having measles actually test negative and have an alternative cause for their symptoms
- Antibiotics are not routinely recommended, but may be needed for secondary otitis media or pneumonia
- Consider admission if dehydrated or evidence of pneumonia

BOX 8.1 MEASLES CONTACTS

The following groups are at high risk of complications. If they have had a significant contact with someone with measles, they may need post-exposure prophylaxis with immunoglobulin arranged through the Health Protection Team (the rules are complex; see UKHSA, 2024):

- Immunosuppressed
- Pregnant
- Infant aged <1 year

References

Munro, A. 2023. The misery: return of measles. https://alasdairmunro.substack.com/p/the-misery-return-of-measles

NICE CKS. 2022. Measles. https://cks.nice.org.uk/topics/measles

UKHSA. 2022. Investigation, diagnosis and management of exposure to viral rash illness in pregnancy. www.gov.uk/government/publications/viral-rash-in-pregnancy

UKHSA. 2023. London at risk of measles outbreaks with modelling estimating tens of thousands of cases. www.gov.uk/government/news/london-at-risk-of-measles-outbreaks-with-modelling-estimating-tens-of-thousands-of-cases

UKHSA, 2024. National measles guidelines. https://assets.publishing.service.gov.uk/media/65a7a806867cd800135ae9bb/national-measles-guidelines-january-2024.pdf

🏴 MENINGOCOCCAL SEPTICAEMIA

- Very rare in the UK today (see Figure 8.1) and declining due to vaccination
- A medical emergency with 10% mortality
- May occur at any age, but babies are the most susceptible

Typical presentation

- The history will be **short** – hours or days, not weeks
- Fever (but absence of fever or a good response to an antipyretic does **not** exclude meningitis)
- Symptoms may initially be non-specific and may include:
  - Flu-like symptoms with sore throat, headache and muscle/joint pain (especially leg pain)
  - Prostration (difficulty in standing up)
  - Gastrointestinal symptoms such as nausea, vomiting or diarrhoea, off their food
  - Confusion or drowsiness
  - Photophobia
  - In babies, high-pitched cry
  - Rash (not always present or may not develop until a late stage, so absence of rash does not exclude meningitis)

Examination

- The person looks ill, often irritable
- General signs of sepsis (see Chapter 2) include rapid heart rate, fast respiratory rate and CRT >2 s in children (or low BP in adults). Babies may have a stiff body or could be agitated, floppy or unresponsive
- In babies aged <3 months with bacterial meningitis, 50% have no fever (Okike et al., 2018)
- Babies may be too unwell to cry, or the cry may be abnormal, like a cat
- Fontanelle (if not yet closed) may be bulging
- 'Neck stiffness' is often listed as a sign of meningitis, but in a relatively well person with discomfort on turning the head, muscular inflammation or tender cervical lymphadenopathy are much more likely causes. In meningeal irritation, neck flexion may be limited, but this is a very late sign
- To test for neck stiffness in a child, ask them to 'kiss their knees'
- The classic rash is purpuric (dull purplish red macules that do not blanch on pressure), but there may be a non-specific rash in the early stages, or no rash at all

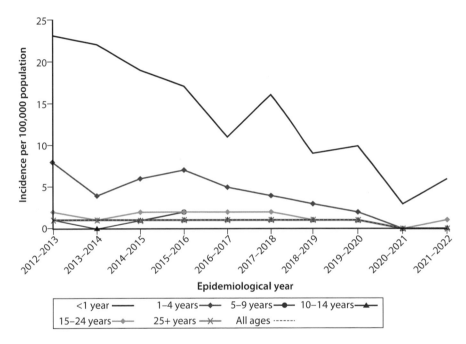

Figure 8.1 Meningococcal septicaemia: rates have fallen in the UK. Incidence of invasive meningococcal disease in England: 2012/13 to 2021/22. (Source: UKHSA, 2023. Contains public sector information licensed under the Open Government Licence v3.0.)

Action

If meningitis/meningococcal septicaemia suspected:

🚩 Give benzylpenicillin IV/IM (<1 year, 300 mg; 1–9 years, 600 mg; 10 years to adult, 1.2 g) and admit very urgently under Medical/Paediatrics

References

NICE. 2015. CG102. Meningitis (bacterial) and meningococcal septicaemia in under 16s: recognition, diagnosis and management. www.nice.org.uk/guidance/cg102

Okike, I.O., Ladhani, S.N., Johnson, A.P., et al. and neoMen Study Group. 2018. Clinical characteristics and risk factors for poor outcome in infants less than 90 days of age with bacterial meningitis in the United Kingdom and Ireland. *Pediatr Infect Dis J*; 37(9):837–43. https://doi.org/10.1097/INF.0000000000001917 *The classic features of meningitis were uncommon. The presentation in young infants was often non-specific, and only half of cases presented with fever.*

UKHSA. 2023. Invasive meningococcal disease in England: annual laboratory confirmed reports for epidemiological year 2021 to 2022. www.gov.uk/government/publications/meningococcal-disease-laboratory-confirmed-cases-in-england-in-2021-to-2022/invasive-meningococcal-disease-in-england-annual-laboratory-confirmed-reports-for-epidemiological-year-2021-to-2022

Skn

RASH WITH FEVER

1. Non-specific viral infection
2. Slapped cheek (fifth disease, parvovirus B19)
3. Hand, foot and mouth disease
4. Scarlet fever

NON-SPECIFIC VIRAL INFECTION

A generalised rash is a feature of many viral infections. There are thousands of different types of virus, and the pattern of rash that they cause is not consistent, so it is usually impossible to name the virus. It may reassure the person/parent to know if there have been similar cases in the neighbourhood. Sometimes a specific cause can be identified from the collection of features, such as the herpes virus of roseola infantum, but in the absence of any specific treatment, such diagnoses are rarely helpful.

Usually, it does not matter that you cannot identify the virus, unless the person is pregnant or has been in contact with a pregnant woman. Rubella is now very rare in the UK; at the time of writing the last confirmed case was in 2019, and pregnant women in the UK are no longer being tested for immunity (UKHSA, 2022a). Parvovirus is much more common.

History

- Often accompanied by symptoms such as runny nose, dry cough, loose stools or fever
- The rash may take many forms; however, it is likely to be bilateral

Examination

- Temperature
- CRT in children aged <12 years/BP in adults and older children
- Heart rate
- Respiratory rate
- Targeted examination based on any symptoms – e.g., chest, abdomen, ears
- Consider scarlet fever (see later in this chapter); if suspected, check throat
- If no fever, consider an allergic reaction

Self-care

- No treatment available for non-specific viral infection, other than supportive measures
- No exclusion from school needed

RED FLAG

- Pregnant/pregnant contact (*see UKHSA, 2022b*)

Reference

UKHSA. 2022a. Rubella notifications and confirmed cases by oral fluid testing 2013 to 2022 by quarter. www.gov.uk/government/publications/rubella-confirmed-cases/rubella-notifications-and-confirmed-cases-by-oral-fluid-testing-in-england-2013-to-2014-by-quarter

UKHSA. 2022b. Investigation, diagnosis and management of exposure to viral rash illness in pregnancy. www.gov.uk/government/publications/viral-rash-in-pregnancy

SLAPPED CHEEK (FIFTH DISEASE)

- Caused by parvovirus B19
- Common in children aged 6–10 years, though may occur at any age; 50% of adults have been infected
- Immunosuppressed people and those with haematological disorders may develop bone marrow problems

History

- May have fever, nasal discharge, diarrhoea preceding the onset of the rash
- Joint pains in adults
- Immunosuppressed, bone marrow or blood disorder
- Pregnant

Examination

- Bright red cheek(s)
- May be followed by lacy rash on trunk and limbs, which may last for several weeks

Self-care

- Reassure that it is a mild, self-limiting viral infection
- No specific treatment available
- No exclusion from school needed
- Take paracetamol or ibuprofen[P] if needed for joint pain

> **RED FLAGS**
> - Pregnant (*may cause miscarriage; inform Obstetrics*)
> - Immunosuppressed (*may develop chronic anaemia; check full blood count (FBC) and reticulocytes*)
> - Blood disorders (*may develop aplastic anaemia; check FBC and reticulocytes*)

References

NICE CKS. 2022. Parvovirus B19 infection. https://cks.nice.org.uk/topics/parvovirus-b19-infection/management/pregnant-women

UKHSA. 2022. Investigation, diagnosis and management of exposure to viral rash illness in pregnancy. www.gov.uk/government/publications/viral-rash-in-pregnancy

HAND, FOOT AND MOUTH DISEASE (HFMD)

- Caused by a virus (usually coxsackie A16)
- Mainly affects children aged <10 years

History

- Fever, sore throat and malaise
- Painful blisters emerging on different parts of the body
- Confusion/neurological symptoms

Examination

- Painful vesicles in mouth, then papules on hands and feet, which turn into vesicles. Groins, knees and buttocks may also be affected

Self-care

- Reassure that it is not related to foot and mouth disease in animals
- No specific treatment available
- Advise that symptoms will get better on their own in 7–10 days
- Outbreaks are common in nurseries, childcare centres and schools. No exclusion is necessary unless they are too unwell to attend
- Take paracetamol or ibuprofen[P] if needed for pain
- Maintain fluid intake and seek help if dehydration suspected

90   The Minor Illness Manual

- Eat a soft diet if painful mouth ulcers present
- Nails may be shed several months later

 RED FLAGS

> - Pregnant woman who is also immunosuppressed or with delivery expected within 3 weeks (*low risk of severe illness; discuss with Obstetrics*). Outside this period, reassure the woman that there is no risk to the fetus
> - Neurological symptoms; complications have been associated with a particular strain (Saguil et al., 2019) (*admit urgently under Paediatrics*)

References

NICE CKS. 2020. Hand, foot and mouth disease. https://cks.nice.org.uk/topics/hand-foot-mouth-disease

Saguil, A., Kane, S.F., Lauters, R., et al. 2019. Hand-foot-and-mouth disease: rapid evidence review. *Am Fam Physician*; 100(7):408–14. https://fmhub.org/wp-content/uploads/2021/08/hand-foot-and-mouth-disease.pdf

SCARLET FEVER

- Caused by group A beta-haemolytic streptococcus (GABHS)
- Over 37,000 cases in England and Wales during the winter of 2022/23
- Usually, most cases occur in February/March
- Commonest in children (peak at age 4)
- Complications are rare but include invasive group A streptococcal (iGAS) infection, secondary infections (e.g., pneumonia) and late complications (e.g., rheumatic fever, glomerulonephritis)
- There is a greater risk of sepsis occurring if there are breaches in the skin, e.g., from a wound or co-existing chickenpox

History

- Sore throat and cervical lymphadenopathy
- Fever (typically >38.3°C), malaise and headache
- Rash starting 12–24 hours after initial symptoms; starting on the chest and abdomen before spreading to the rest of the body
- Nausea and vomiting
- 🚩 Immunosuppressed
- 🚩 Structural heart disease
- 🚩 Previous rheumatic fever

Examination

- Blanching, rough, red pinpricks (which feel like sandpaper). Rash peels after 7 days
- Skin folds are deep red in colour
- Flushed face, pale around the mouth
- 'Strawberry tongue'; a white coating may form on the tongue that then peels, leaving a red and swollen tongue
- Red throat with macules over the hard and soft palates

Action

- Take a throat swab if the person is allergic to penicillin, is in contact with vulnerable people or if an outbreak is suspected (though a negative swab does not exclude the diagnosis)

Self-care

- Over the years, the mortality from scarlet fever has dropped from 25% to 0.1%. Most of this reduction occurred before the development of antibiotics

- Infectious until 24 hours after starting antibiotics – particularly avoid contact with immunosuppressed people and those with structural heart problems, previous rheumatic fever, open wounds or chickenpox
- Without antibiotics, people remain infectious for up to 3 weeks after symptoms have appeared
- Wash hands frequently; avoid sharing cutlery, cups and towels; put used tissues in bin immediately
- Safety-netting: seek further advice if worsening or no improvement after 7 days

Prescription

- If scarlet fever is clinically suspected, antibiotics should be prescribed without waiting for swab results
- Prescribe phenoxymethylpenicillin for 10 days (500 mg four times a day for an adult; see BNFC for children's doses). If a child cannot tolerate the taste of phenoxymethylpenicillin solution, use amoxicillin
- If allergic to penicillin and not pregnant, the current advice from the UKHSA (2023) is to use azithromycin[PIQ] for 5 days (500 mg once daily for adults) or clarithromycin[PIQ] for 10 days (500 mg twice a day for adults)
- If allergic to penicillin and pregnant, erythromycin[Q] for 10 days is recommended (250–500 mg four times a day)
- Notify the Health Protection Team

RED FLAGS

- Structural heart disease, e.g., heart valve problem (*consider urgent admission under Medical/Paediatrics*)
- Immunosuppressed (*consider urgent admission under Medical/Paediatrics*)
- At high risk of invasive complications due to, for example, chickenpox, wounds, recent pregnancy (*monitor carefully for sepsis, with condition-specific safety-netting advice and follow up in 24-48 hours*)
- Previous rheumatic fever (*refer to experienced colleague; at high risk of recurrence*)

Skn

References

NHS England. 2023. Group A Streptococcus: reinstatement of NICE sore throat guidance for children and young people and withdrawal of NHS England interim guidance. www.england.nhs.uk/wp-content/uploads/2022/12/PRN00247_Group-A-Streptococcus-reinstatement-of-NICE-sore-throat-guidance-for-children-and-young-people-and-wi.pdf

NICE CKS. 2023. Scarlet fever. https://cks.nice.org.uk/topics/scarlet-fever

UKHSA. 2023. Guidelines for the public health management of scarlet fever outbreaks in schools, nurseries and other childcare settings. https://assets.publishing.service.gov.uk/government/uploads/system/uploads/attachment_data/file/1148200/guidelines-for-public-health-management-scarlet-fever-outbreaks-january-2023_.pdf

ACUTE GENERALISED ITCHY RASH

1. Chickenpox
2. Urticaria
3. Scabies
4. Pityriasis rosea
5. Eczema (see later Miscellaneous section)

CHICKENPOX

- Caused by the varicella zoster virus (also called herpes zoster)
- Incubation period of 10–21 days
- Highly infectious: significant exposure is regarded as over 5 minutes face-to-face or 15 minutes in the same room (*As a clinician, are you protected by previous infection or vaccination?*)
- Not currently part of the UK childhood vaccination programme, but may be introduced soon

History

- May cause fever, headache and malaise (tends to be more marked in adults)
- Then scattered itchy spots developing one at a time, turning into vesicles

🏴 Immunosuppressed

🏴 Pregnant

Examination

- Separate itchy papules at different stages of development, turning to vesicles which usually crust over within 5 days. The crusts will fall off after 1–2 weeks

Self-care

- It is important to avoid scratching, which creates the risk of secondary bacterial infection
- Crotamiton[PB] lotion OTC (keep in fridge, avoid application to nipple area if breastfeeding) may be used to reduce itching. Cooling gels are popular, although there is little evidence to support their use. Calamine lotion has a drying effect, and is marked as 'less suitable' in the BNFC; the oily form may be preferable, though little research is available (Joy, 2022)
- Chlorphenamine[PBI] is useful at night because of its sedative action, but sedation may be unacceptable (for adults, 4 mg at bedtime, repeated after 4 hours if necessary. See BNFC for children's doses)
- Non-sedating antihistamines are probably ineffective
- Avoid ibuprofen as it increases the risk of secondary bacterial infection (Quaglietta et al., 2021; Stone et al., 2018)
- Porridge oats in fine mesh fabric (e.g., tights or sock) held under running bath water may be soothing

Action

- Previously thought to be most infectious in the 24 hours before spots appear, but this is now disputed (Marin et al., 2021). Infectious until all lesions crusted over (usually 5 days). Avoid contact with vulnerable people (see below)
- Chickenpox is a notifiable disease in Northern Ireland

Prescription

Some people with the infection may benefit from anti-viral treatment:

- Prescribe higher-dose aciclovir to the immunosuppressed (800 mg five times a day for 7 days for adults)
- Prescribe higher-dose aciclovir if onset of rash <24 hours ago and either of the following:
  - Age ≥14 years
  - Severe symptoms

For contacts of people with the infection (UKHSA, 2023):

- Arrange varicella zoster immunoglobulin (VZIG) for neonates who have been exposed within 7 days of delivery
- Prescribe aciclovir for those who are not immune and are pregnant or immunosuppressed. Note that the dosage is different from the treatment of chickenpox, and that the course should start on day 7 after exposure. The rules are complex; consider seeking specialist advice (UKHSA, 2023)

RED FLAGS

- Immunosuppressed (*give aciclovir; seek specialist advice*)
- Pregnant or <4 weeks after childbirth (*see UKHSA, 2022a; seek specialist advice*)
- Baby aged <4 weeks (30% mortality) (*needs IV aciclovir; admit urgently under Paediatrics*)
- Breathless/confused/severe headache/petechial rash (*pneumonia, encephalitis and thrombocytopenia are possible complications of chickenpox; pregnant women are at highest risk. Admit urgently under Medical/Paediatrics*)
- At risk of Mpox because of recent travel to West Africa or contact with a known case (*refer to Sexual Health; see UKHSA, 2022b*)
- Suspected secondary bacterial infection (*risk increased if the person is taking an oral corticosteroid or an NSAID such as ibuprofen*). Some lesions become painful rather than itchy and may weep purulent fluid; a second phase of fever develops (*consider urgent admission under Medical/Paediatrics if any sign of sepsis. If treating in primary care, take a swab from any weeping lesion for bacterial culture, and prescribe as for cellulitis*)

References

Joy, N. 2022. Calamine lotion. *J Skin Sex Transmitted Dis*; 4(1)83–6. https://jsstd.org/calamine-lotion *Calamine contains zinc oxide/carbonate and ferric oxide. Evaporation provides the lotion its soothing and antipruritic effect but is also drying.*

Marin, M., Leung, J., Lopez, A.S., et al. 2021. Communicability of varicella before rash onset: a literature review. *Epidemiol Infect*; 149:E131 https://doi.org/10.1017/S0950268821001102 *Transmission before rash onset seems unlikely, although the possibility of pre-rash respiratory transmission cannot be entirely ruled out.*

NICE CKS. 2022. Chickenpox. https://cks.nice.org.uk/topics/chickenpox/

Quaglietta, L., Martinelli, M., and Staiano, A. 2021. Serious infectious events and ibuprofen administration in pediatrics: a narrative review in the era of COVID-19 pandemic. *Ital J Pediatr*; 47(1):20. https://doi.org/10.1186/s13052-021-00974-0 *Pre-hospital use of ibuprofen may increase the risk of complicated pneumonia in children.*

Stone, K., Tackley, E., and Weir, S. 2018. BET 2: NSAIs and chickenpox. *Emerg Med J*; 35(1):66. https://doi.org/10.1136/emermed-2017-207366.2 *It is advisable to avoid NSAID use in cases of primary varicella due to the potential increased risk of severe bacterial skin infections.*

UKHSA. 2022a. Guidance on the investigation, diagnosis and management of viral illness, or exposure to viral rash illness, in pregnancy. https://assets.publishing.service.gov.uk/government/uploads/system/uploads/attachment_data/file/1116128/viral-rash-in-pregnancy-guidance.pdf

UKHSA. 2022b. Mpox (monkeypox): background information. www.gov.uk/guidance/monkeypox

UKHSA. 2023. Guidelines on post exposure prophylaxis (PEP) for varicella/shingles. www.gov.uk/government/publications/post-exposure-prophylaxis-for-chickenpox-and-shingles

URTICARIA

This is a rash triggered by the immune system either appropriately (infection), inappropriately (allergy) or for an unknown reason (idiopathic). It is caused by dilation of capillaries and the release of histamine from mast cells, causing leakage of plasma into the skin. It is also called 'hives' or 'nettle rash' (the botanical name of the nettle is *Urtica*).

History

- Usually an itchy rash that comes and goes over a few hours
- Accompanied by burning or itching
- Try to identify possible triggers:
  - Drugs (e.g., aspirin, penicillins, NSAIDs, ACE inhibitors)
  - Viral infection (including COVID-19)
  - Food allergy (e.g., milk, eggs, peanuts, tree nuts and shellfish)
  - Gastrointestinal symptoms (associated with *H. pylori*)
  - Bites and stings
  - Heat or cold (e.g., 'prickly heat')
  - Vigorous exercise
  - Pressure
  - Psychosocial stress ('stress rash')

🏴 Any symptoms suggesting severe allergic reaction, angioedema or anaphylaxis (see earlier section on Anaphylaxis)

🏴 Wheals last >24 hours and leave a mark (possible underlying vasculitis)

Examination

- Raised bumps/patches in many shapes and sizes. These can look pink/red on someone with white skin, but the colour of the rash may be more difficult to see on brown or black skin

Self-care

- Usually self-limiting without treatment, but for people with symptoms requiring treatment:
  - Oral (not topical) antihistamines: loratadine[PB] or cetirizine[PB] (10 mg once daily for adults) or fexofenadine[PBC] (120 mg once daily for adults; note that the 180 mg dose is licensed only for chronic idiopathic urticaria). If one of these proves ineffective, try an alternative. Children aged <12 years should take cetirizine[PB] or

fexofenadine[PBC] twice daily. For adults, if the effect of a once-daily antihistamine does not last, the daily dose may be divided in two

- Chlorphenamine[PBI] may be added if sedation is desirable/acceptable (4 mg every 4–6 hours if required; maximum 24 mg per day for adults)

- Avoid any identified triggers

Prescription

- If symptoms are severe, consider prescribing a short course of an oral steroid (prednisolone[PI], 40 mg daily for up to 7 days in adults)

- Allergy specialists may recommend increasing the dose of non-sedating antihistamine up to four times the level recommended in the British National Formulary (BNF). This dosage is unlicensed but may be considered on specialist advice, or by a practitioner with appropriate competence and experience

- Consider prescribing a leukotriene receptor antagonist (e.g., montelukast[PB] [10 mg once daily for adults]) in addition to the antihistamine if needed

- H2-antihistamines may provide additional benefit (*unlicensed indication;* e.g., famotidine[PBCQ], 20 mg daily for adults). For more information on this unusual use of these medicines, see the relevant entry under Prescribing Insights in the Members' section of the NMIC website

RED FLAGS

- Any suspicion of anaphylaxis (*get help and administer IM adrenaline; send very urgently to hospital*)
- Suspicion of angioedema (*if significant, treat as anaphylaxis*)
- Pregnant (*refer to experienced colleague, see CKS topic 'Itch in pregnancy', NICE CKS, 2022a*)
- Painful/persistent (*seek specialist advice or refer to Dermatology*)
- Urticaria in children with food allergy triggers may herald future anaphylaxis (*consider referral to Allergy Clinic*)

References

British Association of Dermatologists. 2020. Patient leaflet on urticaria and angioedema. www.bad.org.uk/pils/urticaria-and-angioedema

Hazell, T. 2022. Urticaria. https://patient.info/doctor/urticaria-pro

NICE CKS. 2022a. Itch in pregnancy. https://cks.nice.org.uk/topics/itch-in-pregnancy

NICE CKS. 2022b. Urticaria. https://cks.nice.org.uk/topics/urticaria

Powell, R.J., Leech, S.C., Till, S., et al. 2015. BSACI guideline for the management of chronic urticaria and angioedema. www.bsaci.org/guidelines/bsaci-guidelines/chronic-urticaria-and-angioedema-2

SCABIES

- Caused by a mite that burrows under the skin, most commonly on the web space between fingers. On average, 12 mites are present

- Transmission usually requires prolonged skin contact, although it is thought to be possible through shared towels and bedding. More common in migrants and in tropical countries (Delaš Aždajić et al., 2022)

- Long incubation period – up to 8 weeks for the rash to appear

- Not acquired from domestic pets (their form of scabies cannot reproduce on humans)

- Common in institutions such as care homes, nurseries and migrant centres

History

- Widespread severe itching, worse at night. May affect the nipples or scrotum

- Sleeping partners or other family members may be affected

Examination

- Burrows may be visible – bumpy grey lines 2–15 mm long, most often found on sides of fingers, finger webs, edges of hands, wrists and feet
- Spreading variable allergic rash usually develops after 2–6 weeks

Self-care

- Permethrin dermal cream should be applied simultaneously to all household and sexual contacts from the previous 2 months. This should be repeated after 7 days. Larger people may require 2 × 30 g packs. Do not use the liquid 1% creme rinse, which is inadequate for treating scabies. At the time of writing, there were problems with the availability of all scabies treatments
    - A prescription is required for babies aged <2 months (*unlicensed indication*)
    - Despite what the product leaflet may say, apply this to the whole body (BNF, 2023), including face, neck, scalp and ears (avoid contact with eyes)
    - Be sure to cover finger and toe webs and under nails
    - Do not apply just after a bath or shower as this may increase absorption into the blood
    - Wash off after 12 hours (i.e., apply in evening and leave on overnight)
    - Reapply treatment if washed off before this time (e.g., to hands)
- Machine wash clothes, towels and bedding at a high temperature (60°C or above) on the day of treatment. Laundry that cannot be washed at a high temperature should be sealed in a plastic bag for at least 72 hours
- Sedating antihistamines (e.g., chlorphenamine[PBI]) give best relief of itch, but sedation is long-lasting and may be unacceptable (4 mg at bedtime for adults, repeated after 4 hours if necessary)
- It is debatable whether non-sedating antihistamines are effective
- Crotamiton[PB] may help relieve itch and has some insecticidal activity. Topical corticosteroids may be used once the mites have been eradicated
- Successful treatment results in no new burrows or rash appearing. **However, itching may persist for 6 weeks. It is important that the person is made aware of this!**
- If resistant to treatment, then may need referral to Dermatology for treatments including oral ivermectin[PBC]
- Special precautions are needed when outbreaks occur in migrant centres or care homes (UKHSA, 2023)

References

British Association for Sexual Health and HIV (BASHH). 2016. UK national guideline on the management of scabies. www.bashhguidelines.org/media/1137/scabies-2016.pdf

Centers for Disease Control and Prevention. 2020. Scabies frequently asked questions. www.cdc.gov/parasites/scabies/gen_info/faqs.html *Useful information for someone diagnosed with scabies.*

Delaš Aždajić, M., Bešlić, I., Gašić, A., et al. 2022. Increased scabies incidence at the beginning of the 21st century: what do reports from Europe and the world show? *Life*; 12(10):1598. https://doi.org/10.3390/life12101598 *The greatest scabies burdens were recorded for East and Southeast Asia.*

UKHSA. 2023. UKHSA guidance on the management of scabies cases and outbreaks in long-term care facilities and other closed settings. www.gov.uk/government/publications/scabies-management-advice-for-health-professionals/ukhsa-guidance-on-the-management-of-scabies-cases-and-outbreaks-in-long-term-care-facilities-and-other-closed-settings

PITYRIASIS ROSEA

- Occurs mainly in those aged 10–35; more common in women
- Cause is not known, though reactivation of herpes virus types 6 and 7 has been described (Drago et al., 2009)

History

- Malaise, fever or lymphadenopathy before the rash appears
- Itching is often present with rash. This is usually mild but may occasionally be intense

Examination

- Usually starts with a larger initial 'herald' patch (a 2-5 cm oval-shaped area of pink or red scaly skin), often on trunk
- 2–14 days later, the more widespread rash develops with numerous salmon-coloured, oval patches, around 1 cm in diameter, appearing over a period of days. These have a ring of scale on the outer edge
- In people with darker skin, the patches can be grey, brown or black
- Patches line up symmetrically with their long axes aligned with the ribs on the trunk and upper limbs ('Christmas tree' rash in the T-shirt and shorts area). In children the face and scalp may be affected
- Consider an alternative diagnosis: guttate psoriasis affects a similar age group, but the patches are smaller, rounder and pinker (see Guttate Psoriasis section in this chapter)

Self-care

- Reassure; no specific treatment is required
- Explain that the rash may get worse before it gets better; new crops may occur for several weeks
- Rash will last 2–12 weeks then disappear; there may be some hyper- or hypo-pigmentation of the affected skin for several months, but there will be no scarring
- In dark-skinned people, the marks may take longer to fade
- Not contagious
- Recurs in ~25% of people (Yüksel, 2019)
- Emollients (e.g., Oilatum) may be helpful for itching
- Hydrocortisone ointment if itching severe

Prescription

If symptoms are severe, aciclovir may be prescribed (*unlicensed indication*) at a dose of 800 mg five times a day for adults (Contreras-Ruiz et al., 2019). *CKS state that high-quality evidence is lacking, and that this should be instigated in secondary care.*

RED FLAG

- Pregnant (*concern about miscarriage* [Wenger-Oehn et al., 2022]; *discuss with Obstetrics*)

References

British Association of Dermatologists. 2019. Pityriasis rosea www.bad.org.uk/pils/pityriasis-rosea

Contreras-Ruiz, J., Peternel, S., Gutiérrez, C.J., et al. 2019. Interventions for pityriasis rosea. *Cochrane Database Syst Rev*; 10:CD005068. https://doi.org/10.1002/14651858.CD005068.pub3 *When compared with placebo or no treatment, oral aciclovir probably leads to good rash improvement.*

Drago, F., Broccolo, F., and Rebora, A., 2009. Pityriasis rosea: an update with a critical appraisal of its possible herpesviral etiology. *J Am Acad Dermatol*; 61(2):303–18. https://doi.org/10.1016/j.jaad.2008.07.045

NICE CKS. 2020. Pityriasis rosea. https://cks.nice.org.uk/topics/pityriasis-rosea

Wenger-Oehn, L., Graier, T., Ambros-Rudolph, C., et al. 2022. Pityriasis rosea in pregnancy: a case series and literature review. *J Dtsch Dermatol Ges*; 20(7):953–9. https://doi.org/10.1111/ddg.14763

Yüksel, M. 2019. Pityriasis rosea recurrence is much higher than previously known: a prospective study. *Acta Derm Venereol*; 99(7):664–7. https://doi.org/10.2340/00015555-3169

PURPLE RASHES

Purple rashes are usually caused by leaking of blood from the vessels just under the skin; therefore, they do not blanch with pressure or when covered by a glass (the 'tumbler test'). Pinpoint rashes are described as petechial, larger areas as purpuric. Such rashes may be caused by:

- Pressure changes, e.g., 'love bites', violent vomiting or coughing, excessive scratching or friction, attempted strangulation

- Platelet abnormalities, e.g., leukaemia, thrombocytopenia, dual antiplatelet therapy after myocardial infarction, aspirin in older people
- Vasculitis, e.g., Henoch–Schönlein purpura (HSP), which mainly affects children
- Very rarely, meningococcal septicaemia. Of 1329 children attending a paediatric A&E in the UK with fever and a non-blanching rash, only 1% had meningococcal disease (Waterfield et al., 2021)

 RED FLAG CONDITION

BOX 8.2 PURPLE RASH

Someone with an unexplained purple rash requires urgent assessment:

- Sepsis suspected: *admit very urgently under Medical/Paediatrics*
- HSP suspected: *admit urgently under Paediatrics*
- Otherwise: *arrange urgent FBC and refer to experienced colleague*

References

Waterfield, T., Maney, J.A., Fairley, D., et al., 2021. Validating clinical practice guidelines for the management of children with non-blanching rashes in the UK (PiC): a prospective, multicentre cohort study. *Lancet Infect Dis*; 21(4):569–77. https://doi.org/10.1016/S1473-3099(20)30474-6

LOCALISED BACTERIAL INFECTIONS

1. Impetigo
2. Boils
3. Cellulitis
4. Ingrowing toenail
5. Paronychia

IMPETIGO

A common superficial bacterial infection of the skin. Can affect all ages, but commoner in young children.

History

- May be secondary to wound or viral lesion
- May be systemically unwell if infection is severe (but then check carefully for cellulitis)
- Slowly spreading sore areas, not usually symmetrical across the midline
- 🚩 Immunosuppressed

Examination

There are two types of impetigo that can be either localised (usually around the mouth and nose in children) or widespread:

- **Non-bullous** (75%) is caused by *Staphylococcus aureus* or *Streptococcus* or both. Golden crusted lesions, typically 2 cm in diameter, resembling glued-on cornflakes. May be mildly itchy
- **Bullous** (25%, commoner in children aged <2 years) is caused by *Staphylococcus aureus*. Fluid-filled lesions, typically >5 mm in size

Self-care

- Will heal without scarring, unless picked
- Wash off crusts with soapy water
- Stay out of school until lesions crusted, or 48 hours after starting antibiotics

Skn

- Advise hygiene measures to reduce spreading, e.g., wash hands regularly, hot wash of clothing, do not share facecloths or towels and avoid contact with immunosuppressed people
- If localised non-bullous impetigo and person not immunosuppressed, treat with topical antiseptic. This is currently first line because of concerns about antibiotic resistance. NICE (2020) recommends hydrogen peroxide 1% cream (Crystacide[B] [OTC], applied two or three times a day for 5 days. Cautions: avoid the eyes; bleaches fabric)
- Safety-netting: seek further advice if worsening or no improvement after 7 days

Prescription

- If localised non-bullous impetigo for which topical hydrogen peroxide has failed or is unsuitable, or widespread non-bullous impetigo, prescribe either topical antibiotic (sodium fusidate 2% ointment applied two or three times a day for 5 days) or oral antibiotic; flucloxacillin (500 mg four times a day for 5 days for adults), or, for those allergic to penicillin, clarithromycin[PIQ] (250–500 mg twice daily for 5 days for adults)
- If bullous impetigo, or systemically unwell or immunosuppressed, prescribe oral antibiotic as above
- If no improvement after initial treatment, send a skin swab and step up treatment: if previously using topical antibiotic, switch to oral antibiotic; and if already taking oral antibiotic, extend the course pending swab results
- Consider also treating inside nostrils with Naseptin if recurrent facial impetigo
- Avoid mupirocin[P], which should be reserved for treatment of methicillin-resistant *Staphylococcus aureus* (MRSA)
- Do not offer combination treatment with a topical and oral antibiotic
- Advise the person to seek help if worsening or no improvement after 7 days

RED FLAGS

- Bullous impetigo in infants aged <1 year (*possible staphylococcal scalded skin syndrome; admit urgently under Paediatrics*)
- Painful, non-healing ulcer (*syphilis, cancer, cutaneous diphtheria in a migrant; refer urgently to experienced colleague and/or Health Protection Team*)

References

Chaplin, S. 2016. Topical antibacterial and antiviral agents: prescribing and resistance. *Prescriber*; 27:29–36. https://wchh.onlinelibrary.wiley.com/doi/pdf/10.1002/psb.1480

Hoffmann, T.C., Peiris, R., Glasziou, P., et al. 2021. Natural history of non-bullous impetigo: a systematic review of time to resolution or improvement without antibiotic treatment. *Br J Gen Pract*; 71(704), e237–e242. https://doi.org/10.3399/bjgp20X714149 *Symptoms resolve in some people by about 7 days without using antibiotics, with about one-quarter of people not improving.*

Levi, L.I., Barbut, F., Chopin, D., et al. 2021. Cutaneous diphtheria: three case-reports to discuss determinants of re-emergence in resource-rich settings. *Emerg Microbes Infect*; 10(1):2300–302. https://doi.org/10.1080/22221751.2021.2008774 *Migration, travel and vaccine scepticism are key factors not only for diphtheria re-emergence, but for the future of most preventable diseases.*

NICE. 2020. NG153. Impetigo: antimicrobial prescribing. www.nice.org.uk/guidance/ng153

NICE CKS. 2022. Impetigo. https://cks.nice.org.uk/topics/impetigo/

BOILS AND CARBUNCLES

- A boil is an infection of a single hair follicle, usually caused by *Staphylococcus aureus*
- A carbuncle is a larger lesion caused by several boils joining together. It is more painful than a boil, and the person may be systemically unwell

History

- Duration
- Fever or pain
- Discharge
- Are these recurrent?
- Any contacts with similar boils?
- Risk factors and/or symptoms of diabetes (thirst/polyuria/tiredness) (See Box 8.3)
- 🚩 Immunosuppressed

Examination

- Temperature, BP, heart rate and respiratory rate if systemically unwell
- Fluctuation (sensation of fluid moving between two fingers placed on either side – imagine a balloon full of water)
- Cellulitis – is the surrounding skin hot, red and tender?
- Enlarged lymph nodes (suggest underlying cellulitis)

Tests

If the infection is recurrent, severe or affecting other family members:

- Swab lesion, nose and axilla to identify staphylococcal carriage (affects around 20% of population, commoner in healthcare workers), and ask the lab to check for Panton–Valentine leukocidin *Staphylococcus aureus* (PVL-SA) (British Association of Dermatologists, 2019)
- Check for immunosuppression:
    - FBC
    - HbA1c or FPG (see Box 8.3)
    - Consider HIV test

Self-care

- Apply heat to encourage pointing (e.g., warm flannel) four times daily
- Cover with sterile gauze
- Wash hands after touching the boil
- Do not share towels or flannels
- Wash and tumble dry bedding, towels and underclothes daily
- Avoid swimming until healed
- If getting frequent boils, consider decolonisation treatment with chlorhexidine 4% body wash daily for 5 days (and use as shampoo on days 1, 3 and 5)

BOX 8.3 CHECKING FOR DIABETES

There is currently no national screening programme in the UK for diabetes. Instead, guidance advises testing those who are identified as being at high risk, ideally through use of a validated risk assessment tool. Such tools include the Leicester Diabetes Risk Score, which has been adopted by Diabetes UK as the 'Know Your Risk' tool.

- If someone presents with classical symptoms of diabetes, such as thirst, polyuria and weight loss, then caution is necessary. Check a fingerprick glucose and check the blood/urine for ketones
- Consider whether this might be a presentation of type 1 diabetes and discuss with an experienced colleague. Missing a case of type 1 diabetes can be catastrophic, potentially resulting in diabetic ketoacidosis. A question to consider is whether this fits as type 2 diabetes or does it seem a surprise? Don't discount the possibility of type 1 diabetes based on age or BMI alone. If in doubt, call your local diabetes specialist team and talk it though. If suspecting type 1 diabetes, then send the person in to hospital. If fingerprick glucose is raised and there are blood/urinary ketones, **this is type 1 diabetes and an emergency unless proven otherwise**
- If there are classical symptoms of diabetes but type 1 is not suspected, then get an HbA1c urgently. This doesn't require fasting, although it is unreliable in pregnancy or any condition affecting blood cell turnover (such as anaemia). FPG is an alternative; one result in the diabetes range is needed to make the diagnosis
- If there are no classical symptoms of diabetes, then two results in the diabetes range are needed to make the diagnosis. As above, HbA1c is usually preferred, but FPG can be used if HbA1c is not clinically appropriate
- Note that, at the thresholds of diagnosis, test results may not be concordant. For example, someone may have an HbA1c which is within the diabetes range while also having a FPG which is not within the diabetes range. To avoid confusion, it is advisable to use only one type of test in an individual when checking for diabetes
- Inform the person that you are testing for diabetes, as this diagnosis would have significant implications (e.g., for their life insurance)

References

NICE. 2017. PH38. Type 2 diabetes: prevention in people at high risk. www.nice.org.uk/guidance/ph38
NICE. 2022. NG17. Type 1 diabetes in adults: diagnosis and management. www.nice.org.uk/guidance/ng17

Action

- Magnesium sulphate paste is traditionally used, although there is a lack of evidence to support it
- Incision and drainage may be needed if fluctuant
- Advise the person to watch for symptoms of cellulitis
- Prescribe antibiotic if indicated (see Box 8.4)
- Treat nasal colonisation topically according to swab (mupirocin[P] reserved for MRSA)

 BOX 8.4 ANTIBIOTIC FOR BOILS

Prescribe an antibiotic only if:

- Unwell with fever or cellulitis
- High-risk group (immunosuppressed, diabetes)
- On the face
- Carbuncle

Antibiotic choice

If a swab was taken, treat according to sensitivity. If MRSA or PVL-SA isolated, these need special treatment; take advice from a microbiologist. Otherwise, if an antibiotic is indicated, prescribe a 5-7 day course of:

- Flucloxacillin (500mg four time daily for adults)
- Clarithromycin[PIQ] if allergic to penicillin (500 mg twice daily for adults)

> **RED FLAGS**
>
> - Facial boil causing cellulitis (*can become life-threatening; admit urgently under Medical/Paediatrics*)
> - Apparent boil in anogenital area or natal cleft (between buttocks) (*may be Bartholin's cyst, Crohn's disease or pilonidal abscess; consider referral to Surgical or Gynaecology*)
> - Carbuncle or large/fluctuant boil requiring incision and drainage (*admit under Surgical if procedure not available in primary care*)
> - Recurrent boils in axillae and groins (*possible hidradenitis suppurativa; seek specialist advice or refer to Dermatology*)

References

British Association of Dermatologists. 2019. PVL (Panton–Valentine leukocidin) staphylococcus aureus. www.bad.org.uk/pils/pvl-panton-valentine-leukocidin-staphylococcus-aureus/

NICE CKS. 2022. Boils, carbuncles, and staphylococcal carriage. https://cks.nice.org.uk/topics/boils-carbuncles-staphylococcal-carriage/

CELLULITIS

A potentially serious infection that may lead to sepsis. A bacterial infection of the deeper layers of the skin, usually caused by *Streptococcus pyogenes* (two-thirds of cases) or *Staphylococcus aureus* (one-third of cases). It is more common in people with diabetes; there is an increase of 12% in the odds of cellulitis for every 11 mmol/mol elevation in HbA1c (Zacay et al., 2021). Cellulitis is often misdiagnosed (Santer et al., 2018); consider other diagnoses such as DVT. Bilateral cellulitis is very unlikely (Chuang et al., 2022); consider other possibilities, e.g., varicose eczema or inflammation of skin stretched by oedema.

History

- Duration and onset
- Nature of any wound or break in the skin
- Pain
- Unilateral localised swelling and heat (bilateral symptoms are rarely due to cellulitis)
- 🚩 Fever/malaise/rigors
- 🚩 Immunosuppression (especially intravenous substance use or diabetes)

Examination

- Temperature
- Heart rate
- Respiratory rate
- CRT in children aged <12 years/BP in adults and older children
- Well-defined area is red, hot, swollen, hard and tender, with possible vesicles
- Colour (cellulitis appears scarlet initially)
- Discharge
- Localised lymphadenopathy
- If a leg is affected, get the person to lie flat and raise the leg to 45° for 1–2 minutes. If the redness significantly reduces, cellulitis is said to be unlikely (Santer et al., 2018)
- 🚩 Tracking (lymphangitis)

Tests

- Take swab **only** if the skin is broken and:
    - there is a penetrating injury *or*
    - there has been exposure to water-borne organisms *or*
    - the infection was acquired outside the UK
- If history of recurrent skin infections, or symptoms/risk factors of diabetes, consider tests for HIV and diabetes (HbA1c or FPG, see Box 8.3)

Self-care

- Keep limb elevated (if applicable)
- Mark boundary with indelible, soft-tipped, disposable pen (such as those used for minor surgery) – ask the person to seek help if area is enlarging beyond boundary (but advise them that this may happen temporarily in the first 24 hours of antibiotic treatment)
- Take paracetamol if needed for pain
- Use an emollient after 48 hours

Action

- Admit to hospital if any red flags (see Red Flags box that follows)
- Assess the severity using the Eron score (see Table 8.1). Class III or IV cellulitis will require urgent admission to hospital
- Arrange IV antibiotics in primary care **only** if person is unable to swallow or tolerate oral medication (NICE, 2019)
- Check portal of entry. Wound cleaning and dressing as appropriate
- If not warranting admission to hospital, prescribe antibiotic for 5–7 days (longer course may be needed in lymphoedema) (see Table 8.2) and review after 48 hours
- If the person has diabetes, start 'sick-day rules' and optimise glucose control (see Box 1.2 in Chapter 1)
- If recurrent cellulitis, consider prophylactic antibiotic (Dalal et al., 2017)
- Once settled, manage any factors which may predispose to breaks in the skin (e.g., eczema; see later section)

Table 8.1 The Eron classification system for cellulitis

Class I	Systemically well, no uncontrolled comorbidity
Class II	Systemically unwell or comorbidity (e.g., peripheral arterial disease, chronic venous insufficiency or morbid obesity)
Class III	Significant systemic upset, for example acute confusion, tachycardia, tachypnoea, hypotension, or unstable comorbidity
Class IV	Sepsis or necrotising fasciitis

Table 8.2 Oral antibiotic choice for cellulitis

Presentation	Antibiotic	Penicillin allergy
Typical cellulitis with no unusual features	Flucloxacillin (500–1000 mg* four times a day for adults for 5–7 days)	Clarithromycin[P][Q] (500 mg twice a day for adults for 5–7 days)
Post chickenpox	As above. Dual antibiotics are no longer recommended (NICE, 2019)	As above
Background of lymphoedema	As above but for 14[†] days	As above but for 14[†] days
Facial cellulitis	Co-amoxiclav (500/125 mg three times a day for adults for 7 days)	Clarithromycin[P][Q] (500 mg twice a day for adults for 7 days) and metronidazole[Q] (400 mg three times a day for adults for 7 days)
Following wound in water	Consult microbiologist	Consult microbiologist

* Use flucloxacillin 1000 mg (1 g) four times daily (*unlicensed indication*, but listed in BNF) for people with impaired circulation (e.g., diabetes or venous insufficiency) (NICE, 2019).
[†] British Lymphology Society, 2022.

RED FLAGS

Consider urgent admission under Medical/Paediatrics if:

- Unable to swallow/keep down oral antibiotic
- Alternative serious diagnosis cannot be excluded (e.g., DVT, septic arthritis)
- Class III or IV or rapidly deteriorating cellulitis
- Age <1 year or frail
- Immunosuppressed/diabetes or other reason for high risk (*e.g., artificial joint*)
- Significant lymphoedema
- Facial cellulitis
- Lymphangitis ('*tracking*')
- Pointing abscess (*needs incision and drainage/referral to Surgical*)
- Worsening despite treatment, or not responding to initial treatment after 3 days

References

Aebi, C., Ahmed, A., and Ramilo, O. 1996. Bacterial complications of primary varicella in children. *Clin Infect Dis*; 23(4):698–705. https://doi.org/10.1093/clinids/23.4.698 *The most likely cause of secondary infection of chickenpox is group A beta-haemolytic streptococcus (59% of cases), with* Staphylococcus aureus *being the second most likely (28%).*

British Lymphology Society. 2022. Guidelines on the management of cellulitis in lymphoedema. www.thebls.com/documents-library/guidelines-on-the-management-of-cellulitis-in-lymphoedema *Evidence for 14-day course.*

Chuang, Y.C., Liu, P.Y., Lai, K.L., et al. 2022. Bilateral lower limbs cellulitis: a narrative review of an overlooked clinical dilemma. *Int J Gen Med*; 15:5567–5578. https://doi.org/10.2147/IJGM.S356852 *In the absence of specific risk factors such as skin trauma, bilateral involvement is usually rare.*

Dalal, A., Eskin-Schwartz, M., Mimouni, D., et al. 2017. Interventions for the prevention of recurrent erysipelas and cellulitis. *Cochrane Database Syst Rev*; 6:CD009758. https://doi.org/10.1002/14651858.CD009758.pub2 *For people with at least two episodes of cellulitis in the previous 3 years, antibiotic prophylaxis (usually phenoxymethylpenicillin, 250 mg twice daily) reduces the number of recurrences by 50%.*

NICE. 2019. NG141. Cellulitis and erysipelas: antimicrobial prescribing. www.nice.org.uk/guidance/ng141

NICE CKS. 2023. Cellulitis – acute. https://cks.nice.org.uk/topics/cellulitis-acute/ *Note that CKS guidance differs from NICE NG141 with regard to lymphoedema and the role of IV antibiotics.*

Santer M., Lalonde A., Francis N.A., et al. 2018. Management of cellulitis: current practice and research questions. *Br J Gen Pract* 68 (677): 595–6. https://doi.org/10.3399/bjgp18X700181

Zacay, G., Hershkowitz Sikron, F., and Heymann, A.D., 2021. Glycemic control and risk of cellulitis. *Diabetes Care*; 44(2):367–72. https://doi.org/10.2337/dc19-1393

INGROWING TOENAIL

Here the sides of the toenail have grown into the surrounding skin. The big toe is most commonly affected. The nail curls and pierces the skin, which becomes red, hot, swollen and tender.

History

- Duration
- Discharge
- Previous episodes
- Background/symptoms/risk factors for diabetes

Examination

- Check for evidence of cellulitis – pus, spreading redness or fever (N.B. inflammation around the ingrowing corner of the nail does not indicate infection)
- Discharge
- Granulation tissue

Test

- Swab any discharge

Self-care

- Soak toe in warm salty water for 10 minutes (1 teaspoon of salt in 500 ml of water)
- With a cotton bud, push skin fold downwards and away from ingrown nail. Start at root of the nail and move outwards
- Repeat daily for a few weeks
- As end of nail grows forward, push tiny pledget of cotton wool under it to help nail grow over skin
- Change cotton wool daily
- Cutting the nails too short or cutting in at the edges encourages the condition. Allow the nail to grow forward until clear of end of toe, and cut nail straight across
- When feet are sweaty, it is easier for the nail to pierce the skin and embed itself. Keep feet clean and change socks regularly, using cotton socks rather than synthetics
- Wear comfortable shoes that fit properly

Action

- Refer to podiatry if persistent/recurrent
- If localised cellulitis (pus, fever, spreading redness), see previous section on Cellulitis

 RED FLAG

- Immunosuppressed/diabetes with cellulitis (*consider admitting urgently under Medical/Paediatrics*)

Reference

Tidy, C. 2023. Ingrowing toenails. https://patient.info/foot-care/ingrowing-toenails-ingrown-toenails

PARONYCHIA

A superficial infection of the skin fold around a nail, usually caused by *Staphylococcus aureus*. Common in all age groups; three times more common in women than men.

History

- Typically affects only one nail
- Localised pain and tenderness
- Risk factors include manicuring, frequent hand washing, finger sucking and nail biting, ingrown nail and trauma

Examination

- Pain and swelling at the side/base of one finger
- Nail fold is red, hot, tender and swollen. Pus may be seen
- Check for signs of cellulitis (see previous section)

Self-care

- Reassure that most cases resolve in 2–4 days with treatment
- Advise moist warm compresses for 10–15 minutes, three times daily, to help with pain and increase blood supply to the area
- Take paracetamol or ibuprofen[P] for pain relief
- Keep the affected areas clean and dry
- Address any risk factors identified in the history

Action

- If fluctuant, consider micro-incision and drainage. If micro-incision and drainage is not feasible or indicated:
  - Topical sodium fusidate 2% (three times daily for 7 days) for mild infection with no risk factors for severe illness (e.g., immunosuppression), *or*
  - Prescribe an oral antibiotic for 5–7 days: flucloxacillin (250–500 mg four times daily for adults) or, if allergic to penicillin, clarithromycin[PIQ] (250–500 mg twice daily for adults)
- Chronic paronychia (develops slowly and lasts for weeks) often needs treatment with antifungal medication

Reference

NICE CKS. 2022. Paronychia – acute. https://cks.nice.org.uk/topics/paronychia-acute/

OTHER LOCALISED RASHES

1. Cold sores
2. Shingles
3. Warts and verrucae
4. Molluscum contagiosum
5. Fungal infections
6. Nappy rash

COLD SORES

Caused by recurrence of herpes simplex virus (usually HSV-1).

History

- Often recurrent on same site (not always the lip)
- Tingling in skin before appearance of the sore
- Triggers include stress, ultraviolet (UV) light, pre-menstruation, minor trauma to the area, and other infections such as colds
- 🏴 Immunosuppressed

Examination

- Crops of vesicles on the border of the lip, tongue or mouth that break down into small red areas with yellowish membrane
- Check for evidence of cellulitis (see earlier section)

Self-care

- Aciclovir cream is available OTC. It is not routinely recommended but may be helpful if used within 48 hours of cold sore appearance (the sooner the better). At first sign, apply to lesions five times a day (approximately every 4 hours), for 5–10 days
- If on lip, avoid kissing
- Do not share objects that have touched the area
- Take care not to touch eyes or genitalia after touching cold sore
- Sunblock may help prevent recurrences
- Avoid non-essential contact with babies aged <4 weeks until sore has healed (risk of herpes simplex encephalitis). Mothers should minimise the risk of transferring virus from the cold sore to the baby

Prescription

- If immunosuppressed, recurrent or severe symptoms, consider oral aciclovir (200–400 mg five times daily in adults; see BNF for dosage advice) from the time of onset of prodromal symptoms before vesicles appear (if possible) until lesions have healed, for a minimum of 5 days

RED FLAGS

- Lesion not resolving after 10 days (*consider alternative diagnosis, e.g., syphilis*)
- Immunosuppressed (*at increased risk of complications; refer to experienced colleague*)
- Pregnant and near term (*theoretical risk to baby; discuss with Obstetrics*)

References

Chi, C.C., Wang, S.H., Delamere, F.M., et al. 2015. Interventions for prevention of herpes simplex labialis (cold sores on the lips). *Cochrane Database Syst Rev*; 8:CD010095. https://doi.org/10.1002/14651858.CD010095.pub2

NICE CKS. 2023. Herpes simplex – oral. https://cks.nice.org.uk/topics/herpes-simplex-oral

SHINGLES

Caused by recurrence of dormant varicella zoster virus (also called herpes zoster; the virus which causes chickenpox), often after a period of debility or psychosocial stress. The lifetime incidence is around 25%. It may occur in children but is commoner and more likely to cause long-term pain in those aged >50. Unlikely to recur (about 5%; Kim et al., 2019); people who have been diagnosed with recurrent shingles in the same area usually actually have herpes simplex. In the UK, vaccination against shingles is being rolled out from age 65 and from age 50 in the immunosuppressed.

History

- Location – affects only one side of the body. If the rash crosses the midline by more than two thumb widths, then it is not shingles
- Starts with macules and papules that develop into painful vesicles, weeping infectious fluid, over 3–5 days
- These crust over and heal after 2–4 weeks
- Severity – the pain (if present) may be burning, stabbing or throbbing
- Malaise, mild fever and burning or tingling pain in the area may occur up to 4 days before the rash appears
- ⚑ Immunosuppressed

Examination

- Affects the area of skin supplied by one nerve root (dermatome); commonest on the chest
- Note which nerve root is affected (see Figures 8.2 and 8.3)
- Local lymph nodes may be enlarged
- ⚑ Rash involves the eye or nose

Self-care

- Keep the rash dry
- Creams and lotions are best avoided because of the risk of spreading skin bacteria into the blistered area
- Adhesive dressings are not recommended
- Infectious until all vesicles have crusted over (usually 5–7 days). Avoid non-essential contact with babies aged <1 month, pregnant women without immunity (i.e., no previous infection with chickenpox or vaccination) and anyone who is immunosuppressed
- Fluid from the rash cannot give anyone shingles but could give chickenpox to someone without immunity. However, the risk of infection is very low if the rash is covered, and routine exclusion from school and work is not necessary
- In pregnancy, shingles carries no known risk to mother or baby
- Malaise or pain may require rest and time off work
- Avoid ibuprofen – increased risk of secondary bacterial infection (Mikaeloff et al., 2008)
- Seek advice again if the rash flares up or fever develops (this may be secondary bacterial infection needing an antibiotic)

Prescription

- Aciclovir tablets (800 mg five times daily for adults) if within 72 hours of onset of rash and any of the following:
  - Immunosuppressed (10-day course; see also Red Flags box below)
  - Age >50 (7-day course)
  - Affecting area other than the trunk (7-day course)
  - Anything more than mild symptoms (7-day course)
  - Nose or eye affected (7-day course; also prescribe aciclovir eye ointment, five times daily; see Red Flags box below)
- For pain not controlled by ordinary analgesics, offer an analgesic suitable for neuropathic pain, e.g., amitriptyline[PCIQ] or gabapentin[PC] (see CKS topic 'Post-herpetic neuralgia', NICE CKS, 2022)

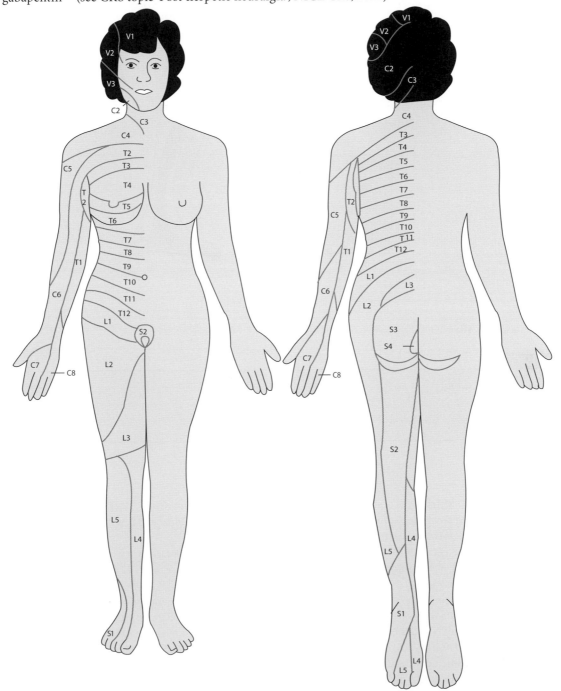

Figure 8.2 Dermatome diagram. Each area is labelled with the spinal nerve that carries sensation from the skin to the spinal cord. The areas overlap to some extent, and an individual person may vary from normal. C: Cervical; L: Lumbar; S: Sacral; T: Thoracic; V: Fifth cranial nerve (trigeminal).

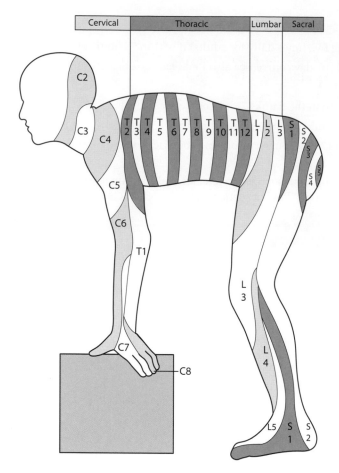

Figure 8.3 Dermatomes on all fours. (Image credit: DoctorOfMedicine.)

The dermatomes of the limbs are much easier to understand when you consider that we evolved from animals who walked on all four limbs.

 RED FLAGS

- Nose or eye affected (*prescribe oral and topical aciclovir [eye ointment]; send urgently to hospital with referral to Ophthalmology [Tuft, 2020]*)
- Immunosuppressed person with severe symptoms (*may need IV antivirals; seek specialist advice*)

References

Apok, V., Gurusinghe, N.T., Mitchell, J.D., et al. 2011. Dermatomes and dogma. *Pract Neurol*; 11(2):100. https://doi.org/10.1136/jnnp.2011.242222 *The term 'dermatome' generally refers to an area of skin innervated by a particular neural element, specifically nerve root, dorsal root ganglion or spinal segment.*

Kim, Y.J., Lee, C.N., Lee, M.S., et al. 2019. Recurrence rate of herpes zoster and its risk factors: a population-based cohort study. *J Korean Med Sci*; 34(2):e1. https://doi.org/10.3346/jkms.2019.34.e1 *The recurrence rate is 12.0 per 1000 person-years. Older women are at the highest risk.*

Mikaeloff, Y., Kezouh, A., and Suissa, S. 2008. Nonsteroidal anti-inflammatory drug use and the risk of severe skin and soft tissue complications in patients with varicella or zoster disease. *Br J Clin Pharmacol*; 65(2):203–9. https://doi.org/10.1111/j.1365-2125.2007.02997.x *Use of NSAIDs is associated with an elevated risk of severe skin and soft-tissue complications of varicella zoster virus infection. For shingles, the baseline risk was 0.6%, which increased to 1% in NSAID users.*

NICE CKS. 2022. Post-herpetic neuralgia. https://cks.nice.org.uk/topics/post-herpetic-neuralgia/

NICE CKS. 2023. Shingles. https://cks.nice.org.uk/topics/shingles

Tuft, S. 2020. How to manage herpes zoster ophthalmicus. *Community Eye Health*; 33(108):71–2. www.ncbi.nlm.nih.gov/pmc/articles/PMC7205171/ *The evidence of the benefit of adding in aciclovir eye ointment is insubstantial, but it will produce much higher concentrations of the drug in the anterior eye and provide some lubrication.*

WARTS AND VERRUCAE

- Typical warts are raised pale swellings and may have a surface like a cauliflower
- Verrucae are flattened areas with underlying black dots
- Caused by strains of human papillomavirus (HPV)

Self-care

- Contagious – take steps to avoid self- or cross-infection. People with a verruca should use a waterproof plaster for swimming and avoid sharing towels
- Most disappear by themselves with time, but may take 2–3 years
- Avoid scratching or picking them
- Generally best left untreated. See the decision aid on patient.info (https://patient.info/news-and-features/warts-and-verrucca-treatment-options)
- Salicylic acid (OTC) – limited evidence for effectiveness:
  - May cause chemical burns
  - Do not apply to the face
  - Do not use in people with diabetes, peripheral vascular disease or reduced sensation
  - Proper application is important:
    - Soak in warm water for 5–10 minutes
    - Remove hard skin with an emery board
    - Avoid paring or applying the treatment to the surrounding skin
    - Treat daily for at least 12 weeks
- Liquid nitrogen[c] (cryotherapy) – limited evidence for effectiveness:
  - Not for children aged <10 years (painful)
  - Not suitable for people with diabetes, poor circulation or reduced sensation
  - May also cause dramatic blood blistering, temporary numbness and scarring
  - 4–6 treatments may be needed
  - OTC products do not lower the skin temperature to the same degree
- Duct tape – limited evidence for effectiveness but little risk of harm (Goldman, 2019):
  - Cover the wart with duct tape for 6 days. Make sure it is the opaque type (Samlaska, 2011)
  - If tape falls off, apply a fresh piece
  - Remove tape, soak wart in water and debride with emery board
  - Leave the wart uncovered overnight and apply a fresh piece of tape next day
  - Continue treatment for up to 2 months
- Banana skin – no evidence for effectiveness but little risk of harm:
  - Anecdotally, the application of a banana skin (with the white inside part taped against the wart) each night for 2 weeks has often been reported to be effective, but it seems highly unlikely that a clinical trial on this treatment would ever be funded. It does have the advantage of being virtually free

RED FLAGS

- Anogenital warts (*refer to Sexual Health*)
- Single wart in the elderly or immunosuppressed (*raised crusted lesion on head/neck/hand may be a squamous cell carcinoma; USC referral to Dermatology*)

References

Goldman, R.D., 2019. Duct tape for warts in children: should nature take its course? *Can Fam Physician*; 65(5):337–8. www.cfp.ca/content/65/5/337.long

Kwok, C.S., Gibbs, S., Bennett, C., Holland, R., and Abbott, R., 2012. Topical treatments for cutaneous warts. *Cochrane Database Syst Rev*; 9:CD001781. https://doi.org/10.1002/14651858.CD001781.pub3

Skn

Samlaska, C., 2011. Clear duct tape is not duct tape. *Br J Dermatol*; 165(2):432–3. https://doi.org/10.1111/j.1365-2133.2011.10299.x *Make sure to get the proper opaque stuff, which has a polyisoprene-based adhesive.*

Sterling, J.C., Gibbs, S., Haque Hussain, S.S., et al. 2014. British Association of Dermatologists' guidelines for the management of cutaneous warts. *Br J Dermatol*; 171(4): 696–712. https://onlinelibrary.wiley.com/doi/10.1111/bjd.13310 *Not revised since 2014, from which we conclude that there is no significant new evidence.*

Tidy, C. 2020. Warts and verrucas. https://patient.info/skin-conditions/warts-and-verrucas-leaflet *Includes a decision aid.*

MOLLUSCUM CONTAGIOSUM

This is a poxvirus infection that produces clusters of round, raised, pearly-white lesions (sometimes with a darker central dimple), usually on the trunk and limbs of children. In adults, it may also be a sexually transmitted infection. It is best left untreated as it resolves completely, without scarring, after several months. If itching is a problem, treat with emollients or hydrocortisone ointment. Sometimes secondary bacterial infection may occur.

References

Heo, J.Y., Park, T.H., and Kim, W.I., 2022. The efficacy and safety of topical 10% potassium hydroxide for molluscum contagiosum: a systematic review and meta-analysis. *J Dermatol Treat;* 33(3):1682–90. https://doi.org/10.1080/09546634.2021.1898527 *10% potassium hydroxide appears to be effective, although care must be taken to avoid normal skin. Note however that the (expensive) potassium hydroxide solution available OTC is only 5%.*

van der Wouden, J.C., van der Sande, R., Kruithof, E.J., et al. 2017. Interventions for cutaneous molluscum contagiosum. *Cochrane Database Syst Rev*; 5:CD004767. https://doi.org/10.1002/14651858.CD004767.pub4 *This review found no significant evidence for any intervention, including potassium hydroxide.*

FUNGAL INFECTIONS (TINEA)

Can affect:

- Foot (athlete's foot, tinea pedis) – may be in the toe web (most common) or on the sole (scaly or blistering)
- Body (ringworm, tinea corporis) and groin (tinea cruris)
- Nails (onychomycosis or tinea unguium)

History

- If on the foot, body or groin, an itchy localised red rash, slowly enlarging over several weeks
- Treatments tried
- Any domestic pets with itchy skin conditions
- Risk factors for body or groin fungal infections include diabetes, hot humid environments, wearing tight-fitting clothing, obesity and hyperhidrosis
- Nail infections tend to be in toenails rather than fingernails and are more common in older people

Examination

- Feet: affected foot may have white or red fissured scaling in the skin web between the toes. It typically starts between the fourth and fifth toe and spreads inwards. The dry type presents with scaling, thickening and redness of the sole and outer parts of the foot. The vesico-bullous type presents with multiple small vesicles and blisters, mainly on the arches and soles of the foot
- Skin: eczema-like patches. Not usually symmetrical across the midline. Often a scaly, inflamed edge with central area appearing normal
- Nails: affected nails may be thickened and discoloured – usually starting at the edges and spreading inward. It is unusual for all of the nails to be affected

Self-care

- Explain that it is an infection acquired from other humans or animals
- Scratching pets should be checked by a vet
- Wash the affected area daily and dry thoroughly
- Wash clothes, towels and bed linen frequently

- Wear loose-fitting clothes made of cotton or a material designed to wick moisture away from the skin. For nail infections, wear clean socks every day and avoid tight-fitting footwear
- Terbinafine cream[PBC] (OTC) twice daily for 7–14 days is first line for fungal skin infections. A prescription will be needed for anyone aged <16, pregnant (safety data are reassuring; Andersson et al., 2020) or breastfeeding (avoid application to the mother's chest; LactMed, 2018)
- Second line: clotrimazole cream 1% (OTC) twice daily for 4–6 weeks (continue for 1–2 weeks after rash has resolved)
- Third line: undecenoic (synonyms: undecylenic, undecanoic) acid cream (Mycota, OTC) twice daily for 4–6 weeks
- But if first treatment has failed, reconsider the diagnosis
- If itching is severe, hydrocortisone 1% cream may be applied once a day for a maximum of 7 days in addition to the antifungal. However, it should not be used alone because of its immunosuppressant effect
- For nail infections, amorolfine[PBC] 5% nail lacquer (OTC, expensive) once weekly for 6–12 months (cure rate only 15%–30%). If successful, the infected nail may not change, but new nail growth (from the base) will appear normal
- Urea enhances the effect of antifungal medicines on nail infections (Pan et al., 2013). Evidence reviews have not identified any trial in which urea alone was effective in treating fungal nail infections (Foley et al., 2020). However, many such preparations are sold OTC
- There is some evidence to support daily application to the nail of Vicks VapoRub[B] (Derby et al., 2011)
- There is no reliable evidence to support the use of (expensive) laser treatment (Foley et al., 2020)

Action

- If rash/nail infection persists despite an adequate course of topical treatment, reconsider diagnosis and take skin scrapings from the scaly edge or 'dust' from under the nail (do not refrigerate the sample; the results may take up to three weeks). Oral treatment (e.g., Terbinafine[PBCI]) may be needed

Prescription

Note that NHS England (2018) identified lymphoedema and previous cellulitis as exceptions to the OTC prescribing restrictions for fungal infections; topical antifungals may be prescribed in these situations.

References

Andersson, N.W., Thomsen, S.F., and Andersen, J.T. 2020. Evaluation of association between oral and topical terbinafine use in pregnancy and risk of major malformations and spontaneous abortion. *JAMA Dermatol*; 156(4):375–83. https://doi.org/10.1001/jamadermatol.2020.0142 *Among pregnancies exposed to oral or topical terbinafine, no increased risk of major malformations or spontaneous abortion was identified.*

British Association of Dermatologists. 2017. Patient leaflet on fungal infections of the nails. www.bad.org.uk/pils/fungal-infections-of-the-nails

Dars, S., Banwell, H.A., and Matricciani, L., 2019. The use of urea for the treatment of onychomycosis: a systematic review. *J Foot Ankle Res*; 12(1):22. https://doi.org/10.1186/s13047-019-0332-3 *Topical urea, **as an adjunct** to topical and oral antifungal treatment regimens, may improve the efficacy of treatment.*

Derby, R., Rohal, P., Jackson, C., et al. 2011. Novel treatment of onychomycosis using over-the-counter mentholated ointment: a clinical case series. *Am Board Fam Med*; 24(1): 69–77. https://doi.org/10.3122/jabfm.2011.01.100124 *The ingredients in Vicks VapoRub (thymol, menthol, camphor and oil of eucalyptus) have shown efficacy against dermatophytes in vitro; 83% of the 18 participants in this trial had a positive response.*

Foley, K., Gupta, A.K., Versteeg, S., et al. 2020. Topical and device-based treatments for fungal infections of the toenails. *Cochrane Database Syst Rev*; 1:CD012093. https://doi.org/10.1002/14651858.CD012093.pub2 *Terbinafine had the best cure rate and side effect profile.*

Gil, M.F.C. 2022. Onychomycosis: a review of current pharmacological and non-pharmacological treatment options. https://repositorio-aberto.up.pt/bitstream/10216/143779/2/576824.pdf *Developments in modern technology may have a lot to offer in the treatment of onychomycosis, but currently evidence is lacking.*

LactMed. 2018. Terbinafine. www.ncbi.nlm.nih.gov/books/NBK501397 *Topical terbinafine has not been studied during breastfeeding. Because only about 1% is absorbed after topical application, it is considered a low risk to the nursing infant. Avoid application to the nipple area and ensure that the infant's skin does not come into direct contact with the areas of skin that have been treated. Only water-miscible cream, gel or liquid products should be applied to the breast because ointments may expose the infant to high levels of mineral paraffins via licking.*

NHS England. 2018. Conditions for which over the counter items should not routinely be prescribed in primary care: guidance for CCGs. www.england.nhs.uk/publication/conditions-for-which-over-the-counter-items-should-not-routinely-be-prescribed-in-primary-care-guidance-for-ccgs/

Pan, M., Heinecke, G., Bernardo, S., et al. 2013. Urea: a comprehensive review of the clinical literature. *Dermatol Online J*; 19(11). https://doi.org/10.5070/D31911020392 *Combination therapies consisting of urea with a variety of antifungal agents have been found to partially cure onychomycosis in some patients. By softening the nail bed, urea facilitates greater penetration of antifungal medicines.*

Public Health England. 2017. Fungal skin and nail infections: diagnosis and laboratory investigation. https://assets.publishing. service.gov.uk/government/uploads/system/uploads/attachment_data/file/619770/Fungal_skin_and_nail_infections_guidance.pdf

NAPPY RASH

Acute inflammation of the skin in the nappy area, which affects up to 25% of nappy-wearing infants at any given time. It is typically caused by contact with irritants (urine and faeces) or by fungal infection (generally *Candida*). Secondary bacterial infection is rare but serious.

History

- Duration
- Type of nappy, changing routine, cleansers used
- Distress on changing nappy
- Itching
- Creams already tried
- Other areas affected (makes nappy rash unlikely)
- Recent broad-spectrum antibiotic use, including by breastfeeding mother (may predispose to *Candida* infection)
- 🚩 Fever
- 🚩 Reduced oral intake

Examination

- Well-defined red and shiny or scaly areas
- Check for satellite spots (sharply marginated bright red patches or plaques around the perianal skin suggestive of *Candida*). Look for oral thrush, which often co-exists (and treat if found – see Chapter 5)
- Sparing of the skin folds suggests an irritant cause, whereas skin-fold involvement suggests *Candida*
- 🚩 Inflammation around the anus suggests streptococcal infection
- 🚩 If systemically unwell, suspect secondary bacterial infection and check temperature, heart rate, respiratory rate and CRT

Self-care

- Leave nappy off when possible
- Clean and change nappy as soon as wet or soiled. Parents on a tight budget may find it difficult to buy adequate supplies of disposable nappies
- Use high-absorbency nappies
- Use water or fragrance-free and alcohol-free baby wipes. The wipes with the fewest ingredients are least likely to be associated with nappy rash (Phipps et al., 2021)
- Dry gently after cleaning – avoid vigorous rubbing
- Bathe once daily
- Do not use soap or bath additives. Consider soap substitute, for example Hydromol Bath and Shower (OTC)
- Barrier creams should not be used routinely as they can prevent the nappy from absorbing liquid away from the skin but, if rash is present, apply one such as Metanium (OTC), Medihoney (OTC) or dexpanthenol 5% (OTC) at each nappy change. (These recommendations are based on anecdotal evidence, as there are no relevant published studies)
- *Candida* infection is common in nappy rash that has been present for >48 hours (Benitez Ojeda and Mendez, 2023). The presence of satellite spots, distress and the involvement of the skin creases make this more likely. If suspected, recommend clotrimazole 1% cream for 3 weeks and avoid barrier cream

RED FLAGS

- Secondary bacterial infection is rare (*if suspected, take swab and prescribe flucloxacillin or, if allergic to penicillin, clarithromycin*[PIQ])
- Primary streptococcal proctitis may cause severe inflammation around the anus (Gualtieri et al., 2021) (*if suspected, take swab and prescribe amoxicillin or, if allergic to penicillin, clarithromycin*[PIQ]). The differential diagnosis includes sexual abuse; *refer to experienced colleague*

References

Benitez Ojeda, A.B., and Mendez, M.D. 2023. Diaper dermatitis. *StatPearls*. www.ncbi.nlm.nih.gov/books/NBK559067/

Gualtieri, R., Bronz, G., Bianchetti, M.G., et al. 2021. Perianal streptococcal disease in childhood: systematic literature review. *Eur J Pediatr*; 180(6):1867–74. https://doi.org/10.1007/s00431-021-03965-9 *Perianitis is an infection with a distinctive presentation and a rather long time to diagnosis. There is a need for a wider awareness of this condition among healthcare professionals.*

Phipps, F.M., Price, A.D., Ackers-Johnson, J., et al. 2021. 698 mothers and babies, 38 390 nappy changes: what did we learn? *Br J Midwifery*; 29(3):150–7. https://doi.org/10.12968/bjom.2021.29.3.150 *Wipe formulation is a significant factor in prevention or reduction of nappy rash during the first 8 weeks of life. The fewer ingredients, the better.*

Van Gysel, D., 2016. Infections and skin diseases mimicking diaper dermatitis. *Int J Dermatol*; 55:10–13. https://doi.org/10.1111/ijd.13372 *A useful overview of the differential diagnosis.*

MISCELLANEOUS

1. Eczema
2. Seborrhoeic dermatitis
3. Guttate psoriasis
4. Head lice
5. Suspected skin cancer
6. Umbilical granuloma
7. Acne

ECZEMA

This condition accounts for 30% of all skin consultations in primary care. It occurs when the lipid layer that covers the skin becomes thin, causing water loss.

- A genetically determined deficiency in filaggrin, a protein in the skin, significantly increases the risk of eczema in 'atopic families', whose members often also suffer from asthma and hay fever
- Emotional or environmental factors may trigger a flare; the role of bacterial infection in exacerbations has recently been challenged (NICE, 2021)
- It is a long-term, relapsing condition; it is important for the person/parent to appreciate this
- The term 'dermatitis' is used for eczema due to a known trigger

History

- Duration
- Previous episodes
- Suspected cause/trigger (solvents, nickel, detergents, latex)
- Distribution (usually symmetrical – flexures, face, hands)
- Itching (if absent, eczema is unlikely)
- Previous treatments and effects
- Occupation (hairdressers are at high risk)
- Fever/discharge/pain/blisters (suggest infection)

Examination

- Poorly defined inflamed scaly patches
- May be dry and cracking
- Usually symmetrical (if not, look for trigger, e.g., nickel)
- In babies, mainly on the face, or outside surface of elbows and knees. In children and adults, mainly in the flexures (inside surface of elbows and knees)
- 🚩 If possibility of infection, check temperature, heart rate, respiratory rate and BP in adults/CRT in children
- 🚩 Portal of entry for infection
- 🚩 Inflamed/weeping/blistered/signs of cellulitis

Tests

- Swab if discharging
- Scrapings for fungal testing if diagnosis in doubt, or treatment unsuccessful

Self-care

- Education is key to the management of eczema; www.eczemacareonline.org.uk is a useful resource
- Treatments can control, but not cure. In children, usually improves with time
- Avoid scratching – rub with fingertips or soft paintbrush
- Keep cool and avoid synthetic fibres
- Dietary changes and dust mite avoidance are not recommended
- Use emollients (commonly called moisturisers) three or four times daily. Most effective after a bath or shower ('soak and smear'). Stroke them on liberally, do not rub in. Emollients should be obtained OTC for mild irritant dermatitis or mild dry skin, but may be prescribed for eczema
  - Up to 600 g of emollient per week may be needed. It should still be used even when the skin has cleared
  - There is no evidence to favour one type of emollient (Ridd et al., 2022; van Zuuren et al., 2017), but people often have strong preferences. The best emollient is the one which will actually be used. Oilatum or Cetraben would be reasonable first choices – be guided by your local formulary. Do not recommend aqueous cream, which may cause skin irritation (MHRA, 2013)
  - Try small tubes first, to avoid wasteful mistakes
  - Tubes or pump dispensers are preferred to pots, to avoid contamination from fingers
  - Ointments work better than creams if greasiness is tolerated; they contain fewer additives
  - Do not routinely recommend emollients containing additives (e.g., urea, antiseptic)
  - If there is an adverse reaction to an emollient, it is likely that an additive is the cause. Swap to one which does not contain sensitisers, e.g., Diprobase Advanced Cream (see Table 8.3)
  - Emollients carry a fire risk if they are absorbed into fabrics, even if they do not contain paraffin (MHRA, 2018). If the person is at high risk (e.g., smoker), your local fire service can arrange a free 'Safe and Well' home visit
  - Many emollients may be used as soap substitutes, or these may be bought separately, for example Hydromol Bath and Shower, Oilatum Shower Gel
- Bath additives are ineffective (Santer et al., 2018)
- Avoid detergents (e.g., bubble bath – even if marketed for babies). If hands are affected, use cotton-lined rubber gloves for washing up
- If itching is troublesome, consider (OTC) fexofenadine[PBC] (120 mg daily for adults) or chlorphenamine[PBI] at night if sedation is acceptable (4 mg at bedtime, repeated after 4 hours if necessary, for adults). The benefits of antihistamines are small (Matterne et al., 2019; Tay et al., 2021)

Table 8.3 Sensitisers in emollients (cetosteryl group includes cetyl alcohol and steryl alcohol)

	Cetosteryl alcohol	Other
Aproderm colloidal oat cream	Present	
Aveeno cream	Present	Benzyl alcohol
Cetraben ointment	Present	Phenoxyethanol
Diprobase Advanced		
Doublebase gel		Triethanolamine
E45 cream	Present	Parabens, lanolin
Epimax ointment	Present	
Hydromol ointment	Present	
Oilatum cream	Present	Benzyl alcohol, sorbic acid, propylene glycol
Zerobase ointment	Present	Chlorocresol

Action

- If not responding, reconsider diagnosis (may be fungal) and also consider a reaction to sensitiser in emollient. See Box 8.5 for further management
- Flares of eczema may cause crusting and weeping; this does not usually indicate bacterial infection and evidence does not support the use of an antibiotic unless the person is systemically unwell (NICE, 2021)

Prescription

Skn

> **BOX 8.5 TREATING FLARES OF ECZEMA**
>
> - If systemically unwell, see Red Flags box below
> - Use a topical steroid ointment (e.g., Eumovate or hydrocortisone 1%) once daily until 48 hours after the redness has settled. It may be applied to broken skin
> - Fingertip units are a useful measure (McKechnie, 2023)
> - Topical steroids **stronger than hydrocortisone** may cause atrophy and thinning of the skin after prolonged use. Tiny blood vessels become visible, for which no treatment is available. The skin of the face is the most sensitive, the palms and soles least sensitive. Children's skin is more sensitive than adults' – seek advice before using any stronger steroid than hydrocortisone 1% in children or on the face (see Table 8.4)
> - Topical steroids can be used in pregnancy and breastfeeding, but aim to use the lowest-potency steroid to the smallest area of skin necessary. If breastfeeding, either avoid application to the nipple area or clean thoroughly before putting baby to the breast. Only water-miscible cream should be applied to the breast because ointments may expose the infant to high levels of mineral paraffins via licking (Noti et al., 2003; LactMed, 2021)
> - 1% hydrocortisone cream and ointment may be bought OTC (for considerably less than the prescription charge), but the packs carry warnings not to use the product if pregnant, for children aged <10 years, or on the face or genital area, and the pharmacist is not allowed to sell them for these purposes. If the person has been assessed by a clinician and a prescription issued, these warnings no longer apply, but the pharmacist is still technically not permitted to sell the cream OTC
> - Arrange a review appointment to step down steroid treatment. Consider maintenance therapy of using steroid only at weekends, to reduce likelihood of further flares (Lax et al., 2022)

- For mild infection, prescribe topical sodium fusidate 2% (three times daily for 7 days)
- For more severe infection, or if at high risk of severe illness, prescribe oral flucloxacillin for 5–7 days (250–500 mg four times daily for adults) or, if allergic to penicillin, clarithromycin[PIQ] for 5–7 days (250–500 mg twice daily for adults)

Table 8.4 Topical preparations for eczema

Preparation	Steroid potency
Emollients	Zero
Hydrocortisone 1%	Low
Eumovate	Moderate
Betnovate	High

RED FLAGS

- Bacterial infection of eczema (*difficult to diagnose with certainty, but requires prompt antibiotic treatment if the person is systemically unwell*)
- Eczema herpeticum is a rare but life-threatening herpes virus infection. It usually affects the head and neck area of a child with eczema and presents with areas of rapidly worsening, painful eczema with clustered vesicles and small, uniform, punched-out erosions. The child may be feverish and distressed (*admit urgently under Paediatrics*)

References

Axon, E., Chalmers, J.R., Santer, M., et al. 2021. Safety of topical corticosteroids in atopic eczema: an umbrella review. *BMJ Open*; 11(7):e046476. http://dx.doi.org/10.1136/bmjopen-2020-046476 *There was no evidence of harm when topical steroids were used intermittently 'as required' to treat flares or 'weekend therapy' to prevent flares. However, long-term safety data were limited.*

Cardona, I.D., Stillman, L., and Jain, N. 2016. Does bathing frequency matter in pediatric atopic dermatitis? *Ann Allergy Asthma Immunol*; 117(1):9–13. https://doi.org/10.1016/j.anai.2016.05.014 *No strong evidence, but daily bathing is probably best, if used with 'soak and smear' emollients.*

LactMed. 2021. Mineral oil. www.ncbi.nlm.nih.gov/books/NBK501885 *Mineral oil paraffins (e.g.,Vaseline) are not metabolised by the body; they accumulate in body fat. The consequences are unclear, but it seems wise to limit a baby's exposure.*

Lax, S.J., Harvey, J., Axon, E., et al. 2022. Strategies for using topical corticosteroids in children and adults with eczema. *Cochrane Database Syst Rev*; 3:CD013356. https://doi.org/10.1002/14651858.CD013356.pub2 *Weekend (proactive) topical steroid therapy was associated with a drop in the relapse rate from 58% to 25%.*

Li, A.W., Yin, E.S., and Antaya, R.J. 2017. Topical corticosteroid phobia in atopic dermatitis, a systematic review. *JAMA Dermatol*; 153(10):1036–42. https://doi.org/10.1001/jamadermatol.2017.2437 *Negative feelings and beliefs about topical steroids are common and lead to undertreatment.*

Matterne, U., Böhmer, M.M., Weisshaar, E., et al. 2019. Oral H1 antihistamines as 'add-on' therapy to topical treatment for eczema. *Cochrane Database Syst Rev*; 1:CD012167. https://doi.org/10.1002/14651858.CD012167.pub2 *This review found little conclusive evidence to establish the effectiveness of H1 antihistamines as add-on therapy to topical treatment for eczema.*

McKechnie, D. 2023. Fingertip units for topical steroids. https://patient.info/treatment-medication/steroids/fingertip-units-for-topical-steroids

MHRA. 2013. Aqueous cream: may cause skin irritation, particularly in children with eczema, possibly due to sodium lauryl sulfate content. *Drug Safety Update*; 6(8):A2. www.gov.uk/drug-safety-update/aqueous-cream-may-cause-skin-irritation

MHRA. 2018. Emollients: new information about risk of severe and fatal burns with paraffin-containing and paraffin-free emollients. www.gov.uk/drug-safety-update/emollients-new-information-about-risk-of-severe-and-fatal-burns-with-paraffin-containing-and-paraffin-free-emollients

NICE. 2021. NG190. Secondary bacterial infection of eczema and other common skin conditions: antimicrobial prescribing. www.nice.org.uk/guidance/ng190

NICE. 2023. CG57. Atopic eczema in under 12s: diagnosis and management. www.nice.org.uk/guidance/cg57

Noti, A., Grob, K., Biedermann, M., et al. 2003. Exposure of babies to C15–C45 mineral paraffins from human milk and breast salves. *Regul Toxicol Pharmacol*; 38(3):317–25. https://doi.org/10.1016/s0273-2300(03)00098-9 *In a worst-case situation, daily intake of mineral oil products from breast-care products by babies is estimated to reach 40 mg/kg.*

Ridd, M.J., Santer, M., MacNeill, S.J., et al. 2022. Effectiveness and safety of lotion, cream, gel, and ointment emollients for childhood eczema: a pragmatic, randomised, phase 4, superiority trial. *Lancet Child Adolesc Health*; 6(8):522–32. https://doi.org/10.1016/S2352-4642(22)00146-8 *This review found no difference in effectiveness between the four main types of emollients for childhood eczema.*

Santer, M., Ridd, M.J., Francis, N.A., et al. 2018. Emollient bath additives for the treatment of childhood eczema (BATHE): multicentre pragmatic parallel group randomised controlled trial of clinical and cost effectiveness. *BMJ*; 361:k1332. https://doi.org/10.1136/bmj.k1332 *They don't work.*

Sharma, R., Abrol, S., and Wani, M. 2017. Misuse of topical corticosteroids on facial skin. A study of 200 patients. *J Dermatol Case Rep*; 11(1):5–8. https://doi.org/10.3315/jdcr.2017.1240 *Prolonged use of topical corticosteroids on facial skin was recommended by non-professional persons. The adverse events ranged from transient to permanent.*

Tay, C.J., Zhao, X., Allen, J.C., et al. 2021. Effectiveness of antihistamines for itch and sleep disturbance in atopic dermatitis: a retrospective cohort study. *Itch*; 6(2):e47. https://doi.org/10.1097/itx.0000000000000047 *Second-generation antihistamines improved itch and sleep disturbance scores better than first-generation antihistamines.*

van Zuuren, E.J., Fedorowicz, Z., Christensen, R., et al. 2017. Emollients and moisturisers for eczema. *Cochrane Database Syst Rev*; 2:CD012119. https://doi.org/10.1002/14651858.CD012119.pub2 *No clear evidence to favour any type of emollient.*

SEBORRHOEIC DERMATITIS

This is a type of skin inflammation in areas with many sebaceous glands. It occurs in babies aged 2 weeks to 6 months and in older children and adults. It is affected by hormone balance and stress, but the yeast *Malassezia* is also implicated.

History

- Duration
- Areas affected:
  - In older children and adults, it typically affects the scalp (dandruff is the non-inflamed form), nasolabial folds, ears, eyebrows and chest
  - In infants, it typically affects the scalp (cradle cap), face, ears, neck and nappy area
- Itch

Examination

- Red/pink patches that are scaly and flaky
- Oily, dense scaling or crusting (white or yellow)
- In darker skin, the affected areas may appear hypo- or hyper-pigmented
- Usually symmetrical

Self-care

- In babies, reassure the parent/carer that infantile seborrhoeic dermatitis is not serious, is unlikely to bother the baby and typically resolves spontaneously within a few months
- To manage cradle cap, apply warm olive oil or baby oil and keep on for several hours, then wash with a coal tar shampoo and brush gently to remove scales. If this is ineffective, consider trying clotrimazole 1% cream
- In adults and children aged ≥12 years with scalp involvement (usually presenting as dandruff), ketoconazole[c] 2% shampoo may be used (twice weekly for at least 4 weeks). Leave on for at least 5 minutes before rinsing off
- In adults, advise that it is a chronic condition and long-term maintenance treatment is needed, although some may need treatment only for flares
  - On the skin, use an azole cream, e.g., clotrimazole 1% (OTC) two to three times daily for at least 4 weeks. Antifungal shampoo (e.g., ketoconazole[c] 2%) may also be used as body wash
  - Use emollient soap substitutes, e.g., Hydromol Bath and Shower or Oilatum Shower Gel
- Given that stress may exacerbate symptoms and lead to flares, efforts to manage stress may be beneficial (although evidence is lacking)

Action

- If self-care measures have failed, review diagnosis and consider adding hydrocortisone 1% ointment

Reference

Hazell, T. 2022. Seborrhoeic dermatitis. https://patient.info/doctor/seborrhoeic-dermatitis-pro

GUTTATE PSORIASIS

Psoriasis is a common long term inflammatory condition affecting the skin, joints and nails. Most forms do not present acutely, but guttate psoriasis may mimic other acute rashes, for example pityriasis rosea (which has larger, browner patches). Guttate psoriasis usually starts in children or young adults and may develop 2–3 weeks after a streptococcal or viral infection.

- Small (<1 cm) round or oval, scaly papules that may be pink or red
- Many scattered lesions, mainly on the trunk and upper limbs
- May also occur on the face, ears and scalp
- Usually resolves spontaneously, but may take 3–4 months
- Emollients and topical steroids may improve itching
- Antibiotic treatment is of no benefit

Reference

NICE CKS. 2022. Guttate psoriasis. https://cks.nice.org.uk/topics/psoriasis/management/guttate-psoriasis/

HEAD LICE

Common in children, this infestation requires head-to-head contact for transmission.

History

- Nits (hatched egg cases)
- Lice seen
- Scratching
- Outbreaks at schools/institutions

Examination

- Examine head for nits and live lice using a detection plastic comb, for example Bug Buster
- Louse eggs adhere to hair tightly, whereas dandruff falls off easily
- Look for enlarged occipital lymph nodes

Self-care

- Check all of household and treat only those in whom live lice have been found
- Wet combing with conditioner is the best method of checking because it immobilises the lice
- Use one of the following methods (all should be obtained OTC):
  - First line: dimeticone lotion – best evidence of effectiveness, and resistance is unlikely because of its mode of action (it is a silicone-based lubricant that physically blocks the excretory system of lice); apply once weekly for two doses, rub into dry hair and scalp, allow to dry naturally, shampoo after minimum 8 hours or overnight. Caution: flammable
  - Wet combing using the Bug Buster comb weekly
  - Malathion[B] 0.5% aqueous liquid (apply once weekly for two doses, rub into dry hair and scalp, allow to dry naturally, shampoo after minimum 12 hours)
- Reassure that head lice are not associated with poor hygiene
- Warn that nits (eggs) may still be visible after treatment
- Advise that there is no need to wash clothing and bedding at high temperature

Reference

NICE CKS. 2021. Head lice. https://cks.nice.org.uk/topics/head-lice/

SUSPECTED SKIN CANCER

Most moles develop in early childhood and adolescence, and there is a gradual decrease in their number in old age. Not unreasonably, malignant melanoma is a concern behind many consultations, for which most people need reassurance. Many lesions which people call moles are, in fact, seborrhoeic keratoses that are superficial (appearing stuck-on), golden brown in colour with a scaly, greasy surface. They are harmless and, in contrast with true moles, are much more common in the elderly.

Not all skin cancers are pigmented. Basal cell carcinomas (rodent ulcers) are pearly lesions most commonly found on the face, whereas squamous cell carcinomas are usually raised and crusted and are typically found on the head, neck or hand of someone with immunosuppression.

History

- What is worrying them?
- Duration
- Itch/change in sensation
- Inflammation/oozing
- Family history
- History of significant sun exposure/use of sun beds
- ⚑ Enlarging/changing shape/changing colour/new mole (70% of melanomas arise in a new mole)
- ⚑ Scabbing over but not healing
- ⚑ Immunosuppressed (*increased risk of squamous cell carcinoma*)
- ⚑ Pigmented lesion under a nail without history of trauma (see Red Flags box below)

> **⚑ RED FLAGS**
>
> Melanoma under the nail (*USC referral to Dermatology*) may present with:
>
> - Spreading brown or black streaks in the nail without any known injury
> - Bruise on the nail that does not heal or move up as the nail grows
> - Nails that thin, crack, distort or separate from the nail bed
> - Darkening skin next to the nail
> - A nail that bleeds or develops a nodule

Examination

- Colour
- Diameter
- ⚑ Feel for induration (hardness)
- ⚑ Ulceration
- ⚑ Rolled edge may suggest basal cell carcinoma
- ⚑ Small visible blood vessels on surface (easily seen with illuminated magnification) – associated with basal cell carcinoma
- ⚑ Scaling/crusting with red base – suspicious of squamous cell carcinoma
- ⚑ Major features of mole (two points each – see Red Flags box below for interpretation):
  - Change in size
  - Irregular shape
  - Irregular colour
- ⚑ Minor features of mole (one point each – see Red Flags box below for interpretation):
  - Largest diameter ≥7 mm
  - Inflammation
  - Oozing
  - Change in sensation

Self-care

- Advise the person to watch the area, ideally measure or photograph it with a ruler adjacent, and seek help if they notice any of the following (ABCDE):
  - Asymmetrical
  - Border irregular
  - Colours (more than one)
  - Diameter (enlarging)
  - Elevated

RED FLAGS

- Pigmented lesion scoring ≥3 points (*USC referral to Dermatology*)
- New lesion in someone with immunosuppression (*USC referral to Dermatology*)
- Suspected squamous cell carcinoma (*USC referral to Dermatology*)
- Pigmented lesion under a nail (*USC referral to Dermatology*)
- Suspected basal cell carcinoma (*routine referral to Dermatology unless particular concern*)

References

NICE. 2021. NG12. Suspected cancer: recognition and referral. www.nice.org.uk/guidance/ng12/chapter/Recommendations-organised-by-site-of-cancer#skin-cancers

Seebacher, N. A. 2022. Melanoma of the nail unit. https://dermnetnz.org/topics/melanoma-of-the-nail-unit

UMBILICAL GRANULOMA

This common cherry-like swelling on a newborn baby's umbilical stump was previously treated with topical silver nitrate. Concerns about chemical burns with this treatment have led to trials using home treatment with salt:

- Apply enough table salt to cover the granuloma surface
- Cover the area with a gauze swab and keep it in place for 10–30 minutes
- Clean the site using a clean gauze swab soaked in warm water
- Repeat the procedure twice a day for 5 days

References

Al Saleh, A. 2016. Therapeutic effect of common salt on umbilical granuloma in infants. *Int J Med Sci Public Health*; 5(5): 911–15. www.ejmanager.com/mnstemps/67/67-1452639453.pdf.

Institute of Health Visiting. 2022. Understanding umbilical granuloma. https://ihv.org.uk/for-health-visitors/resources-for-members/resource/ihv-tips-for-parents/transition-to-parenthood-and-the-early-weeks/umbilical-granuloma/

ACNE VULGARIS

This is one of the commonest skin conditions in the UK, affecting up to 95% of adolescents. It commonly causes psychological distress and may persist into adult life. The causes are not well understood. Three factors seem to play a part: plugs in the hair follicles (comedones), increased sebum production and a change in the bacterial flora. It may be worsened by hormone changes, e.g., puberty, the menstrual cycle, polycystic ovarian syndrome (PCOS) and the use of anabolic steroids.

History

- Distribution
- Previous treatments and results
- Is it leaving scarring?
- Psychological impact
- Taking an oral contraceptive?
- Pregnant, or planning a pregnancy?

Examination

- Mild acne: blackheads (open comedones) and whiteheads (closed comedones)
- Moderate acne: inflamed papules and pustules
- Severe acne: pustules, nodules, scarring and pigmentation

Self-care

- There are many myths about acne – it is not infectious and there is no evidence that acne is caused by poor hygiene or by eating too much chocolate, although there is observational evidence that foods which cause significant rises in blood glucose may be linked to its development
- Treatment does not heal existing lesions but prevents new ones, so it may take at least 12 weeks to be visibly effective
- Wash no more than twice daily with lukewarm water using 'non-comedogenic' synthetic detergents with a pH similar to the skin (e.g., Sebamed, CeraVe). Soap is too alkaline
- Do not scrub or pick at the skin
- Avoid cosmetics as much as possible, and remove them completely at night
- If skin is dry, use a water-based emollient (i.e., a cream or lotion rather than an ointment)
- Mild acne should first be treated with OTC preparations, unless there are exceptional circumstances
- Treat the whole spot-bearing area, not just the spots
- Benzoyl peroxide[CB] (Acnecide) is the OTC treatment with the best evidence of effectiveness. Unfortunately, only 5% strength is currently available, which some people find too irritating. If this is the case, advise to leave on for 30–60 minutes before washing off, then gradually increase the duration of treatment as tolerated
- The British Association of Dermatologists' website (www.acnesupport.org.uk) gives very useful information

Prescription

Many different options are available on prescription (see NICE NG198 for more details); the chosen strategy should be tried for **at least 12 weeks** before reassessment. Dual therapy should **always** be used, with either a combination of two topical treatments or topical plus oral therapy.

Refer people with severe acne to Dermatology – and while waiting, initiate treatment as for Moderate acne below.

Mild acne
Offer a 12-week course of one of these options:

- Adapalene/benzoyl peroxide (Epiduo[PBC]) (women should use effective contraception)
- Tretinoin/clindamycin (Treclin[PBC]) (women should use effective contraception)
- Benzoyl peroxide/clindamycin (Duac[PBC])

Moderate acne
Offer a 12-week course of one of these options:

- Oral doxycycline[PBC] *or* lymecycline[PBC]

  plus

- Epiduo[PBC] (women should use effective contraception) *or* azelaic acid (Skinoren[PBC])
- There is insufficient evidence to support any one tetracycline over another, but minocycline[PBC] is best avoided because of its higher risk of adverse reactions. **Tetracyclines cannot be used in pregnancy**, and any woman of reproductive age requires effective contraception if using this treatment
- For all acne prescriptions except benzoyl peroxide/cllindamycin, advise protecting skin from UV light
- Do not recommend monotherapy with an oral antibiotic, or a combination of a topical antibiotic and an oral antibiotic
- For women, a combined oral contraceptive (COC) pill could also be considered as an alternative to an oral antibiotic. This should only be prescribed by an appropriate clinician

- The Primary Care Dermatology Society (PCDS) suggests using COCs with a lower oestrogen content such as Eloine or Mercilon as first line (due to a better safety profile than co-cyprindiol)
- If those COCs are not effective, co-cyprindiol[PBC] may be used. It is licensed for moderate to severe acne not responding to topical treatment or oral antibiotics and may be particularly suitable for women with PCOS. It carries a higher venous thromboembolism (VTE) risk than standard COCs (at least double) and should be stopped once the acne has been clear for 3–4 months

Directions and doses for adults

- Apply all topical treatments after washing
  - Apply benzoyl peroxide[CB] once or twice daily
  - Apply adapalene[PBC] thinly in the evening
  - Apply azelaic acid[PBC] twice daily
  - Apply Epiduo[PBC] thinly in the evening
- Doxycycline[PBC], 100 mg once daily
- Lymecycline[PBC], 408 mg twice daily

References

Hastuti, R., Mustifah, E.F., Ulya, I., et al. 2019. The effect of face washing frequency on acne vulgaris patients. *J Gen Proced Dermatol Venereol Indones*; 3(2):35–40. https://doi.org/10.19100/jdvi.v3i2.105 *People with acne can be advised to wash their faces once a day. Three times is too often.*

Meixiong, J., Ricco, C., Vasavda, C., et al. 2022. Diet and acne: a systematic review. *JAAD Int*; 7:95–112. https://doi.org/10.1016/j.jdin.2022.02.012 *High glycaemic index, increased glycaemic load, and carbohydrate intake may cause a modest yet significant increase in acne.*

NICE. 2023. NG198. Acne vulgaris: management. www.nice.org.uk/guidance/ng198

Primary Care Dermatology Society. 2023. Acne: acne vulgaris. www.pcds.org.uk/clinical-guidance/acne-vulgaris#management

Scott, A.M., Stehlik, P., Clark, J., et al. 2019. Blue-light therapy for acne vulgaris: a systematic review and meta-analysis. *Ann Fam Med*; 17(6):545–53. https://doi.org/10.1370/afm.2445 *More research is needed.*

Walsh, T.R., Efthimiou, J., and Dréno, B. 2016. Systematic review of antibiotic resistance in acne: an increasing topical and oral threat. *Lancet Infect Dis*; 16(3):e23–e33 https://doi.org/10.1016/S1473-3099(15)00527-7 *The benefit-to-risk ratio of long-term antibiotic use should be carefully considered and, in particular, single antibiotic use should be avoided when possible.*

CHAPTER 9

Abdomen

Many conditions can present with abdominal pain. Some of these are more serious than others; taking a good history, performing a clinical examination and proactively identifying red flags are essential for picking out those requiring prompt management or further assessment. The cause of the pain may not always be initially apparent; if there are no immediate concerns, safety-netting is key.

ABDOMINAL PAIN

History

- Site and radiation
- Duration
- Intermittent/continuous
- Character: stabbing/dull/cramping
- Previous episodes (diagnosis and outcome)
- Previous abdominal surgery
- Vaginal discharge or bleeding
- Medication (*many drugs can cause abdominal pain side effects such as diarrhoea, vomiting, urinary retention*)
- Associated features:
  - Fever
  - Constipation/diarrhoea/bloating
  - Vomiting/nausea/loss of appetite
  - Dysuria/frequency/urgency
  - Upper respiratory tract infection in children (*may cause abdominal pain due to enlarged lymph nodes*)
- OTC preparations tried
- 🚩 Possibility of pregnancy (*may be ectopic*)
- 🚩 Vaginal discharge or bleeding (*possible ectopic pregnancy or pelvic inflammatory disease [PID]*)
- 🚩 Pain worse with coughing (*suggestive of peritonitis [indicating serious infection in abdomen, e.g., appendicitis]*)
- 🚩 Type 1 diabetes with recent missed insulin doses and/or high blood glucose (*possible diabetic ketoacidosis*)
- 🚩 Type 2 diabetes and taking an SGLT2 inhibitor (e.g., dapagliflozin) (*possible ketoacidosis*)
- 🚩 Recent increased thirst/urination (*suggestive of new-onset diabetes*)
- 🚩 Unintentional weight loss (*various possible causes including inflammatory bowel disease [IBD] and bowel cancer*)
- 🚩 Pain or swelling in testicles or groin (*possible torsion, infection or hernia*)
- 🚩 Rectal bleeding (*possible IBD or bowel cancer*)

Examination

- Temperature
- Heart rate and respiratory rate
- CRT in children aged <12 years/BP in adults and older children
- Examine abdomen:
  - Record site of any pain. Is there tenderness or guarding?
  - Check for masses (especially palpable bladder) or distension
  - Check groins for any swellings (such as hernias/lymph nodes)
  - Check loins for tenderness (suggestive of kidney inflammation)
- In children, examine throat (streptococcal and viral throat infections can cause abdominal pain)

Tests

- Consider testing urine with multi-reagent dipstick (most will include tests for nitrites, leucocytes, blood, protein, glucose and ketones; to avoid contaminating the whole sample, pour a little urine on the test strip)

  - Nitrites (in particular), leucocytes, blood and protein may indicate infection (but there are exceptions; see later section on Cystitis [Lower Urinary Tract Infection])

  - Blood, without other indicators of infection, may be due to menstruation, kidney stones or many other possible diagnoses

  - Ketones may be due to fasting. However, in someone with known diabetes or symptoms of diabetes, they raise suspicion of diabetic ketoacidosis (>2+ on dipstick is highly suggestive; if present, check capillary blood ketones)

- If period is due or late, check pregnancy test

- Consider sending midstream urine (MSU) for culture if urinary tract infection (UTI) suspected (unless uncomplicated cystitis)

- Consider sending stool sample if food poisoning suspected or otherwise indicated (see later section on Diarrhoea and Vomiting)

- Test immediate fingerprick glucose if known diabetes or new-onset diabetes suspected (a result of >11 mmol/l indicates that diabetes is likely)

RED FLAGS

- If unable to make a firm diagnosis of dyspepsia, UTI or gastroenteritis (*many possible causes; refer to experienced colleague*)
- Positive pregnancy test (*ectopic pregnancy may cause severe lower abdominal pain, usually one-sided, in a woman whose period is late or just due. She may not have vaginal bleeding. Send urgently to hospital with referral to Gynaecology*)
- Severe pain causing difficulty climbing on to examination couch, or exacerbated by coughing (*suggests peritonitis [inflammation of the inner lining of the abdomen, usually due to a serious infection, e.g., appendicitis]; admit urgently under Surgical*)
- Guarding/rigid abdomen (*suggests peritonitis; admit urgently under Surgical*)
- Enlarged bladder with inability to pass urine despite strong urge (*acute urinary retention; inform Urology and send urgently to A&E for catheterisation*)
- Pain or swelling in testicles or groin (*possible torsion, infection or hernia; send urgently to hospital with referral to appropriate specialty*)
- Arrange urgent investigations including blood tests and faecal immunochemical test (FIT) with view to USC referral for possible bowel cancer if persistent abdominal pain and any of:
  - Age ≥50
  - Age ≥40 with unexplained weight loss
  - Abdominal mass
  - Rectal bleeding
  - Change in bowel habit
- Possible new-onset diabetes/type 1 diabetes (particularly if recent missed insulin doses)/type 2 diabetes on an SGLT2 inhibitor, with any of: vomiting, diarrhoea, lethargy, confusion, fruity-smelling breath, deep breathing or dehydration (*check fingerprick blood glucose [may be normal if type 2 diabetes on an SGLT2 inhibitor] and check ketones. A blood ketone level >3 mmol/l strongly suggests diabetic ketoacidosis. Also consider this diagnosis in anyone with type 1 diabetes who is unwell even if lower ketone level; admit urgently under Medical/Paediatrics*)

GASTROENTEROLOGY

1. Dyspepsia/indigestion
2. Diarrhoea and vomiting
3. Constipation
4. Irritable bowel syndrome

DYSPEPSIA/INDIGESTION

Over recent years, there has been increasing recognition of the complex interactions between the gut and brain and the problems linked with dysfunction of these pathways. A key example is functional dyspepsia, which is now thought to be the predominant cause of dyspepsia symptoms and estimated to affect 7% of the population.

According to the British Society of Gastroenterology (Black et al., 2022), the diagnosis of functional dyspepsia can be made if there is an 8-week history of one or more of the following: fullness after eating, early satiation (fullness while eating) or epigastric pain/burning, with no concerning features or evidence of other causes likely to explain the symptoms. People with functional dyspepsia may also have lower gastrointestinal (GI) symptoms (e.g., irritable bowel syndrome [IBS]).

Functional dyspepsia is not dangerous in itself but the symptoms can be long-lasting, difficult to manage and have a significant impact on quality of life. Current routine investigations, which tend to look only at the structure of the upper GI system rather than its complex interactions and functioning, are normal in this condition.

Therefore, one of the key considerations when assessing someone with symptoms of dyspepsia is whether there are any features suggesting that this is something other than functional dyspepsia – in other words, who should be investigated further? Around a quarter of people with dyspepsia have an underlying cause such as a stomach ulcer, *Helicobacter* infection, reflux, medication side effects or stomach cancer.

History

- What does the person mean by the words they use (such as heartburn, indigestion or reflux)?
- Duration
- Site of symptoms (dyspeptic symptoms are typically in the upper centre of the abdomen; pain in the right upper quadrant may suggest gallstones)
- Is it better or worse with eating?
- Feeling of fullness during or after eating (can they finish a normal-sized meal? Does it impact their plans/activities after eating?)
- Symptoms/features suggesting reflux (retrosternal pain, tasting acid in the mouth, worse when lying down, sore throat, dry cough)
- Vomiting/nausea
- Belching/bloating
- Loss of appetite
- Diet, eating habits and any trigger foods (e.g., irregular meals, large meals at night, fatty foods can cause digestive symptoms)
- Psychosocial stress
- Nicotine and alcohol consumption
- Medication history (particularly those that increase risk of GI bleed, such as non-steroidal anti-inflammatory drugs [NSAIDs; e.g., ibuprofen, naproxen], anticoagulants [e.g., warfarin, apixaban], antiplatelet drugs [e.g., aspirin, clopidogrel], selective serotonin reuptake inhibitors [SSRIs; e.g., fluoxetine, sertraline], prednisolone, spironolactone)
- Previous episodes and how these were treated
- OTC preparations tried
- 🚩 Difficulty swallowing (*possible oesophageal cancer*)
- 🚩 Worse with exercise (*may be ischaemic heart disease*)
- 🚩 Unexplained weight loss (*suggestive of cancer*)
- 🚩 Persistent change in bowel habit (*various possible causes including IBD and cancer*)
- 🚩 Vomiting of 'coffee grounds' (*suggestive of GI bleed*)
- 🚩 Dark, tarry stools (melaena) (*suggestive of GI bleed*)

Examination

- Examine abdomen
  - Confirm site of pain

- Record site of any tenderness or guarding
- Check for masses or distension
- If any suspicion of GI bleed, check heart rate and BP

Tests

- Although Public Health England has recommended a more targeted approach, the British Society of Gastroenterology recommends arranging *Helicobacter pylori* (*H. pylori*) testing in everyone with dyspeptic symptoms. Depending on your area, this may be a breath test or stool test
  - *H. pylori* testing is unreliable if they have taken a proton pump inhibitor (PPI) in the previous 2 weeks or an antibiotic in the previous 4 weeks. If taking a PPI, they will need a 2-week washout period before testing
  - H2-antihistamines (e.g., famotidine[PBCQ], nizatidine[PC]) have much less effect than PPIs on the sensitivity of breath or stool testing, and there is conflicting evidence on whether they have any effect at all. People taking a PPI can be switched to these medicines if testing for *H. pylori* is required and they cannot cope without any treatment for 2 weeks; pragmatically, many testing labs suggest that these medicines should be stopped 48 hours before the test is performed
  - Antacids can be continued (apart from preparations containing bismuth such as Pepto-Bismol, which need to be stopped 4 weeks before testing)
- Depending on features, consider:
  - FBC (for anaemia and platelet count [raised platelet count suggests investigation for possible cancer is needed; low platelet count predisposes to bleeding])
  - Ferritin (for iron-deficiency anaemia – which is typically related to bleeding)
  - Liver function tests (LFTs) (if gallstones or liver issue possible)
  - IgA-TTG (for coeliac disease – note that this is valid only if there has been gluten in the diet for the 6 weeks prior to the test)
- If the symptoms are suggestive of gallstones rather than dyspepsia (pain after eating in right upper quadrant of abdomen, has not responded to PPI), then request ultrasound scan of abdomen (discuss with a suitable colleague if you cannot request directly)

Self-care

- Avoid any identified triggers such as fatty foods
- Regular physical activity
- If overweight, try to manage weight
- If smoker/vaper, consider quitting or cutting down
- Reduce alcohol intake
- Stop NSAIDs, if possible
- If taking aspirin or other gastric irritant medicines, see a suitably experienced colleague to discuss alternatives
- For mild symptoms, try OTC antacids (though avoid in kidney disease); Mucogel[CI] or Gaviscon Advance[CI]
- Some PPIs can be bought OTC (though they are expensive)
- Stress management – self-referral to local NHS talking therapies service

Prescription

- If *H. pylori* is detected, then eradication treatment should be prescribed. For initial management, offer triple therapy. Doses for adults, to be taken twice daily for 1 week:
  - Omeprazole[Q] 20 mg (or lansoprazole[PBCIQ] 30 mg) *plus*
  - Amoxicillin 1 g (or metronidazole 400 mg if allergic to penicillin) *plus*
  - Clarithromycin[PIQ] 500 mg
- If symptoms recur or there is suspicion of treatment failure, *refer to an experienced colleague*
- If *H. pylori* is not detected and there are no concerning features, then diet and lifestyle changes should generally be tried first before medication

- If a prescription is necessary (perhaps because self-management has not been effective or there are exceptional circumstances), then prescribe omeprazole^Q for 1 month (20 mg daily for adults) and arrange review appointment. Do not add this to the repeat medication list; there are many problems associated with long-term PPIs
- Interestingly, PPIs (and H2-antihistamines) tend to be effective for managing functional dyspepsia as well as that driven by underlying disease. Use the lowest effective dose unless there is specific reason to do otherwise

RED FLAGS

- Epigastric/chest discomfort related to exercise (*may be ischaemic heart disease; refer to experienced colleague, may need urgent referral or, if unstable, urgent admission under Medical*)
- On anticoagulant (*at high risk of GI bleed and needs urgent investigation; refer to experienced colleague*)
- Fever and tenderness in right upper quadrant (*suspected acute cholecystitis – infection of gallbladder; admit urgently under Surgical*)
- Jaundice (*suspected biliary obstruction; admit urgently under Surgical*)
- 'Coffee-ground' or bloodstained vomit or black, tarry stools (*GI bleed; admit urgently under Medical*)
- Difficulty in swallowing (*possible oesophageal cancer; USC referral to Gastroenterology*)
- Persistent change in bowel habit (*various possible causes including IBD and cancer; refer to experienced colleague*)
- Aged ≥55 with weight loss and dyspepsia, reflux or upper abdominal pain (*possible gastric or oesophageal cancer; USC referral to Gastroenterology*)
- Aged ≥55 without weight loss but with any of the following: treatment-resistant dyspepsia, upper abdominal pain with anaemia, raised platelet count, nausea/vomiting (*need to rule out gastric or oesophageal cancer [but diagnosis less likely than for bullet point above]; direct access upper GI endoscopy or refer to experienced colleague*)

References

Black, C.J., Paine, P.A., Agrawal, A., et al. 2022. British Society of Gastroenterology guidelines on the management of functional dyspepsia. *Gut*; 71(9):1697. https://doi.org/10.1136/gutjnl-2022-327737 *Recommends testing everyone with dyspepsia symptoms for* H. pylori.

Malfertheiner, P., Megraud, F., O'Morain, C.A., et al. 2017. Management of *Helicobacter pylori* infection—the Maastricht V/Florence consensus report. *Gut*; 66(1):6–30. *Explains the evidence behind the different 'washout' periods required for different classes of acid-suppressing medication before* H. pylori *testing.*

NICE. 2023. NG12. Suspected cancer: recognition and referral. www.nice.org.uk/guidance/ng12

Public Health England. 2019. Test and treat for *Helicobacter pylori* (HP) in dyspepsia. Quick reference guide for primary care: for consultation and local adaptation. https://assets.publishing.service.gov.uk/government/uploads/system/uploads/attachment_data/file/828593/HP_Quick_Reference_Guide_v18.0_August_2019_change_highlighted.pdf

DIARRHOEA AND VOMITING

Viruses cause gastroenteritis much more often than food poisoning; rotavirus and adenovirus are common in children, norovirus in adults. Diarrhoea is the main symptom. Note that this section deals only with acute presentations (<4 weeks) and that a viral cause is much less likely in chronic presentations.

An understanding of the person's usual bowel habits is helpful. Take care to use language that the person can understand. The terms 'motions', 'stools' or 'faeces' may be unfamiliar; 'poo', however, is widely understood (Wilcox, 2019).

History

- Duration
- Severity (number of episodes in last 24 hours, stool consistency)
- Fever
- Fluid balance and urine output (frequency and volume)
- Contacts with similar symptoms, especially if they started on the same day
- Suspect foods (undercooked or out of date) and time taken before symptoms appeared
- Recent tropical travel or farm visit

Abd

- Occupation – food handler/carer/health professional
- Sorbitol/maltitol consumption (sweeteners used in diet foods and chewing gum that may cause diarrhoea)
- Reptile at home (*risk of salmonella infection*)
- Potentially causative medication, e.g., broad-spectrum antibiotics, laxatives, metformin, colchicine, orlistat
- Taking PPI (*increased risk of Clostridioides difficile [C. difficile] infection*)
- Medications that may be affected by the illness, e.g., prednisolone, warfarin, anti-epileptic drugs, ACE inhibitors, SGLT2 inhibitors, combined oral contraceptives, gastro-resistant/enteric-coated drugs
- 🚩 Preceding constipation
- 🚩 Blood (red, brown or black) in stool/vomit
- 🚩 Green vomit
- 🚩 Hospital admission in previous 8 weeks
- 🚩 Broad-spectrum antibiotics in previous 8 weeks
- 🚩 Previous bowel disease or gastric bypass
- 🚩 Immunosuppressed
- 🚩 Possibility of pregnancy

Examination

- Temperature
- Heart rate and respiratory rate
- CRT in children aged <12 years/BP in adults and older children
- Other signs of dehydration:
    - Lethargy
    - Dry tongue/mouth
    - Dry skin not reshaping after a soft pinch
    - Sunken, non-reflective eyes
    - Sunken fontanelle in children aged <2 years
- Abdominal examination, looking for rigidity or guarding
- Consider rectal examination if overflow suspected (see Red Flags box)

Test

- Arrange stool culture if motions are still liquid and any of the following apply:
    - Duration ≥7 days
    - Suspected food poisoning
    - An outbreak is suspected (e.g., petting farm, swimming pool)
    - Known contact with someone infected with *Giardia, C. difficile Escherichia coli* (*E. coli*) O157 (this is an example of Shiga toxin-producing *E. coli* [STEC]),
    - Febrile/systemically unwell
    - Blood or pus in stool
    - Immunosuppressed
    - Recent broad-spectrum antibiotic therapy (also request *C. difficile* test if not included routinely)
    - Recent hospital admission (also request *C. difficile* test if not included routinely)
    - Recent travel to tropical area (also request ova, cysts and parasites – this usually requires three samples to be sent at least 24 hours apart. The samples should **not** be refrigerated)
- Consider stool culture if any of the following apply:
    - Pregnant
    - On PPI
    - Food handler/carer/healthcare staff/in contact with vulnerable people (check with HPT)

- Advice regarding stool sampling:
  - The person should use a clingfilm-lined container and, using the 'scoop' in the specimen bottle or a disposable spoon, collect 5 ml of sample from this
  - Write name on the specimen bottle, or affix label, before giving out
  - Note that <5% of samples identify a bacterial cause
- Also check urine dipstick and MSU in children aged <5 years with persistent or recurrent diarrhoea or vomiting (see later section on Urology in this chapter)

Self-care

- If appropriate, reassure that acute diarrhoea and vomiting is rarely serious in primary care and usually has a viral cause (which generally resolves in 5–7 days)
- Dehydration is rare over 6 months of age
- Do not return to work/school/day care until free of symptoms for 48 hours
- If cryptosporidium is diagnosed, do not swim in public pools for 2 weeks
- Provide safety-netting advice, including the symptoms/signs of dehydration
- Advice regarding eating and drinking:
  - Sip extra fluids, e.g., 200 ml for each loose stool in adults
  - Avoid orange juice and fizzy drinks, but isotonic still sports drinks are a good option. Gatorade contains potassium, which replaces losses from both the gut and the kidneys (renal excretion of potassium increases after vomiting to maintain acid–base balance). Half-strength apple juice (which also contains potassium) has been shown to be preferable to oral rehydration solution (ORS) in children aged ≥2 years with mild gastroenteritis (Freedman et al., 2016)
  - Advise against replacing fluid losses with plain water or homemade recipes
  - Supplement with purchased ORS if:
    - Child <2 years, especially if <6 months or premature
    - Diarrhoea >5 times in 24 hours
    - Vomiting >2 times in 24 hours
    - Frail, malnourished or elderly
  - Fasting is not recommended. A normal diet should be resumed as soon as symptoms permit. Warn about the gastro-colic reflex of the lower gut being stimulated by food received in the stomach (often mistaken by people as food 'going straight through')
  - Babies should continue normal feeds. There is no need to restrict dairy products unless diarrhoea is prolonged and lactose intolerance is suspected (Box 9.1)
- Hygiene advice
  - Take care when washing hands after using toilet/changing nappy
  - Remember to use the clean hand (i.e., not the one which has been used for wiping) to flush the toilet and turn on the taps
  - Close the toilet lid before you flush
  - Toilet seats, handles, taps and toilet door handles should be cleaned at least daily with hot water and detergent. Also use disinfectant or bleach to clean toilets
  - Soiled clothing should be washed separately at the highest temperature it will tolerate
  - Alcohol gel is no substitute for handwashing; it does not protect against norovirus and *C. difficile*
- Self-care with OTC medication
  - Paracetamol may be taken for stomach cramps
  - Avoid NSAIDs (gut irritants)
  - Loperamide[PCQ] may be taken by adults if diarrhoea is disabling, but should not be used to drive premature resolution of symptoms to enable return to work. Avoid if there is fever, blood in the stool, *C. difficile* or severe malaise. 'The body has evolved for our survival, and not for our comfort'

- 'Probiotics probably make little or no difference to the number of people who have diarrhoea lasting 48 hours or longer, and we are uncertain whether probiotics reduce the duration of diarrhoea', concluded a recent Cochrane review regarding their use in acute infective diarrhoea (Collinson et al., 2020). However, there is evidence of benefit in antibiotic-associated diarrhoea (note that the evidence for safety in people with immunosuppression is currently unclear) (Goodman et al., 2021)

> **BOX 9.1 LACTOSE INTOLERANCE**
>
> Occasionally, after a bout of gastroenteritis, small children may develop a temporary inability to digest lactose, which may delay the resolution of their diarrhoea. If this is suspected, suggest using lactose-free milk (e.g., SMA LF) and a lactose-free diet for up to 6 weeks.

Prescription (none for most people)

- Buccal prochlorperazine[PBCQ] (adult dose: 3–6 mg up to twice daily; tablets to be placed high between upper lip and gum and left to dissolve) may be helpful to stop vomiting in adults who are at risk of dehydration or need to take essential medication, but carries the rare risk, particularly in young adults, of an oculogyric crisis
- Antibiotics should not be used unless a specific bacterial/protozoal cause has been identified through culture and a specific treatment is indicated

Action

- Advise about medication, for example loss of protection from oral contraceptive, or reduced effectiveness of critical medication (see Red Flags box)
- Consider stopping PPI, which reduces the natural defences against GI infection
- People with diabetes should be advised to follow sick-day rules (which include stopping metformin and SGLT2 inhibitors [e.g., canagliflozin, dapagliflozin] when unwell; see Box 1.2 in Chapter 1)
- If at risk of dehydration or low BP, advise temporarily stopping the DAMN drugs to reduce the risk of acute kidney injury (AKI):
  - **D**iuretic/**D**igoxin
  - **A**ngiotensin-converting enzyme (ACE) inhibitor/**A**ngiotensin receptor blocker (ARB)
  - **M**etformin/**M**ethotrexate
  - **N**SAID
- Notify HPT, and inform the person that you are doing so, if:
  - Food poisoning suspected because of history
  - Blood or pus in stool
  - Bacterial or protozoal infection confirmed by culture

RED FLAGS

- Duration ≥4 weeks (*many possible causes; refer to experienced colleague*)
- Dehydration (*admit urgently under Medical/Paediatrics*)
- Severe illness (*consider sepsis; admit urgently under Medical/Paediatrics*)
- Multimorbidity/frailty/immunosuppressed (*high risk for serious illness or unusual microbial cause; consider admitting urgently under Medical*)
- Taking an oral corticosteroid long-term (*at risk of adrenal crisis; consider IM hydrocortisone and/or admitting urgently under Medical/Paediatrics*)
- Taking other essential medication, e.g., anticonvulsants, antiplatelet agents, medication for Parkinson's disease, glucose-lowering drugs (*refer to experienced colleague*)
- Bowel disease, for example ulcerative colitis, Crohn's disease, diverticular disease (*seek urgent specialist advice, e.g., IBD nurse*)
- Green vomit (*suggests bowel obstruction; admit urgently under Surgical*)
- Significant blood loss: red or brown vomit/red or black stools (*likely GI bleed; admit urgently under Medical/Paediatrics*) (*note that a child with bloody diarrhoea after a farm visit may have a virulent form of E. coli called STEC*)
- Early pregnancy (*ectopic pregnancy may cause vomiting and diarrhoea without vaginal bleeding; send urgently to hospital with referral to Gynaecology*)
- Abdominal rigidity or guarding (*suggests peritonitis; admit urgently under Surgical*)
- Previous constipation (*possible faecal impaction and overflow; arrange rectal examination*)
- Possible new-onset diabetes/type 1 diabetes (particularly if recent missed insulin doses)/type 2 diabetes on an SGLT2 inhibitor, with any of: vomiting, diarrhoea, lethargy, confusion, fruity-smelling breath, deep breathing or dehydration (*check fingerprick blood glucose [may be normal if type 2 diabetes on an SGLT2 inhibitor] and check blood ketones. A blood ketone level >3 mmol/l strongly suggests diabetic ketoacidosis. Also consider this diagnosis in anyone with type 1 diabetes who is unwell even if lower ketone level; admit urgently under Medical/Paediatrics*)

Abd

References

Collinson, S., Deans, A., Padua-Zamora, A., et al. 2020. Probiotics for treating acute infectious diarrhoea. *Cochrane Database Syst Rev*; 12:CD003048. https://doi.org/10.1002/14651858.CD003048.pub4

Freedman, S.B., Willan, A.R., Boutis, K., et al. 2016. Effect of dilute apple juice and preferred fluids vs electrolyte maintenance solution on treatment failure among children with mild gastroenteritis: a randomized clinical trial. *JAMA*; 315(18):1966–74. https://doi.org/10.1001/jama.2016.5352

Goodman, C., Keating, G., Georgousopoulou, E., et al. 2021. Probiotics for the prevention of antibiotic-associated diarrhoea: a systematic review and meta-analysis. *BMJ Open*; 11(8):e043054. https://doi.org/10.1136/bmjopen-2020-043054 *This meta-analysis found that co-administration of probiotics (*Lactobacillus *and* Bifidobacterium *species) with antibiotics reduced the risk of antibiotic-associated diarrhoea by 37%.*

Masukume, G. 2011. Nausea, vomiting, and deaths from ectopic pregnancy. *BMJ*; 343:d4389. https://doi.org/10.1136/bmj.d4389 *More than a third of women who died because of ectopic pregnancy in the United Kingdom between 1997 and 2011 had nausea, vomiting and diarrhoea, but no vaginal bleeding.*

NICE. 2009. CG84. Diarrhoea and vomiting caused by gastroenteritis in under 5s: diagnosis and management. www.nice.org.uk/guidance/CG84

Public Health England. 2020. UK standards for microbiology investigations; gastroenteritis and diarrhoea. https://assets.publishing.service.gov.uk/government/uploads/system/uploads/attachment_data/file/930517/S_7i2_FINAL-UKSMI.pdf *Stool sampling recommendations.*

Think Kidneys. 2018. Primary care. www.thinkkidneys.nhs.uk/aki/resources/primary-care/ *Advice on avoiding and managing acute kidney injury*

Wilcox, S. 2019. Pee and poo and the language of health. https://digital.nhs.uk/blog/transformation-blog/2019/pee-and-poo-and-the-language-of-health

CONSTIPATION

Though this has been defined by NICE as 'defecation that is unsatisfactory because of infrequent stools (fewer than three times a week), difficult stool passage or seeming incomplete', it is arguably better to define constipation as a change from a person's usual bowel pattern towards less frequent stools.

History

- Duration; is it habitual?
- How often bowels opened
- Consistency of motion
- Difficulty passing stools/straining
- Abdominal pain
- Fluid intake
- Physical activity levels
- Symptoms of hypothyroidism, e.g., fatigue, cold intolerance, weight gain (if so, arrange thyroid function tests)
- Potentially causative medication (e.g., opioids, iron, PPIs, medicines with anticholinergic effects [e.g., oxybutynin, chlorphenamine, amitriptyline])
- 🏴 Vomiting
- 🏴 Previous abdominal surgery
- 🏴 Blood in stool, on toilet paper or in toilet pan
- 🏴 Unintentional weight loss

Examination

- Check abdomen for tenderness and masses
- Consider arranging rectal examination if unclear whether the person has faecal impaction/loading

Self-care

- Stop any constipating medicine, if possible
- Adequate fluid intake (for an adult, 1.5 to 2 litres per day, including food)
- Recommend regular physical activity, particularly if they are generally sedentary
- Consider resting feet on a step while sitting on the toilet, and leaning forward with elbows on knees to relax the puborectalis muscle (Modi et al., 2019)
- Increase intake of whole grains, apples, apricots, prunes and dried fruit. Dried fruits are high in sorbitol, a natural laxative
- Try Beverley–Travis natural laxative mixture: take 1 cup each of raisins, pitted prunes, prune concentrate, dried figs, dates and currants. Combine contents together in grinder or blender to a thickened consistency. Store in fridge. Dose: 2 tablespoons twice a day. Increase or decrease dose according to consistency and frequency of bowel movements

Laxatives

- In children, do not use dietary measures alone. Prescribe macrogol[CP] (*the BNFC lists limitations of the licensing for children of various ages*). See NICE guideline CG99 (2017) for more information
- In adults, short-term, infrequent constipation caused by changes in lifestyle or diet should generally be managed through self-care and OTC laxatives if necessary
- Bulk-forming laxatives such as ispaghula husk are first-line treatment for adults (one sachet twice daily; dose to be given in water, preferably after meals, morning and evening but avoid taking just before sleeping), except for constipation caused by opioids (see below). An adequate fluid intake is important
- If it does not respond adequately, prescribe macrogol[CP] (adult dose: one to three sachets daily in divided doses, usually for up to 2 weeks; maintenance therapy dose is one or two sachets daily)
- If stools are soft but still difficult to pass, add a stimulant laxative such as senna[C] (adult dose: 7.5–15 mg at bedtime, increased if necessary up to 30 mg) or bisacodyl[C] (adult dose: 5–10 mg at night, increased if necessary up to 20 mg)
- Treatment may need to continue for several weeks and should be accompanied by adequate fluid intake for optimal effectiveness

- Adults with faecal loading need high-dose oral macrogol[CP] (initially four sachets on first day, then increased in steps of two sachets daily; total daily dose to be drunk within a 6-hour period. After disimpaction, switch to maintenance laxative therapy if required; maximum eight sachets per day) or, for faster resolution, glycerol suppositories (4 g for adults) or an enema

- For opioid-induced constipation, use docusate orally (adult dose: up to 500 mg daily in divided doses, adjusted according to response) with a stimulant laxative such as senna[C] (adult dose: 7.5–15 mg at bedtime, increased if necessary up to 30 mg)

RED FLAGS

- Severe constipation associated with vomiting, distension and/or previous abdominal surgery (*possible bowel obstruction; admit urgently under Surgical*)
- Symptoms from first few weeks of life in a child (*possible Hirschsprung's disease; refer urgently to Paediatrics*)
- Rectal/anal mass (other than faeces) or ulceration (*possible rectal cancer; USC referral to lower GI*)
- *Arrange FIT to inform referral pathway* (i.e., whether USC referral needed) if:
  - Unexplained change in bowel habit
  - Mass in abdomen other than a loaded descending colon
  - Age <50 with rectal bleeding **and** either unexplained weight loss or abdominal pain
  - Age ≥50 with rectal bleeding **or** unexplained weight loss or abdominal pain
  - Iron-deficiency anaemia, or anaemia even without iron deficiency if age ≥60

References

Ghossein, N., Kang, M., and Lakhkar, A.D. 2022. Anticholinergic medications. *StatPearls*. StatPearls Publishing. www.ncbi.nlm.nih.gov/books/NBK555893/

Hale, E.M., Smith, E., St James, J., et al. 2007. Pilot study of the feasibility and effectiveness of a natural laxative mixture. *Geriatr Nurs*; 28(2):104–11. *Evidence for the Beverley–Travis mixture.*

Modi, R.M., Hinton, A., Pinkhas, D., et al. 2019. Implementation of a defecation posture modification device. *J Clin Gastroenterol*; 53(3):216–9. https://doi.org/10.1097/MCG.0000000000001143

Müller-Lissner, S., Bassotti, G., Coffin, B., et al. 2017. Opioid-induced constipation and bowel dysfunction: a clinical guideline. *Pain Med*; 18(10):1837–63. https://doi.org/10.1093/pm/pnw255

NICE. 2023. DG56. Quantitative faecal immunochemical testing to guide colorectal cancer pathway referral in primary care. www.nice.org.uk/guidance/dg56

NICE. 2017. CG99. Constipation in children and young people: diagnosis and management. www.nice.org.uk/guidance/cg99

NICE. 2023. NG12. Suspected cancer: recognition and referral. www.nice.org.uk/guidance/ng12

NICE CKS. 2023. Constipation. https://cks.nice.org.uk/topics/constipation/

IRRITABLE BOWEL SYNDROME

You may see people with seemingly acute constipation or, more commonly, diarrhoea where the symptoms appear to have a trigger. This may be a period of psychosocial stress (e.g., examinations), certain foods (often expressed as a concern about 'gluten allergy') or related to the menstrual cycle. On further exploration, the pattern of symptoms in response to the identified trigger(s) may go back several years. This is very likely to be due to irritable bowel syndrome (IBS).

IBS is extremely common and thought to affect around 10%–20% of the population. It is a functional disorder: the bowel itself appears normal; instead, interactions between the gut and brain are implicated. Symptoms include passing mucus, bloating, altered stool passage (e.g., urgency) and abdominal pain which tends to be relieved by passing a stool. Diarrhoea or constipation, or a mixture, can predominate and the aforementioned triggers are common. It is important to appropriately reassure that, in IBS, sensitivities to particular foods are not allergies. Tests for food allergies (including IgG blood tests) are widely offered outside the NHS but are illogical and not evidence-based. The presence of IgG simply shows that you have been exposed to a particular food (Farooque, 2022).

Features which suggest that IBS is unlikely and/or investigation is warranted (*refer to experienced colleague*) include:

- Unintentional weight loss

- Blood in stool

⚑ Rectal bleeding

⚑ Severe abdominal pain

⚑ Family history of bowel cancer

Management of IBS includes:

- Support with stress management (if appropriate, advise to self-refer to NHS talking therapies)
- Trial of a low FODMAP diet – a video is available online at https://patientwebinars.co.uk/condition/ibs/webinars/webinar-2-the-low-fodmap-diet and an app to guide food choices is available at www.monashfodmap.com/ibs-central/i-have-ibs/get-the-app
- Peppermint oil (which can be prescribed); this tends to be more effective than antispasmodics such as mebeverine, although both may be worth trying

If there is any doubt about the diagnosis or there is a poor response to treatment, *refer to an experienced colleague or seek specialist advice.* Bile acid malabsorption may be the cause of diarrhoea in 1 in 3 people misdiagnosed as having IBS. It is unlikely to respond to usual IBS treatment but can be treated with a low fat diet and/or medication to bind bile acid.

References

Farooque, S. 2022. *Understanding Allergy.* Penguin Life. ISBN: 978-0-241-52788-7

NICE. 2017. CG61. Irritable bowel syndrome in adults: diagnosis and management. www.nice.org.uk/guidance/CG61

Vincent, P. 2023. Bile acid diarrhoea. https://patient.info/digestive-health/irritable-bowel-syndrome-leaflet/bile-acid-diarrhoea

ANAL PROBLEMS

1. Haemorrhoids ('piles')
2. Thrombosed external pile
3. Anal fissure

History

- Bleeding on defaecation:
  - How much blood and where is it seen (e.g., in toilet pan/on paper only)?
  - Bright red (*suggests bleeding near the rectum*) or dark red (*suggests bleeding deeper in large bowel*)
- Pain on defaecation (*suggests anal fissure, or possibly threadworms in children*)
- Itch (*suspect threadworms in children; see next section*)
- Swelling near anus/swelling appearing on straining (may be felt when wiping)
- Background of constipation
- Treatments tried already

⚑ Change in bowel habit

⚑ Unintentional weight loss

⚑ Family history of lower GI cancer

⚑ Abdominal pain

Examination (may be normal if haemorrhoids are internal)

- Any visible swelling on the perianal skin (thrombosed external piles) or protruding through the anus (prolapsed internal piles)
- Any split in perianal skin (anal fissure)
- Any threadworms (see next section)
- If history does not strongly point to a non-cancerous cause and nothing is found on examination, refer to experienced colleague for abdominal and rectal examination (to check for anal/rectal mass)

Tests

- Consider full blood count (FBC) and ferritin, particularly if any indication of more than trivial blood loss
- FIT if any features suggestive of cancer (e.g., change in bowel habit, weight loss, family history of cancer, abdominal pain) or age ≥50 with unexplained rectal bleeding (see Red Flags box)

Self-care

- Note that any blood loss may appear exaggerated when mixed with water in the toilet pan
- Avoid straining if suspected piles or fissure
- High-fibre diet (see earlier section on Constipation) and consider ispaghula husk
- Drink adequate fluids (for an adult, 1.5 to 2 litres per day, including food)
- Advise using moist wipes to clean after defaecation, then pat area dry
- If the pain of thrombosed piles or anal fissure is severe, relief may be obtained by sitting in a warm bath or applying a bag of frozen peas to the area (which will mould to the required shape)
- Anusol[C] (OTC) ointment and/or suppositories may give symptomatic relief for piles (use twice daily, morning and night, plus additional doses after a bowel movement)

Action

- If piles are suspected, preparations containing local anaesthetic can be used to provide pain relief but could cause sensitisation if used for more than a few days. Preparations containing topical steroids may reduce inflammation but can exacerbate any local infection. Prescribe hydrocortisone with lidocaine[CP] ointment (use several times daily) or spray (use up to three times daily) if pain is severe (for no more than 7 days)
- If an anal fissure is not responding after 1 week, consider prescribing rectal glyceryl trinitrate (GTN) 0.4% ointment, applied twice daily for 6–8 weeks. Warn about the possible side effect of headache

RED FLAGS

- Severe pain from external thrombosed piles or prolapsed internal piles (*admit under Surgical for treatment*)
- Child with anal fissure and no obvious cause such as hard stools or known bowel disease (*although unlikely, the possibility of abuse should be considered; refer to experienced colleague*)
- Rectal/anal mass or ulceration (*possible cancer; USC referral to lower GI*)
- *Arrange FIT to inform referral pathway (i.e., whether USC referral needed) if:*
  - Age <50 with rectal bleeding and either unexplained weight loss or abdominal pain
  - Age ≥50 with rectal bleeding or unexplained weight loss or abdominal pain
  - Abdominal mass
  - Iron-deficiency anaemia, or anaemia even without iron deficiency if age ≥60

HAEMORRHOIDS ('PILES')

These are distended venous cushions inside the anal canal, which have a similar appearance to varicose veins. They may prolapse ('come down') on straining, when they may be visible as soft, purple grape-like swellings protruding from the anus. External haemorrhoids may cause bleeding, itching or discomfort. Internal haemorrhoids usually cause no pain and may have no symptoms apart from bleeding.

Risk factors for developing haemorrhoids include constipation, straining, spending a long time sitting on the toilet (one of the many reasons why staying off the phone when using the toilet is advisable!), heavy lifting, chronic cough and conditions that raise intra-abdominal pressure, e.g., pregnancy, childbirth.

THROMBOSED EXTERNAL PILE

This is caused by a sudden swelling of a small blood vessel near the anus (usually after straining). The blood stretches the sensitive skin, which is very painful. It will gradually disperse, but if the person presents early, it is possible for someone with adequate surgical experience to incise it and relieve pain by releasing the blood clot.

Abd

ANAL FISSURE

A split or an ulcer in the anal skin, previously thought to be caused by passing a large, hard stool but now considered more likely to be an ischaemic ulcer. This is a common cause of pain and bleeding on defaecation. Most will heal within 6 weeks, provided that the stools remain soft.

THREADWORMS (PINWORMS)

History

- Children most commonly affected
- Perianal irritation
- Anal pain at night
- Sometimes vaginal itching
- Worms may be seen – like white cotton threads – on skin or in stool

Examination

- Examine the affected area for worms/trauma

Test

- No testing is necessary unless the diagnosis is in doubt
- Your microbiology laboratory may supply a 'pinworm kit' containing a sticky slide. This should be applied to the anus first thing in the morning to pick up the eggs. Some laboratories request a saline-moistened anal swab instead

Self-care

- An appointment is not necessary if the parent is sure of the diagnosis
- Explain that adult threadworms live for only 6 weeks – their eggs must be transferred to the mouth and swallowed for the infection to continue
- No need to exclude from school/day care
- Practical measures are necessary:
  - Change and launder bed linen, underwear, cuddly toys and night clothes
  - Vacuum bedroom carpet and mattress and damp-dust the bathroom
  - Cut fingernails short, and consider cotton gloves at night
  - Do not put fingers in the mouth
  - Wash hands and scrub nails before each meal and after going to the toilet
  - For 2 weeks:
    - Wear close-fitting underwear in bed and change them every morning
    - Bathe or shower the perianal area in early morning to remove eggs laid during the night, and wet-wipe the area at 3-hourly intervals, if possible

Treatment

- Mebendazole[PBC] (OTC) 100 mg single dose for adults (unless pregnant or breastfeeding) and children aged ≥6 months (a prescription will be needed if aged 6 months to 2 years as it is *unlicensed* in this age group). A second dose may be needed 2 weeks later
- Unless there are exceptional circumstances, this medicine should be obtained OTC rather than prescribed
- Treat all household members simultaneously
- If aged <6 months, pregnant or breastfeeding, practical measures alone should be used

References

NICE. 2017. NG12. Suspected cancer: recognition and referral. www.nice.org.uk/guidance/ng12
NICE CKS. 2021a. Anal fissure. https://cks.nice.org.uk/topics/anal-fissure/
NICE CKS. 2021b. Haemorrhoids. https://cks.nice.org.uk/topics/haemorrhoids/
NICE CKS. 2023. Threadworm. https://cks.nice.org.uk/topics/threadworm/

UROLOGY

1. Cystitis
2. Pyelonephritis
3. Balanitis

A UTI may be lower (cystitis) or upper (pyelonephritis). The former is a minor illness affecting the bladder; the latter is a serious infection affecting the kidneys, which may lead to sepsis.

Note that people aged ≥65 with UTI, particularly those in long-term care facilities, may present with only vague symptoms such as lethargy, confusion or reduced mobility.

CYSTITIS (LOWER URINARY TRACT INFECTION)

History

- Duration
- Dysuria (burning when passing urine; *the symptom with greatest predictive value for UTI*)
- Urgency
- Frequency and nocturia
- Suprapubic discomfort/pain
- Cloudy, red-brown or offensive urine
- Incontinence/bed-wetting
- Previous history of kidney disease
- New vaginal discharge or irritation (*if so, symptoms may be vulval rather than urinary*)
- Symptoms associated with sexual intercourse
- Sexual history (see Box 10.1 in Chapter 10)
- Possibility of pregnancy
- In men, symptoms of urinary obstruction (hesitancy, straining, poor stream)
- 🚩 In men, symptoms of prostatitis (fever, perineal pain)
- 🚩 Fever and/or shivering (*suggestive of pyelonephritis*)

Examination

- Temperature
- Heart rate and respiratory rate
- CRT in children aged <12 years/BP in adults and older children
- Check loins for tenderness, which is suggestive of pyelonephritis
- In children, men or anyone with suspected pyelonephritis, examine abdomen and check for palpable bladder
- In young boys, check the penis for redness (see later section on Balanitis)

Tests

Dip testing

- Dip test the urine of adults aged <65, unless they have a catheter or it is a woman with a clear and typical history of uncomplicated cystitis
- Urine dip is of less diagnostic value in people aged ≥65 and should also not be used in people with indwelling urinary catheters
- Urine dip should be used in children if there is suspicion of UTI (but not for children aged <3 months, who should instead be admitted urgently to Paediatrics)
- Nitrites have the greatest predictive value for UTI and are highly supportive of the diagnosis
- Absence of both nitrites and leucocytes suggests that UTI is unlikely, but dip testing should not be used to rule out UTI in men

- Ideally, there should be an interval of at least 4 hours between last passing urine and passing the sample to be dip tested. Shorter intervals are more likely to cause a false-negative nitrite test
- Urinalysis strips are not sterile and contain many different chemicals. If intending to send the sample to the laboratory, it should not be contaminated by immersing a dipstick. Instead, urine should be transferred onto the strip or into a separate container for dipping
- Many urinalysis test strips are not reliable for dipping urine which has been stored in boric acid-containing specimen tubes. Boric acid is a preservative, typically in the form of a white powder, and particularly affects leucocyte analysis. The commonly used Valutest strips are reported to be compatible with boric acid

Urine culture

- Sending urine for culture can support diagnosis if UTI is suspected but there is uncertainty (although the test is not perfect – a negative culture does not rule out UTI), or if there is a particular need to inform antibiotic choice
- Except for uncomplicated cystitis in a woman aged <65, an MSU should be sent for culture (and before an antibiotic is taken), particularly if any of the following apply:
  - Age ≥65 years and UTI is suspected (and would be treated)
  - Has a catheter and UTI is suspected (and would be treated)
  - Pregnant
  - Male
  - Child
  - Immunosuppressed
  - Recurrent UTIs (≥2 episodes in 6 months or ≥3 episodes in 12 months)
  - Higher risk of antibiotic resistance (e.g., antibiotic in last 6 months, history of resistant UTI, previous treatment failure, recent hospital admission, known kidney/urinary tract disease, care home resident, recent travel to a country with increased resistance)
- In children, a clean catch sample should be collected in a sterile container, for example a universal container or gallipot
  - Clean, but non-sterile containers, can be used at home if no sterile container is available, but they are best lined with clingfilm to reduce contamination
  - For young girls who can use a toilet, it may be easier to collect the sample if they sit facing the cistern
  - In babies, wiping the abdomen repeatedly with a cold wet solution encourages urination ('Quick-Wee Method') (Kaufman et al., 2017)

Other

- Consider sexual health testing if suggested by sexual history or other symptoms. In women, these may include a change in vaginal discharge, pain or bleeding during or after sexual intercourse
- At the time of writing, NICE had issued draft guidance calling for further research into new tests which can identify bacteria in a urine sample within minutes and potentially assess sensitivity to different antibiotics. Depending on the evidence, we may see access to such tests in routine practice over the coming years

Self-care

- Advise adequate, but not excessive, fluid intake (for an adult, 1.5 to 2 litres per day, including food). Excessive fluid intake may increase the amount of dysuria and reduce the effectiveness of the immune response and treatment; there is no evidence that it speeds recovery
- Avoid OTC remedies such as Cymalon or CanesOasis which aim to alkalise the urine; there is insufficient high-quality evidence for benefit and they may interfere with antibiotic treatment (Fransen et al., 2017; Kavanagh, 2022)
- Cranberry extract is considered ineffective for the *treatment* of UTI
- If cystitis tends to occur after sexual intercourse, advise emptying bladder immediately after intercourse

Action

- Offer antibiotics for all except minor, uncomplicated UTIs. Note that antibiotic use in uncomplicated UTI is thought to shorten time to recovery by 2 days (median of 7 days vs. 9 days without antibiotics) (Gadalla et al., 2022)
    - Do not wait for the MSU result before starting antibiotics, especially in pregnancy (pregnant women are immunosuppressed; there is a higher risk of lower UTI progressing to upper UTI, and UTI in early pregnancy increases the risk of miscarriage)
    - In children aged 3 months to 3 years, start antibiotics without waiting for MSU result if either nitrite or leucocyte esterase is positive
    - In children aged ≥3 years, start antibiotics without waiting for MSU result if nitrite is positive (or leucocyte esterase is positive and there is good clinical evidence of UTI)
- Plan to review children and pregnant women when MSU result is available
- Growth of >10^3 organisms per ml is accepted as diagnostic of a UTI. If MSU shows that the organism is resistant to the antibiotic prescribed, check whether the symptoms have resolved. Laboratory sensitivity data do not necessarily reflect what happens to the person who, alongside the antibiotic, also has an immune system to fight the infection
- Catheterised bladders are often colonised by bacteria; growth on MSU in this context therefore may not indicate infection requiring treatment. There is no evidence that antibiotics will benefit the person, unless they have at least one of the following: fever, rigors, new pain/tenderness or new/worsening delirium
- Asymptomatic bacteriuria is common in older people (25% of women and 10% of men aged ≥65). Bacteriuria should not be treated in older people unless there is a clinical suspicion of UTI. Asymptomatic bacteriuria is often detected at pre-op assessment; there is no evidence that treating it improves outcomes after orthopaedic surgery (Mayne et al., 2016)
- However, asymptomatic bacteriuria should be treated in pregnancy as it is associated with poor outcomes if left untreated (including pyelonephritis and preterm labour). Pregnancy is the only indication for a post-treatment MSU

Antibiotic choice

Before the MSU result is known, choice depends on local sensitivities. Consult local guidelines or ask your microbiologist about the local resistance pattern. Trimethoprim has high levels of resistance nationally and should not be prescribed if the person has taken it within the previous 3 months.

- Simple cystitis in a non-pregnant adult woman, for 3 days:
    - Nitrofurantoin MR[PBC] *or*
    - Pivmecillinam *or*
    - Trimethoprim[PI] (avoid if recently used, or care home resident, unless infection sensitivity known) *or*
    - Fosfomycin[PC] (less often used, so may not be stocked by local pharmacies)
- Cystitis in a woman with chronic kidney disease (CKD), abnormal renal tract or immunosuppression: consider extending course to 5–7 days (avoid nitrofurantoin if estimated glomerular filtration rate [eGFR] <30 and consider using an alternative antibiotic if eGFR <45; dose reduction is needed for trimethoprim if eGFR <30; avoid fosfomycin if eGFR <10)
- Pregnant woman: nitrofurantoin MR[PBC] for 7 days (unless ≥30 weeks' gestation; if so, use cefalexin instead)
- Men: treat simple cystitis with nitrofurantoin MR[PBC] for 7 days. Note that this would not be adequate if there is a suspicion of prostatic involvement (fever, perineal or lower abdominal or back pain, pain on ejaculation, urethral discharge). Perhaps for this reason, there is a high failure rate of nitrofurantoin treatment in men (25%), which increases with age (Platteel et al., 2023)
- Children: trimethoprim[PI] for 3 days (or cefalexin for 3 days if allergic to trimethoprim). Although nitrofurantoin oral suspension[PB] is recommended by national guidance, the liquid preparation is prohibitively expensive
- Do not use amoxicillin for UTI unless there is an MSU result showing that the organism is sensitive (50% are resistant)

Abd

Doses in adults

- Nitrofurantoin MR[PBC], 100 mg twice daily
- Pivmecillinam, 400 mg initially, then 200 mg three times daily
- Trimethoprim[PI], 200 mg twice daily
- Cefalexin, 500 mg twice daily
- Fosfomycin[PC], 3 g single dose

Prescription warnings

Nitrofurantoin[PBC] may produce neonatal haemolysis if used near term or during breastfeeding if the infant is susceptible. Although the BNF states that it may be used up to 36 weeks' gestation, we are more cautious in only recommending up to 30 weeks because preterm labour is not uncommon and the UTI increases this risk (Baer et al., 2021).

Pivmecillinam is a prodrug of mecillinam, a penicillin, so cannot be used for those allergic to penicillin.

Trimethoprim[PI] has serious interactions with methotrexate, azathioprine, ciclosporin, mercaptopurine and tacrolimus, so be aware when prescribing for a person with a long-term inflammatory condition such as rheumatoid arthritis. Trimethoprim also interacts significantly with phenytoin.

Prophylaxis

- Following resolution of UTI, if prophylaxis is warranted:
  - In post-menopausal women, offer topical oestrogen (*unlicensed indication*) (NICE NG112, 2019)
  - D-mannose[P] (a sugar naturally found in some fruits) supplements are considered safe, although lacking robust evidence for benefit (Cooper et al., 2022)
  - There is some evidence of effectiveness for use of cranberry products in prophylaxis, although not in the elderly, people with bladder-emptying problems or pregnant women (Williams et al., 2023)
  - Methenamine hippurate[C] (1 g twice daily) has been shown to be non-inferior to antibiotics for lower, uncomplicated UTI prophylaxis (Harding et al., 2022). It will require a prescription and is relatively expensive (around £18 a month); the BNF marks it as 'less suitable for prescribing'
  - NICE guidance says 'for women with recurrent UTI who are not pregnant, consider a trial of antibiotic prophylaxis only if behavioural and personal hygiene measures, and vaginal oestrogen (in post-menopausal women) are not effective or not appropriate'. If starting antibiotic prophylaxis, arrange follow-up within 3-6 months
  - Generally single dose prophylaxis, for use when exposed to a trigger, should be tried before daily antibiotic prophylaxis unless there are no identifiable triggers or the person is pregnant or male
  - Consider the most appropriate choice of antibiotic, taking into account previous MSU sensitivities. If offering daily antibiotic prophylaxis, explain the risks of resistance and possible adverse effects with long-term antibiotic use
  - First-line for single dose prophylaxis (for adults) are nitrofurantoin[PBC] 100 mg or trimethoprim[PI] 200 mg. Another option is cefalexin 500 mg
  - First-line for daily prophylaxis (for adults) are nitrofurantoin[PBC] 50-100 mg at night or trimethoprim[PI] 100 mg at night. Another option is cefalexin 125 mg at night
  - Note that if a UTI develops while on antibiotic prophylaxis, a different antibiotic should be prescribed for treatment to that used for prophylaxis

RED FLAGS

- Age <3 months (*high risk of severe illness; admit urgently under Paediatrics*)
- Fever (*suspect pyelonephritis or prostatitis: see next section and consider referring to experienced colleague*)
- Enlarged bladder with inability to pass urine despite strong urge (*acute urinary retention; inform Urology and send urgently to A&E for catheterisation*)
- A man with symptoms of urinary obstruction, e.g., hesitancy, straining or poor stream (*suggests prostatic problem; refer to experienced colleague*)
- A change in the total urine output in 24 hours (*may be diabetes if increased, may be acute kidney injury if decreased; refer to experienced colleague*)
- Child or pregnant woman not responding to antibiotics after 48 hours (*high risk of severe illness; review and change antibiotic or refer to experienced colleague*)
- A child with confirmed UTI may need *referral for imaging*, particularly if:
  - Aged <6 months
  - Infected with an organism which is not *E. coli*
  - ≥3 episodes of lower UTI (or ≥2 episodes of UTI if one was an upper UTI)
- Persistent or unexplained haematuria (*possible bladder cancer; consider USC referral to Urology*)
- Recurrent UTI without an obvious cause, e.g., ≥2 episodes in 6 months or ≥3 episodes in 12 months (*may need investigation; refer to experienced colleague*)

References

Baer, R.J., Nidey, N., Bandoli, G. et al. 2021. Risk of early birth among women with a urinary tract infection: a retrospective cohort study. *AJP Rep*; 11(1):e5–e14. https://doi.org/10.1055/s-0040-1721668 *Risk increased by up to 40%.*

Cooper, T.E., Teng, C., Howell, M., et al. 2022. D-mannose for preventing and treating urinary tract infections. *Cochrane Database Syst Rev*; 8:CD013608. https://doi.org/10.1002/14651858.CD013608.pub2

Delanghe, J., and Speeckaert, M. 2014. Preanalytical requirements of urinalysis. *Biochem Med (Zagreb)*; 24(1):89–104. https://doi.org/10.11613/BM.2014.011 *Boric acid keeps urinary pH below 7, prevents dissolution of pus cells and is associated with false-negative strip-test results (e.g., protein, leucocyte esterase and ketones).*

Fransen, F., Melchers, M.J.B., Lagarde, C.M.C. et al., 2017. Pharmacodynamics of nitrofurantoin at different pH levels against pathogens involved in urinary tract infections. *J Antimicrob Chemother*; 72(12):3366–73. https://doi.org/10.1093/jac/dkx313 *Nitrofurantoin is more effective at lower pH, so the use of OTC products that make the urine more alkaline could interfere with the antibiotic's effectiveness.*

Gadalla, A., Wise, H., Farewell, D., et al. 2022. Antibiotic consumption and time to recovery from uncomplicated urinary tract infection: secondary analysis of observational data from a point-of-care test trial. *Br J Gen Pract*; 72(725):e882. https://doi.org/10.3399/BJGP.2022.0011 *Antibiotic use shortens time to recovery from UTI by 2 days.*

Harding, C., Mossop, H., Homer, T., et al. 2022. Alternative to prophylactic antibiotics for the treatment of recurrent urinary tract infections in women: multicentre, open label, randomised, non-inferiority trial. *BMJ*; 376:e068229. https://doi.org/10.1136/bmj-2021-0068229 *Non-inferiority of methenamine hippurate compared with antibiotics for UTI prophylaxis.*

Kaufman, J., Fitzpatrick, P., Tosif, S., et al. 2017. Faster clean catch urine collection (Quick-Wee method) from infants: randomised controlled trial. *BMJ*; 357:j1341. https://doi.org/10.1136/bmj.j1341 *Quick-Wee is a simple cutaneous stimulation method that significantly increases the 5-minute voiding and success rate of clean catch urine collection.*

Kavanagh, O.N. 2022. Alkalising agents in urinary tract infections: theoretical contraindications, interactions and synergy. *Ther Adv Drug Saf*; 13:20420986221080794. https://doi.org/10.1177/20420986221080794 *A paper highlighting the potential antibiotic interactions of alkalising agents such as OTC preparations for managing UTI.*

Mayne, A.I.W., Davies, P.S.E., and Simpson, J.M. 2016. Screening for asymptomatic bacteriuria before total joint arthroplasty. *BMJ*; 354:i3569. https://doi.org/10.1136/bmj.i3569 *People with asymptomatic bacteriuria have an increased risk of (joint) infection, but current evidence does not support routine antibiotic treatment before arthroplasty.*

Naber, K.G. 2000. Treatment options for acute uncomplicated cystitis in adults. *J Antimicrob Chemother*; 46(Suppl 1):23–7; discussion 63–5. *Antibiotic treatment for 3 days is as effective as longer duration.*

NICE. 2018. NG109. Urinary tract infections (lower): antimicrobial prescribing. www.nice.org.uk/guidance/ng109/

NICE. 2018. NG112. Urinary tract infections (recurrent): antimicrobial prescribing. www.nice.org.uk/guidance/ng112/

NICE. 2022. NG224. Urinary tract infection in under 16s: diagnosis and management. www.nice.org.uk/guidance/ng224

NICE. 2023. Press release. Four innovative tests for diagnosing UTIs could help in the fight against antimicrobial resistance. www.nice.org.uk/news/article/four-innovative-tests-for-diagnosing-utis-could-help-in-the-fight-against-antimicrobial-resistance

O'Kane, D.B., Dave, S.K., Gore, N., et al. 2016. Urinary alkalisation for symptomatic uncomplicated urinary tract infection in women. *Cochrane Database Syst Rev*; 4:CD010745. https://doi.org/10.1002/14651858.CD010745.pub2

Abd

Platteel, T.N., Beets, M.T., Teeuwissen, H.A., et al. 2023. Nitrofurantoin failure in males with an uncomplicated urinary tract infection: a primary care observational cohort study. *Br J Gen Pract*; 73(728):e204. https://doi.org/10.3399/BJGP.2022.0354 *A Dutch study showing a 25% failure rate for nitrofurantoin in uncomplicated UTI in men.*

Public Health England. 2020. Diagnosis of urinary tract infections. Quick reference guide for primary care for consultation and local adaptation. https://assets.publishing.service.gov.uk/media/5f89809ae90e072e18c0ccc2/UTI_diagnostic_flowchart_NICE-October_2020-FINAL.pdf

Scottish Intercollegiate Guidelines Network (SIGN). 2020. SIGN 160. Management of suspected bacterial lower urinary tract infection in adult women: a national clinical guideline. www.sign.ac.uk/media/1766/sign-160-uti-0-1_web-version.pdf

Williams, G., Hahn, D., Stephens, J.H., et al. 2023. Cranberries for preventing urinary tract infections. *Cochrane Database Syst Rev*; 4:CD001321. https://doi.org/10.1002/14651858.CD001321.pub6 *Cranberry products perform as well as prophylactic antibiotics in reducing the recurrence of UTIs.*

PYELONEPHRITIS (UPPER URINARY TRACT INFECTION)

This is a bacterial infection of the kidney, usually caused by infection spreading up the ureters. This may develop following cystitis, but occurs in only 1% of women with simple cystitis (Jansåker et al., 2022). Rising infection is commoner in children who have vesico-ureteric reflux and in pregnancy, when the ureters are dilated. The key difference in presentation compared with cystitis is that someone with pyelonephritis will often feel very ill and appear systemically unwell with fever. It is not a minor illness and should be managed by experienced practitioners.

History

- There may be symptoms of cystitis (see previous section) – but these can be absent (people aged ≥65, particularly those in long-term care facilities, may present with vague symptoms such as lethargy, confusion or reduced mobility)
- Fever/rigors (may be absent in early illness, in older people or if immunosuppressed)
- Loin pain/suprapubic pain
- Nausea/vomiting
- Feeling very unwell/confused
- In babies: fever/reduced fluid intake/offensive or discoloured urine
- 🚩 Immunosuppressed
- 🚩 Kidney disease
- 🚩 Pregnant

Examination

- Temperature
- Heart rate and respiratory rate
- CRT in children aged <12 years/BP in adults and older children
- Check loins for tenderness
- Examine abdomen for palpable bladder

Tests

- Urinalysis for blood, leucocytes and nitrites can be useful to support the diagnosis but is not essential. It should not be used in people aged ≥65 or anyone with an indwelling urinary catheter, as false-positives are very common
- Send MSU before starting treatment (do not wait for results)

Self-care

- Adequate fluid intake (but not excessive)
- Paracetamol for pain relief
- Safety-netting advice

Action

- May need admission to hospital (see Red Flags box)
- If not admitting to hospital, prescribe an antibiotic. Follow your local antimicrobial guidelines if possible; otherwise treat for 7 days with one of the following options (doses for adults):

- Cefalexin, 500 mg three times daily
- Co-amoxiclav, 500/125 mg three times daily

- **Beware a common prescribing error:** nitrofurantoin, pivmecillinam and fosfomycin are **not** suitable for treating pyelonephritis because they do not achieve adequate concentration in the blood or the tissue of the kidney
- Review after 24 hours and again when MSU result is available

RED FLAGS

- Sepsis – including low BP, rapid heart rate, systemically unwell (*admit very urgently under Medical/Paediatrics*)
- Dehydrated (*if not tolerating oral fluids, admit urgently under Medical/Paediatrics*)
- Enlarged bladder with inability to pass urine despite strong urge (*acute urinary retention; admit urgently under Medical/Paediatrics, or inform Urology and send urgently to A&E for catheterisation*)
- Immunosuppressed (*consider admitting urgently under Medical/Paediatrics*)
- Kidney disease (*consider admitting urgently under Medical/Paediatrics*)
- Pregnant (*consider admitting urgently under Medical*)
- Child aged <3 months (*risk of long-term renal scarring; admit urgently under Paediatrics*)
- Child aged ≥3 months (*consider admitting urgently under Paediatrics*)
- *Refer routinely for investigation* if:
  - Male with any episode of pyelonephritis without an obvious cause
  - Female with ≥2 episodes of pyelonephritis

References

Jansåker, F., Li, X., Vik, I., et al. 2022. The risk of pyelonephritis following uncomplicated cystitis: a nationwide primary healthcare study. *Antibiotics*; 11(12). https://doi.org/10.3390/antibiotics11121695 *Only 1% of 750,000 Swedish women with cystitis developed pyelonephritis.*

NICE. 2018. NG111. Pyelonephritis (acute): antimicrobial prescribing. www.nice.org.uk/guidance/ng111

NICE. 2022. NG224. Urinary tract infection in under 16s: diagnosis and management. www.nice.org.uk/guidance/ng224

NICE CKS. 2023. Pyelonephritis – acute. https://cks.nice.org.uk/topics/pyelonephritis-acute/

BALANITIS (INFLAMMATION OF THE GLANS PENIS)

This occurs in males of all ages and may be due to dermatitis, fungal infection or bacterial infection.

History

- Duration
- Swelling of foreskin
- Discharge
- Itch/odour
- Dysuria
- Consider possibility of diabetes: risk factors (family history, ethnicity, obesity) or suggestive symptoms (excessive thirst and polyuria)
- SGLT2 inhibitors (e.g., dapagliflozin, canagliflozin; used in type 2 diabetes, CKD, heart failure) increase the risk of balanitis
- Sexual history (in adults) (see Box 10.1 in Chapter 10)
- 🏴 Immunosuppressed

Examination

- Gently attempt to retract foreskin (not if age <3 years)
- Assess hygiene, look for discharge
- Localised redness or more generalised cellulitis

Tests

- Consider taking a swab if sevcre

Self-care

- Advise gentle cleaning with lukewarm water and thoroughly patting dry
- Avoid exposure to possible irritants such as soap, bubble bath and shower gel
- Do not attempt to pull back the foreskin if it is tight
- If difficulty passing urine because of pain, then advise sitting in bath

Prescription

- Treat according to the suspected cause:
    - Hydrocortisone cream 1% daily for 7 days for irritant dermatitis without signs of infection (e.g., nappy rash)
    - Clotrimazole cream for 14 days for *Candida* infection (apply thinly and evenly, twice daily, and rub in gently)
    - If cellulitis is present or bacterial infection confirmed, flucloxacillin for 7 days (250 mg four times daily in adults) or, if allergic to penicillin, clarithromycin[PIQ] (250 mg twice daily in adults)

RED FLAGS

- Immunosuppressed/severe symptoms (*send urgently to appropriate specialty*)
- Consider diabetes; this may be the first presentation (*check HbA1c or fasting glucose; see Box 8.3, Checking for diabetes, in Chapter 8*)

References

NICE CKS. 2022. Balanitis. https://cks.nice.org.uk/topics/balanitis/

Wray, A.A., Velasquez, J., and Khetarpal, S. 2022. Balanitis. *StatPearls*. StatPearls Publishing. www.ncbi.nlm.nih.gov/books/NBK537143/

CHAPTER 10

Women's health

BOX 10.1 TAKING A SEXUAL HISTORY

- Establish rapport first
- Explain that you need to ask some sensitive questions to establish what is wrong
- Last sexual intercourse, partner's gender (and partner's age if patient aged <18 or vulnerable), sites of exposure, condom use
- Number of sexual partners in the last 12 months
- Previous sexually transmitted infections (STIs)
- Last menstrual period (LMP), contraceptive history
- Establish if there is an impairment of capacity, or any safeguarding issues

For more information, see the British Association for Sexual Health and HIV guideline: www.bashhguidelines.org/media/1241/sh-guidelines-2019-ijsa.pdf

---

VAGINAL DISCHARGE

Vaginal discharge may be a normal physiological occurrence, especially during higher oestrogen states such as ovulation (usually mid-cycle), the luteal phase (the second part of the cycle after ovulation), puberty and pregnancy, and with oestrogen-based therapies such as the combined oral contraceptive pill (COCP) and hormone replacement therapy (HRT). Physiological discharge tends to be clearer with a stretchy consistency around ovulation, then may be thicker and more yellow during the luteal phase, but it is not associated with itching, redness or swelling and does not have an odour.

The two commonest causes of abnormal vaginal discharge in primary care are bacterial vaginosis (BV) and candidiasis.

- BV is more common than candidiasis, but is underdiagnosed. It is caused by an overgrowth of anaerobic bacteria in the vagina at the expense of the normal commensal lactobacteria. It is not sexually transmitted. It is more common in sexually active women, those of black ethnicity, smokers, copper intrauterine contraceptive device (Cu-IUCD[P]) users and those using bubble baths or vaginal douching
- Candidiasis (a yeast infection) is overdiagnosed and overtreated. Up to 20% of women are colonised by *Candida* as a commensal in their vagina (i.e., it causes no symptoms). This rises to 30% in pregnancy. A change in hormone balance, or a course of broad-spectrum antibiotics may trigger yeast multiplication and symptoms. Approximately 75% of women will have an episode of symptomatic vaginal candidiasis in their lifetime
- Other causes are rarer, but it is important not to miss an STI or pelvic inflammatory disease (PID)

History

Often a woman will consult saying that she has 'thrush', but further exploration of symptoms is required as a self-diagnosis of candidiasis or BV is not always reliable.

- Duration
- Characterisation: colour, odour, volume, consistency
- Associated symptoms: itch, soreness, dysuria
- Medication history, including any treatments tried, recent antibiotics (increased risk of candidiasis) and contraceptive use (Cu-IUCD[P] increases the risk of BV)
- The use of vaginal hygiene products such as washes and deodorants
- Recurrent or cyclical symptoms
- Any possibility of pregnancy?
- ⚑ Vulval pain or blisters (*genital herpes*)

🚩 Offensive discharge (*consider retained tampon*)

🚩 Any other worrying symptoms, e.g., unusual bleeding or pelvic pain (*consider STI, PID or cancer*)

🚩 Recent pregnancy or gynaecological procedure (*high risk of sepsis*)

🚩 Immunosuppression

🚩 Increased risk of STI – risk factors include:

- Age <25
- Previous STIs
- Recent new partner
- >1 sexual partner in past year
- Partner has symptoms of STI

🚩 Symptoms suggesting PID:

- Fever
- Abdominal pain/pain during intercourse/dysuria
- Irregular bleeding/post-coital bleeding/bloodstained or brown discharge

See Table 10.1 for features that differentiate the two commonest causes of abnormal vaginal discharge: BV and candidiasis.

Table 10.1 Clinical features associated with BV and candidiasis

Feature	Bacterial vaginosis	Candidiasis
Symptoms	• Thin discharge • Fishy odour • No discomfort or itch	• Thick white discharge • Non-offensive odour • Vulval itch, discomfort, dyspareunia, dysuria • Timing with menstrual cycle
Signs	No inflammation of vulva	Vulval erythema, oedema, fissuring, satellite lesions
Vaginal pH	>4.5	≤4.5

Examination

- If person is unwell, check:
  - Temperature
  - Heart rate
  - Respiratory rate
  - BP
- Palpate the abdomen for any tenderness or masses
- If no red flag symptoms are present, vaginal examination may not be necessary. If an examination is indicated, obtain consent and offer a chaperone
  - Examine the vulva for lesions, discharge, inflammation or ulcers
  - Vaginal pH/swab testing (see next section) can be performed during the examination or by the person themselves afterwards. Ask what they would prefer
  - If the history is suggestive of PID, a bimanual pelvic examination should be performed in order to identify tenderness of the uterus and fallopian tubes and abnormal masses. A speculum examination should also be performed, looking for inflammation of the cervix, vaginal discharge and any foreign bodies, such as tampon or condom
  - If pelvic examination is not in your skill set, consider the best referral option for the situation (e.g., Sexual Health Service, GP colleague, suitably qualified and experienced nurse)
- See Table 10.1 for typical features on examination for BV and candidiasis
- Painful vesicles are suggestive of genital herpes (*offer oral aciclovir and refer to Sexual Health Service. Inform them that infection may not have come from current partner*)

Tests

- Offer vaginal pH testing; see Box 10.2
- High vaginal swabs traditionally have been used to guide the treatment of vaginal discharge, but a national guideline (Lazaro, 2013) states that there is no evidence that they are useful. Their diagnostic yield is poor, with overdiagnosis of candidiasis and underdiagnosis of BV
- Free, confidential home testing for STIs may be available from www.freetest.me
- If possible ectopic pregnancy, perform a point-of-care urine pregnancy test
- If dysuria is present, consider a urine dipstick to help exclude a urinary tract infection

---

BOX 10.2 VAGINAL pH TESTING

- Take a swab or cotton bud and rub it along the lateral wall of the vagina, collecting some discharge. Avoid the cervix and the posterior fornix (because of alkaline cervical secretions)
- Rub the swab immediately on to specific narrow-range pH paper (e.g., Simplex Health range 3.8–5.4). Urine dipsticks are not suitable
- The normal vaginal pH in a woman of reproductive age is ≤4.5 (kept acidic by normal lactobacilli)
- pH may be raised because of:
  - Menstrual blood
  - Semen
  - KY jelly
  - BV, *Trichomonas vaginalis* (TV), gonorrhoea and chlamydia infection
- *Candida* does not affect the vaginal pH
- pH testing kits may be bought OTC

Self-care

- Advise to avoid tight-fitting, synthetic clothing, local irritants such as perfumed products and soap gels, and vaginal douching
- There is no evidence to support the use of yoghurt or probiotics, but they are unlikely to cause harm
- Sex does not need to be avoided unless there is suspicion of an STI, but note that clotrimazole reduces the effectiveness of latex condoms
- Evidence is lacking for effectiveness of acidifying products sold OTC for BV (Lazaro, 2013)
- There are a range of effective OTC treatments for candidiasis; see later section

Action

- Refer to Sexual Health Service if:
  - Symptoms suggest STI and the person is systemically well with no features suggesting PID (see Red Flags box)
  - The diagnosis is uncertain (microscopy of the discharge is the best way to identify the organism)
- The Sexual Health Service can screen for infections and facilitate partner notification (keep a note of their opening hours, including drop-in clinics and an idea of their waiting times)

OTC treatments for candidiasis

- Options (*only OTC for women aged 16-60*) include:
  - Oral fluconazole[PCIQ], 150 mg capsule
  - Clotrimazole, 500 mg pessary
  - Econazole, 150 mg pessary (preferred by some as waxier and less chalky)
  - Clotrimazole 10% internal cream
- These are similarly effective, although the effect of the topical/intravaginal products may be more rapid (Zhang et al., 2022). There are some differences in side effects. Oral treatments may cause nausea, diarrhoea or headaches,

Wom

whereas creams and pessaries may cause skin reactions. Fluconazole[PCIQ] may prolong the ECG QT interval (see section on QT interval in Chapter 14)

- Clotrimazole external cream may be used in addition for women experiencing both internal and external symptoms. Combination packs available OTC are as follows:
  - Clotrimazole 2% external cream and internal 500 mg pessary (e.g., Canesten Thrush Combi)
  - Clotrimazole 2% external cream and 10% internal cream (e.g., Canesten Thrush Combi)

  (Note that the above combination products containing only topical/intravaginal treatments have the same trade name. However, the packets make clear which product is which)

  - Clotrimazole 2% cream and oral fluconazole[PCIQ] 150 mg capsule (e.g., Canesten Thrush Duo)
- It is generally cheaper to buy these combination packs OTC than pay for a prescription, as they carry two prescription charges
- If itching is severe, combination clotrimazole/hydrocortisone cream may be appropriate, but it is not available OTC for vaginal candidiasis (only for fungal foot infections)
- Advise that clotrimazole affects latex condoms
- There is no need to treat the sexual partner, unless they have symptoms

Prescription

Table 10.2 Treatment regimens for bacterial vaginosis and candidiasis
If multiple options, the person's preference should guide treatment choice

Treatment	Bacterial vaginosis	Candidiasis	
First line	• Metronidazole[Q] 400 mg orally, twice daily for 7 days (a single dose of 2 g may be used if not pregnant and compliance is an issue, but relapse rates are higher) *Or* • Metronidazole 0.75% vaginal gel, nightly for 5 nights (40 g)[†] *Or* • Clindamycin vaginal cream, nightly for 7 nights (40 g)[†]	• Fluconazole[PCIQ] 150 mg orally, one dose* *Or* • Clotrimazole 500 mg pessary, one at night*[†]	
Second line	From the first-line options, use a different treatment to that tried already	From the first-line options, use a different treatment to that tried already	
Pregnancy	Treat if symptomatic,[‡] options are as follows: • Metronidazole[Q] 400 mg orally, twice daily for 7 days *Or* • Metronidazole 0.75% vaginal gel, nightly for 5 nights (40 g) *Or* • Clindamycin vaginal cream, nightly for 7 nights (40 g)	• Clotrimazole 500 mg pessaries, one nightly for up to 7 nights (insert manually) *Or* • Clotrimazole 10% vaginal cream, 5 g nightly for up to 7 nights	
Recurrent	• Prescribe alternative first-line treatment • If there is no response to 7-day course of oral metronidazole, discuss with gynaecologist or Sexual Health specialist	Induction: • Fluconazole[PCIQ] 150 mg orally, every 3 days for 3 doses *Or* • Clotrimazole 500 mg pessaries, one nightly for 7–14 nights[†] (depending on response)	Maintenance: • Fluconazole[PCIQ] 150 mg orally, weekly for 6 months *Or* • Clotrimazole 500 mg pessaries, one weekly for 6 months[†] *Or* • Itraconazole 50–100 mg orally, daily for 6 months

* If severe or persistent symptoms, give repeat after 3 days.
[†] Caution that topical clotrimazole, intravaginal clotrimazole and clindamycin all affect latex condoms.
[‡] There is no good evidence to support treating asymptomatic pregnant women, unless they have HIV or other risk factors for preterm birth (*discuss with Obstetrics or Sexual Health*).

RED FLAGS

- Features suggestive of pelvic inflammatory disease (*admit urgently under Gynaecology*):
  - Nausea/vomiting
  - Fever >38°C
  - Systemically unwell/tachycardia
  - Signs of pelvic peritonitis (pain, tenderness and swelling of lower abdomen)
- Systemically unwell and any of the following: pregnant/postpartum/recent termination of pregnancy or gynaecological procedure (*high risk of sepsis; send urgently to hospital with referral to Gynaecology*)

References

Lazaro, N. 2013. *Sexually Transmitted Infections in Primary Care*, 2nd edition. RCGP/BASHH guideline. www.bashhguidelines. org/media/1089/sexually-transmitted-infections-in-primary-care-2013.pdf

NICE CKS. 2018. Bacterial vaginosis. https://cks.nice.org.uk/topics/bacterial-vaginosis/

NICE CKS. 2022a. Pelvic inflammatory disease. https://cks.nice.org.uk/topics/pelvic-inflammatory-disease/

NICE CKS. 2022b. Candida – female genital. https://cks.nice.org.uk/topics/candida-female-genital/

Plummer, E.L., Bradshaw, C., Doyle, M., et al. 2021. Lactic acid-containing products for bacterial vaginosis and their impact on the vaginal microbiota: a systematic review. *PLOS One*; 16(2):e0246953. https://doi.org/10.1371/journal.pone.0246953 *High-quality evidence is lacking.*

Saxon, C., Edwards, A., Rautemaa-Richardson, R., et al. 2020. British Association for Sexual Health and HIV national guideline for the management of vulvovaginal candidiasis (2019). *Int J STD AIDS*; 31(12):1124–44. https://doi.org/10.1177/0956462420943034

Thinkhamrop, J., Hofmeyr, G., Adetoro, O., et al. 2015. Antibiotic prophylaxis during the second and third trimester to reduce adverse pregnancy outcomes and morbidity. *Cochrane Database Syst Rev*; 6:CD002250. https://doi.org/10.1002/14651858. CD002250.pub3 *Antibiotic prophylaxis did not reduce the risk of preterm pre-labour rupture of membranes or preterm delivery (apart from in the subgroup of women with a previous preterm birth who had BV).*

Zhang, L., DeSalvo, R., Ehret, A., et al. 2022. Vulvovaginal candidiasis: a real-world evidence study of the perceived benefits of Canesten. *SAGE Open Medicine*; 10:20503121221085437. https://doi.org/10.1177/20503121221085437 *The time taken for symptomatic relief to be obtained using an oral fluconazole product (1–2 days) was slightly longer than for a Canesten topical/intravaginal product (≤1 day).*

HEAVY MENSTRUAL BLEEDING (MENORRHAGIA)

Wom

This is defined as the need to change menstrual products every 1–2 hours, passage of clots >2.5 cm or, most importantly, 'heavy' periods as reported by the woman. Heavy menstrual bleeding is a common problem, thought to affect around a third of women, with around half of these having no identified underlying cause. It may have a major impact on quality of life; ensure that any intervention seeks to address this, rather than focusing solely on blood loss.

History

- Duration and heaviness of this period (e.g., frequency of changing pad/tampon/menstrual cup)
- Clots/flooding
- Painful periods (see next section)
- Any other bleeding problems, e.g., nosebleeds, easy bruising
- Contraceptive usage (this may be the cause, e.g., a Cu-IUCD[P])
- Missed pills/unprotected sexual intercourse (consider pregnancy, including miscarriage and ectopic pregnancy, in all women with heavy bleeding)
- Cervical screening history
- Usual pattern of menstrual cycle
- Impact on their quality of life
- Any previous treatment
- Thyroid disease/symptoms of thyroid dysfunction (hypothyroidism may cause weight gain, constipation or cold intolerance in addition to menorrhagia)
- Fatigue (may be secondary to anaemia due to blood loss or a symptom of thyroid disease)

- Taking any herbal supplements, such as ginseng, ginkgo and soya (these may alter oestrogen levels and coagulation)
- 🚩 Period after ≥12 months of amenorrhoea
- 🚩 Vaginal bleeding between periods or bleeding after sex

Examination

- If bleeding is currently very heavy, check heart rate and BP
- If there is a history of heavy bleeding **without** any clinically concerning symptoms (e.g., atypical pain, intermenstrual bleeding or post-coital bleeding), a pelvic examination is not necessary unless initial treatment is ineffective, or a levonorgestrel-releasing intrauterine system (IUS^P) is being considered
- If there is a history of heavy bleeding **with** any clinically concerning symptoms (e.g., atypical pain, intermenstrual bleeding or post-coital bleeding), **an examination is required**:
  - Abdominal examination to feel for any masses such as large fibroids and ascites (fluid in the abdomen)
  - Bimanual pelvic examination (including a speculum examination), except in young girls who are not sexually active. If pelvic examination is not in your skill set, consider the best referral option for the situation (e.g., Sexual Health Service, GP colleague, suitably qualified and experienced nurse)
- Look for features suggesting a possible systemic disease such as a possible blood disorder (e.g., pallor or skin bruises) or thyroid disorder

Tests

- FBC and ferritin should be checked in all women with heavy menstrual bleeding
- Consider thyroid function tests if any symptoms or signs of thyroid dysfunction
- Consider clotting screen if there are symptoms or signs of bleeding from other sites, or if there is a family history of a clotting disorder and there has been heavy bleeding since periods first started

Self-care

- Provide information to explain the condition and treatment options. A self-assessment tool is available on the NHS website – www.nhs.uk/conditions/heavy-periods
- Explain that there is no link between passing 'clots' in the menstrual blood and internal thrombosis. People often worry about this
- Ibuprofen^P (200–400 mg three times daily for adults) often reduces menstrual flow significantly. Mefenamic acid has been marketed for menorrhagia and dysmenorrhoea but ibuprofen has a better side-effect profile. The more potent NSAID naproxen^{PBCI} (500 mg initially, then 250 mg up to three times daily for adults) is now available OTC for painful periods

Action

- Drug treatment can be started without investigation in women without any clinically concerning symptoms
- First-line recommended treatment is an IUS^P. If this is favoured but not feasible/available in-house, offer referral to an appropriate local service
- If this is unsuitable/declined, consider:
  - Tranexamic acid^P: start with menstrual bleeding; two 500 mg tablets three times a day for up to 4 days. Do not use if there is a history of convulsions or thromboembolic disease (e.g., DVT or pulmonary embolism), or they are taking an oestrogen-containing contraceptive (due to DVT risk)
  - Hormonal: COCP or a cyclical oral progesterone such as medroxyprogesterone acetate^{PC} or norethisterone^P – see BNF for dosing. Note that the recommended dose of norethisterone^P carries an increased thromboembolic risk which is comparable to that of the COCP. Progesterone-only contraception may suppress menstruation
- If treatment is unsuccessful or declined, *refer to experienced colleague* for further assessment. Further investigation may be needed, e.g., for possible polycystic ovary syndrome
- Iron supplements may be needed if blood loss has been heavy. The recommended dose to treat iron deficiency is 60–120 mg of elemental iron per day (e.g., ferrous fumarate^{CI}, 322 mg on alternate days) for a minimum of 3 months. Many OTC iron supplements contain much lower doses than this. Evidence suggests that iron is best given once every other day (Stoffel et al., 2017). If there is urgency to correct the blood loss, then daily dosing may be tried and the FBC monitored

RED FLAGS

- Persistent intermenstrual or post-coital bleeding (*possible STI or cervical cancer; refer to experienced colleague*)
- Palpable abdominal mass (*possible fibroids or uterine/ovarian cancer; USC referral to Gynaecology*)
- Bleeding after 12 months of amenorrhoea (post-menopausal bleeding) (*possible uterine cancer; USC referral if aged ≥55 or refer urgently to Gynaecology if aged <55*)

References

Mansour, D. 2012. Safer prescribing of therapeutic norethisterone for women at risk of venous thromboembolism. *J Fam Plann Reprod Health Care*; 38(3):148. https://doi.org/10.1136/jfprhc-2012-100345 *Therapeutic doses of norethisterone should now be seen as a combination-like product with oestrogenic and progestogenic properties.*

NICE. 2021a. NG88. Heavy menstrual bleeding: assessment and management. www.nice.org.uk/guidance/ng88

NICE. 2021b. NG12. Suspected cancer: recognition and referral. www.nice.org.uk/guidance/ng12

NICE CKS. 2023. Menorrhagia. https://cks.nice.org.uk/topics/menorrhagia-heavy-menstrual-bleeding/

Stoffel, N., Cercamondi, C., Brittenham, G., et al. 2017. Iron absorption from oral iron supplements given on consecutive versus alternate days and as single morning doses versus twice-daily split dosing in iron-depleted women: two open-label, randomised controlled trials. *Lancet Haematol*; 4(11):e524–33. https://doi.org/10.1016/S2352-3026(17)30182-5 *In iron-depleted women, providing iron supplements daily as divided doses increases serum hepcidin and reduces iron absorption. Providing iron supplements on alternate days and in single doses optimises iron absorption and might be a preferable dosing regimen.*

PAINFUL PERIODS (DYSMENORRHOEA)

Lower abdominal cramping pains, usually before or during the period, are common. However, they can lead to a significant impact on quality of life, including restriction of daily activities and absence from school or work. Period pain can usually be self-managed, but red flags need to be excluded.

History

- Pain: onset in relation to period, severity, type of pain
- Associated symptoms (e.g., nausea/vomiting, headaches, light-headedness, bloating)
- Period history: length, regularity, volume
- What has been tried so far?
- Cu-IUCD[P] (may worsen period pain)
- 🚩 Symptoms suggestive of PID (see Red Flags box in earlier section on Vaginal Discharge)

Examination

- Abdominal examination to feel for any masses such as large fibroids and ascites
- Arrange pelvic examination if PID is suspected (see earlier section on Vaginal Discharge)

Self-care

- Provide information on the condition and treatment options (available at www.womens-health-concern.org/help-and-advice/factsheets)
- Ibuprofen[P] and/or paracetamol to relieve pain. The more potent NSAID naproxen[PBCI] (500 mg initially, then 250 mg up to three times daily for adults) is available OTC for painful periods
- If Cu-IUCD[P] being used then consider removal and using alternative contraception
- Hot water bottle/warm bath
- Massage back and abdomen
- Gentle exercise such as yoga can help relax the muscles and improve the blood supply to the pelvic area
- Smoking cessation advice; smoking is thought to reduce the supply of oxygen to the pelvic area
- Transcutaneous electrical nerve stimulation (TENS) – set to a high frequency (Igwea et al., 2016)

Wom

Prescription

- Consider prescribing an alternative NSAID if OTC treatment is ineffective
  - Naproxen[PBCI] (500 mg initially, then 250 mg up to three times daily for adults). It is not licensed for this indication in children aged <16 years
  - Mefenamic acid[PBI] is an alternative which is licensed in children aged ≥12 (500 mg three times daily)
- Hormonal contraception: there are multiple different types, all of which can help with dysmenorrhoea, although each has its own advantages and disadvantages
- If treatment is unsuccessful or declined, refer to experienced colleague for further assessment. The person may need further investigation, e.g., for endometriosis or fibroids

RED FLAGS

- Systemically unwell/fever on background of abdominal pain/offensive discharge (*possible PID; send urgently to hospital with referral to Gynaecology/Sexual Health*)
- Persistent intermenstrual or post-coital bleeding (*possible STI or carcinoma of cervix; refer to experienced colleague*)
- Palpable abdominal mass/ascites (*possible fibroids or carcinoma of uterus or ovary; USC referral to Gynaecology*)

References

Igwea, S.E., Tabansi-Ochuogu, C.S., and Abaraogu, U.O. 2016. TENS and heat therapy for pain relief and quality of life improvement in individuals with primary dysmenorrhea: a systematic review. *Complement Ther Clin Pract*; 24:86–91. https://doi.org/10.1016/j.ctcp.2016.05.001 *TENS and heat therapy show potential as adjunct remedies in the management of primary dysmenorrhea, but rigorous high-quality trials are still needed.*

NICE CKS. 2018. Dysmenorrhoea. https://cks.nice.org.uk/topics/dysmenorrhoea

INTERMENSTRUAL BLEEDING

Bleeding in between periods is a common presenting symptom and it can lead to significant anxiety. It is important to remember that it can occur with a normal pattern of ovulation, as well as perimenopause. Other possible diagnoses include cervix changes, fibroids, STI, ectopic pregnancy and polycystic ovary syndrome.

History

- Menstrual cycle
- Previous episodes
- Date of last period (primarily to confirm that they are not pregnant early in the consultation; also, vaginal spotting may occur at the time of ovulation)
- Sexual history (see Box 10.1)
- Has the first experience of penetrative sex occurred recently?
- Cervical screening history (usually available from notes)
- Contraceptive method. If on oral contraceptive, then ask about missed pills, vomiting and enzyme-inducing drugs (e.g., carbamazepine, St John's Wort)
- HRT
- ⚑ Fever
- ⚑ Abdominal pain
- ⚑ Offensive discharge
- ⚑ Recent childbirth, termination of pregnancy, gynaecological intervention or miscarriage

Examination

- Not necessary while still bleeding unless red flags present, in which case *send urgently to hospital with referral to Gynaecology/Sexual Health*
- If not currently bleeding:
  - Abdominal examination to feel for any large masses such as fibroids
  - Pelvic examination including bimanual examination (to check for pelvic mass) and speculum examination (to assess cervix for erosion/abnormality/polyp)
  - If pelvic examination is not in your skill set, consider the best referral option for the situation (e.g., Sexual Health Service, GP colleague, suitably qualified and experienced nurse)

Tests

- Consider pregnancy test in women of child-bearing age
- STI screening if available, or refer to local Sexual Health Service

Action

- If missed contraceptive pills/vomiting/diarrhoea, see next section
- If recent first experience of penetrative sex, reassure that some bleeding is common
- If missed HRT tablets, resume tablet taking and make appointment if bleeding persists

RED FLAGS

- Systemically unwell/fever on background of abdominal pain/offensive discharge (*possible PID; send urgently to hospital with referral to Gynaecology/Sexual Health*)
- Recent childbirth, termination, gynaecological intervention or miscarriage (*possible endometritis; send urgently to hospital with referral to Gynaecology*)
- Pregnant (*discuss with Obstetrics/Gynaecology*)
- Abnormal appearance of cervix (*possible cancer, even with a negative smear test; refer to experienced colleague or USC referral to Gynaecology*)

Wom

References

Jarvis, S. 2020. Patient professional article. Intermenstrual and postcoital bleeding. https://patient.info/doctor/intermenstrual-and-postcoital-bleeding

Kovalenko, M., Velji, Z.A., Cheema, J., and Datta, S. 2021. Intermenstrual and postcoital bleeding. *Obstetr Gynaecol Reprod Med*; 31(11):310–16. https://doi.org/10.1016/j.ogrm.2021.09.003

ORAL CONTRACEPTIVES, DIARRHOEA AND VOMITING

The contraceptive effectiveness of oral contraceptives is likely to be reduced by vomiting or severe diarrhoea.

Combined oral contraception pill (COCP):

- Missed-pill instructions (www.nhs.uk/conditions/contraception/miss-combined-pill/) should be followed if vomiting occurs within 3 hours of taking a pill or if severe diarrhoea occurs for >24 hours. If symptoms persist, use a barrier method

Progestogen-only pill (POP):

- If vomiting or severe diarrhoea occurs within a few hours of taking the pill, another pill should be taken as soon as possible. If this replacement pill is not taken within 3 hours (traditional POP), 12 hours (desogestrel POP) or 24 hours (drospirenone POP) of the time at which the original pill was due, missed-pill rules should be followed – see www.nhs.uk/conditions/contraception/the-pill-progestogen-only

Antibiotics and oral contraceptives

The Faculty of Sexual and Reproductive Healthcare (FSRH) issued guidance in 2011 to bring UK clinical practice in line with WHO guidance issued the previous year. In a review of the evidence for an interaction between antibiotics and contraceptives, the FSRH concluded that: 'Overall, the evidence does not support reduced combined oral contraception efficacy with non-enzyme-inducing antibiotics. Additional contraceptive precautions are not required during or after courses of antibiotics that do not induce enzymes. The same advice applies to progestogen-only methods.'

This has remained unchanged in FSRH guidance since 2011. The antibiotics that we recommend for the treatment of minor illness do not induce liver enzymes, so extra contraceptive precautions are not necessary.

Reference

FSRH, and the Royal College of Obstetricians and Gynaecologists (RCOG). 2022. Drug interactions with hormonal contraception. www.fsrh.org/documents/ceu-clinical-guidance-drug-interactions-with-hormonal/

EMERGENCY CONTRACEPTION (EC)

History

- If aged <16, check if Fraser competent, ability to consent to sex and the age of partner (see Box 10.3)
- Date of last period
- Time since unprotected sexual intercourse (UPSI)
- Sexual history (see Box 10.1)
- Risk of STI (if EC is needed, the woman is at some risk of an STI)
- Any previous UPSI in this cycle (may render oral treatment ineffective; consider Cu-IUCD[P])
- Any previous EC in this cycle
- Usual contraceptive method and any problems, e.g., missed pills, late injection
- Ongoing need for contraception
- On enzyme-inducing medication (e.g., carbamazepine, phenytoin, St John's Wort)
- Breastfeeding
- Past history of porphyria or asthma (this is relevant to prescribing)
- ⚑ Risk of having had non-consensual sexual intercourse

BOX 10.3 LEGAL ISSUES AROUND PROVIDING EMERGENCY CONTRACEPTION TO THOSE AGED <16

In the UK, the legal age of consent to sexual activity is 16. One in three young people have had sexual intercourse before the age of 16, but sexual activity under the age of consent is an offence, even if consensual. Offences are considered more serious (statutory rape) when the person is younger than 13. In England and Wales, it is legal to provide contraceptive advice and treatment to young people without parental consent, provided that the practitioner is satisfied that the Fraser criteria for competence are met:

- The young person understands the practitioner's advice
- The young person cannot be persuaded to inform their parents or will not allow the practitioner to inform the parents that contraceptive advice has been sought
- The young person is likely to begin or to continue having intercourse with or without contraceptive treatment
- Unless they receive contraceptive advice or treatment, the young person's physical or mental health (or both) are likely to suffer
- The young person's best interest requires the practitioner to give contraceptive advice or treatment (or both) without parental consent

All available methods of emergency contraception should be offered, regardless of age, as the risk of an unwanted pregnancy outweighs that of the contraceptive.

Always consider whether there are possible safeguarding issues – it is important to be assured that sex has been consensual and is not occurring in an abusive or incestuous relationship. If it is suspected that force has been used or that sexual abuse has occurred, you have a duty to follow national and local safeguarding procedures.

Reference

FSRH. 2019. FSRH clinical guidance: contraceptive choices for young people. www.fsrh.org/ standards-and-guidance/documents/cec-ceu-guidance-young-people-mar-2010/

Self-care
Indication for EC

- EC is advised following intercourse when:
  - No contraception has been used *or*
  - A barrier contraceptive failed *or*
  - The COCP is used but would be less effective because two or more pills were missed (>48 hours late in week 1) *or*
  - The POP is used but would be less effective because it has been >27 hours since the last pill (>36 hours late for desogestrel-only pill) *or*
  - The injectable progestogen is likely to be less effective as the last injection of medroxyprogesterone acetate was ≥14 weeks ago
- If there has been a recent pregnancy, there must be ≥21 days since childbirth or ≥5 days since termination of pregnancy/miscarriage for EC to be indicated
- Different EC methods have different rates of success in preventing pregnancy (Table 10.3)
- An emergency Cu-IUCD[P] is the most reliable option for EC, about 20 times more effective than the oral methods. It provides ongoing contraception and can be fitted up to day 19 of a 28-day cycle
- Oral EC is provided free of charge by Sexual Health Services and general practices, also by all pharmacies in Scotland and Wales and some pharmacies in England and Northern Ireland
- Women aged ≥16 can obtain levonorgestrel[P] and ulipristal[PB] OTC from most UK pharmacies, Contraceptive or Sexual Health services, and other NHS services (may be free of charge – see www.nhs.uk/conditions/contraception/where-can-i-get-emergency-contraception/)
- Oral EC may cause nausea. Seek help if vomiting within 2 hours of taking levonorgestrel[P] or 3 hours of taking ulipristal[PB] (see later section on Cautions)

Table 10.3 Effectiveness of different EC methods in 1000 women at risk (data from nhs.uk)

	No EC	Levonorgestrel	Ulipristal	Copper IUCD
Pregnancies	80	26	18	1

Advice

- Oral EC is unlikely to be effective if taken after ovulation. See FSRH (2020) for more information and a useful algorithm
- After taking EC, many women ovulate later in the cycle. They must be advised of the need for ongoing contraception
- Use condoms, or do not have penetrative sex, until next period
- The next period may be early or late
- Pregnancy test is recommended if next period more than 1 week late
- If pregnancy occurs despite EC, there is no known adverse effect on fetus if pregnancy occurs, but the risk of ectopic pregnancy is possibly increased. Seek advice if lower abdominal pain (different from usual period pain) or period is lighter than usual
- Consider long-term contraception, STI screening and safe-sex advice

Action

- If Cu-IUCD[P] is preferred but it is not possible to provide this immediately:
  - Refer to another service that can provide this
  - Prescribe oral EC to be used straight away (to cover the possibility that the Cu-IUCD[P] cannot be inserted, or the person changes their mind)
- If Cu-IUCD[P] is declined:
  - Ulipristal[PB] 30 mg, within 120 hours (5 days) of UPSI. Avoid if there is a history of severe asthma treated with oral steroids
  - Levonorgestrel[P] 1.5 mg, preferably within 12 hours of UPSI, but no later than 72 hours (3 days). Consider higher dose of 3 mg if weight >70 kg or BMI >26 kg/m2 (*unlicensed indication*). Avoid if there is a history of ectopic pregnancy or porphyria
- The FSRH guideline states that EC providers should advise women that ulipristal[PB] has been demonstrated to be more effective than levonorgestrel[P] (see Table 10.3)
- For women who have used enzyme-inducing drugs in the past 4 weeks and need EC, a Cu-IUCD[P] should be considered. Taking a double dose of levonorgestrel (3 mg) is an option for women who are unable or unwilling to use a Cu-IUCD[P]. A double dose of ulipristal[PB] is **not** recommended
- Advise that the oral EC dose should be taken as soon as possible, as the earlier it is taken, the more effective it is
- Also offer/refer to appropriate colleague for 'quick start' of a long-term method of contraception, but remember that the effect of ulipristal[PB] may be reduced if the woman takes progestogen (including COCP) in the next 5 days

Cautions

- If they vomit within 2 hours of taking EC, give a replacement prescription, and consider offering domperidone[PIQ], 10 mg, to be taken 30 minutes before EC dose
- For complex problems, contact the National Sexual Health Helpline at 0300 123 7123 (Mon–Fri, 9 a.m.–8 p.m.)

References

FSRH. 2020. CEU clinical guidance: emergency contraception.
      www.fsrh.org/documents/ceu-clinical-guidance-emergency-contraception-march-2017/
NHS. 2022. How effective is emergency contraception?
      www.nhs.uk/conditions/contraception/how-effective-emergency-contraception/

DELAYING A PERIOD

A woman whose period is due when she is on holiday, or taking part in a religious or sporting event, may request medication to delay their period. The traditional and licensed treatment is norethisterone[P] 5 mg three times daily, started 3 days before the period is expected to begin. A light period should occur 2–3 days after stopping the course. This may also reset the timing of the menstrual cycle and therefore affect the date of the next period.

Women should be warned about possible side effects, including irregularities in menstrual cycle, breast tenderness, nausea, headache and disturbances in mood and sex drive. Although norethisterone[P] is a progestogen, it is metabolised to ethinyloestradiol, and the higher doses used to delay a period carry an increased risk of VTE comparable to that of the COCP.

Women who request medication to delay a period should therefore be assessed in the same way as those wishing to start the COCP; if at increased risk of VTE, they should instead be prescribed medroxyprogesterone acetate[PC], 10 mg three times daily (*unlicensed indication*). Neither of these medicines are contraceptive at these doses. Flights of >4 hours double the risk of VTE, but the absolute risk is low: one event per 6000 flights.

If a woman is already taking the COCP, their withdrawal bleed may be delayed by omitting the pill-free interval and moving straight on to the next pill packet, but if she is taking a type that contains placebo tablets (i.e., an every day pack), then she will need preparation-specific advice.

References

Izadi, M., Alemzadeh-Ansari, M., Kazemisaleh, D., et al. 2014. Venous thromboembolism following travel. *Int J Travel Med Glob Health*; 2(1):23–30. www.ijtmgh.com/article_33271_686fb55f40959626391cd33b0901c577.pdf

Mansour, D. 2012. Safer prescribing of therapeutic norethisterone for women at risk of venous thromboembolism. *J Fam Plann Reprod Health Care*; 38(3):148. https://doi.org/10.1136/jfprhc-2012-100345

Mansour, D. 2017. Postponing menstruation: choices and concerns. *J Fam Plann Reprod Health Care*; 43(2):160. https://doi.org/10.1136/jfprhc-2016-101438 *Consider carefully the potential VTE risks associated with COCs and norethisterone, especially if long-haul flights or prolonged periods of immobility on coaches or in cars are planned.*

NICE CKS. 2018. DVT prevention for travellers. https://cks.nice.org.uk/topics/dvt-prevention-for-travellers/

MASTITIS

Mastitis is defined as inflammation of the breast with or without infection. In lactating women, blocked milk flow is the main cause; milk leaks into the surrounding tissues, where cytokines cause inflammation. If milk products pass into the bloodstream, they can produce malaise and fever, even if there is no infection. Without effective milk drainage, staphylococcal infection is likely to develop, which may lead to abscess formation.

In non-lactating women, smokers are at highest risk, and the range of possible bacterial infections is wider.

History

- Lactating
- Smoking history
- Fever/malaise/flu-like illness
- Location of pain and character
- Redness of breast
- Is this recurrent?
- Was onset while in hospital? (If so, culture of breast milk would be indicated)
- Nipple discharge
- 🚩 Immunosuppressed

Examination

- Temperature
- Heart rate
- Respiratory rate
- BP

Wom

- Record area of redness – often wedge-shaped
- Examine nipples for inflammation or visible discharge
- 🚩 Check for any suggestion of an abscess (red, fluctuant lump)

Tests

- Breast milk culture if: severe or recurrent, no response to antibiotics within 2 days, hospital-acquired infection or deep burning pain

Self-care

- If lactating:
  - See a breastfeeding advisor to identify and manage predisposing factors such as poor infant attachment, nipple damage and smoking
  - Continue to breastfeed from both sides, offering the affected side first. Reassure that the milk from the affected side will not harm the infant
  - Express any remaining milk
- Ibuprofen[P] or paracetamol to relieve pain
- Treat any nipple problem (e.g., *Candida*)
- Warm compress, warm bath or shower
- Rest (as much as a newborn/infant allows)
- Do not wear a bra at night
- Seek further advice if worsening or not improving after 48 hours

Action

It is not possible to differentiate clinically between infectious and non-infectious mastitis. An infection is more likely if there is a nipple fissure that is infected, or the symptoms do not improve within 24 hours despite effective milk removal in a lactating woman, or the breast milk culture is positive (i.e., grows bacteria)

Antibiotic treatment

 BOX 10.4 ANTIBIOTICS FOR MASTITIS

Prescribe an antibiotic if:

- Severe symptoms
- Immunosuppressed (including diabetes)
- Yellow discharge from nipple
- Not improving within 24 hours despite effective milk removal (consider a delayed prescription)

A course of antibiotic treatment for mastitis (see Box 10.4) should be for **10–14 days**.

- If lactating:
  - Flucloxacillin, 500 mg four times daily *or*
  - If allergic to penicillin and pregnant/postpartum, erythromycin[Q] is recommended (250–500 mg four times daily), otherwise use clarithromycin[PIQ] (500 mg three times daily)
- If not lactating:
  - Co-amoxiclav, 500/125 mg three times daily *or*
  - If allergic to penicillin use metronidazole[Q] (400 mg three times daily) and clarithromycin[PIQ] (500 mg three times daily) or if pregnant/ postpartum, erythromycin (250-500 mg four times daily)

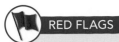

RED FLAGS

- Signs of sepsis or immunosuppressed (*admit urgently under Surgical*)
- Abscess suspected (*ultrasound and aspiration may be needed; admit urgently under Surgical*)
- Underlying mass (*possible breast cancer; USC referral to Breast Clinic*)

References

Health Service Executive. Mastitis. Fact sheet for health care professionals. www.hse.ie/file-library/mastitis-factsheet-for-healthcare-professionals.pdf

NICE CKS. 2023. Mastitis and breast abscess. https://cks.nice.org.uk/topics/mastitis-breast-abscess/

NIPPLE PAIN

Pain during breastfeeding is usually due to problems with attachment of the baby to the breast.

History

- One or both sides affected
- Severity, type and timing of pain
- Use of nipple shield
- Does baby have tongue tie, oral thrush or nappy rash?
- Does nipple blanch during feeds or when it is cold? If so, does it become red afterwards?
- Discharge from nipple

Examination

- Inverted nipples
- Loss of colour in the nipples or areola
- Pink or red colour, flaking, shininess, crusting
- Fissure

Possible causes and their treatment

- Sore and fissured nipples may be due to friction and poor positioning (most common)
  - Problems usually start early; pain occurs during feed and may be severe
  - Self-care: see breastfeeding advisor
- Candidal infection
  - Usually bilateral
  - Delayed until a few weeks after childbirth, unless woman has had recent *Candida* infection
  - Burning and itching
  - Nipples appear pale, fissured or normal
  - Self-care: apply miconazole[1] 2% cream to nipples after each feed for 2 weeks; wipe away any remaining cream before next feed
  - Treat baby with miconazole[1] oral gel (see section on Oral Candidiasis [Thrush] in Chapter 5)
- Blocked duct – small white, yellow or clear spot (bleb) about 1 mm in diameter at the end of the nipple
  - Self-care: bath and rub area with a warm, damp towel; feed from the affected breast frequently; use heat packs for symptom relief; gentle massage of the breast (using a firm movement towards the nipple) while the baby is feeding, to help relieve the obstruction
- Bacterial infection
  - Yellow discharge from nipple
  - Persistent fissure

Wom

- Prescription: topical sodium fusidate 2% (three times daily, apply after feeds, for 7 days) after each feed for 7 days. If severe, prescribe oral flucloxacillin (500 mg four times daily for adults for 5–7 days) or, if allergic to penicillin, clarithromycin[PIO] (500 mg twice daily for adults for 5–7 days)
- Eczema
  - Burning and itching
  - Redness, vesicles, crusting or scaling
  - Base of nipple may be unaffected
  - Self-care: consider allergy to creams or new food given to baby. Avoid using soap and shower gel. Apply hydrocortisone or Eumovate cream twice daily after feeds until recovered; wipe away any remaining cream before next feed. Paraffin-based ointments are not recommended (LactMed, 2021)
- Raynaud's disease of nipple
  - Nipple may blanch during feed or when cold, then become red
  - Intermittent pain persists after feeding, when cold and may be severe
  - Self-care: keep warm. Avoid smoking and caffeine
  - Prescription: nifedipine[PC] capsules, 5 mg three times a day for 2 weeks (*unlicensed indication*). May be continued if necessary

RED FLAG

- Unilateral eczema not responding to treatment (*possible breast cancer; USC referral to Breast Clinic*)

References

LactMed. 2021. Mineral oil. www.ncbi.nlm.nih.gov/books/NBK501885/

NICE CKS. 2022. Breastfeeding problems. https://cks.nice.org.uk/topics/breastfeeding-problems/

CHAPTER 11

Mental health

There is a complex, two-way relationship between physical and psychological wellbeing. Something affecting one will often result in a change in the other, with symptoms potentially worsened or improved accordingly. A diagnosis of depression or anxiety disorder has indeed been shown to have an association with greater presentation rates of minor illnesses – this could relate to generally higher attendance rates, altered illness behaviour or other factors affecting susceptibility to illness.

Mental health problems are very common; one in four adults experiences at least one diagnosable mental health problem every year. A significant proportion of people presenting with minor illness will therefore also have mental health problems. These may be already known or as yet undiagnosed. People may be more inclined to discuss their physical symptoms than those directly relating to mental health.

Non-verbal cues can tell you a lot, but might only be picked up face-to-face. Make sure to ask about how a minor illness is affecting someone and then follow on with enquiries about their concerns and worries. This can give some insight into their current psychological wellbeing. However, also make sure to address their minor illness, or at least make clear that you will be addressing it, before you wade deeply into further enquiry about their mental health; it may otherwise be misconstrued as not taking the physical symptoms seriously or inadvertently suggesting 'it's all in their head'.

You do not need to be an expert in mental health to pick up problems, and it is not necessary to make a definite diagnosis during a single contact in order to provide help. The person may tell you about particular stressors or exacerbating factors; often these relate to relationships, work, finances or housing, for which you may be able to suggest appropriate local or national services. Their ability to cope may be improved by encouraging them to exercise (outdoors if possible) and to learn techniques that enable them to relax.

DEPRESSION

This is a very common condition in which physical or cognitive symptoms, such as abdominal pains, fatigue or forgetfulness, may present initially. It may be an underlying problem or contributor in any consultation. Any age group can be affected; the diagnosis is easily overlooked in older people, although it is often the underlying cause of memory disturbance. Depression in children requires specialist management.

There is ongoing debate about the causes of depression. One theory, stemming from evolutionary psychology (see http://journals.sagepub.com/home/evp), suggests that depression may represent a psychological adaptation in response to life circumstances. Although not established, considering such an explanation may be more helpful to the person with depression than assuming that it is a disease without clear pathophysiology; there is an association between depression and prior stressful life events, especially in childhood (World Health Organization, 2023).

In someone not known to have depression (particularly if they are consulting for an issue ostensibly unrelated to their mental health), a practitioner may initially screen for depression through asking a few simple questions. NICE suggests considering the first two questions from the Patient Health Questionnaire 9 (PHQ-9), asking about 'often being bothered by feeling down, depressed or hopeless' and 'often being bothered by having little interest or pleasure in doing things' within the last month; a 'yes' answer to either should prompt further assessment. These questions have a high sensitivity but less impressive specificity (resulting in false-positives), perhaps due to being closed, somewhat leading enquiries. You may prefer to ask open questions such as 'what are you looking forward to?'

History

Active, empathetic listening is of utmost importance. You may be the first to hear the person's story.

- How long have they felt low?
- Any specific reason or trigger identified (e.g., bereavement, childbirth, relationship difficulties, financial worries, stress at work)
- Core symptoms: feelings of sadness, lack of interest/enjoyment in life – ask 'What are you looking forward to?'

MHe

- Appetite (overeating or undereating) or weight changes
- Sleep disturbance/fatigue (early morning waking is typically described in depression)
- Feelings of worthlessness or guilt
- Loss of concentration/poor memory
- Ask 'How will you know when you're better? What will you be doing that you aren't doing now?'
- Previous episodes and treatment, and what helped them to resolve their problems
- Medication, alcohol intake, recreational drugs
- Risk factors (e.g., previous history of mental health problems, chronic illness, dementia)
- Adequacy of social support, living conditions
- 🚩 Safeguarding issues
- 🚩 Recent childbirth
- 🚩 Thoughts of death
  - Ask 'Have you ever felt that life wasn't worth living?' (passive suicidal ideation)
  - If any such thoughts, ask 'Have you ever felt like ending your own life' (active suicidal ideation) and, if so, 'What has stopped you from acting upon this?' (protective factors)
  - Having a plan for how they would end their life suggests that they are at higher risk
  - Mental health problems are three times more common in women than men, but 74% of the suicides in the UK in 2021 were in men (Mental Health Foundation, 2023)
  - Other risk factors for suicide include substance misuse, recent stressful life event (e.g., bereavement, loss of job, divorce), exposure to another person's suicide, personal/family history of suicide attempts

Examination

- Note their appearance – any signs of self-neglect?
- Speech volume and tone
- Observe body language, especially moist eyes, trembling lower lip, avoiding eye contact

Test

- Ask them to complete the PHQ-9 (https://patient.info/doctor/patient-health-questionnaire-phq-9). For this test, a cut-off of ≥10 has been shown to have the optimal combined sensitivity and specificity in screening for depression (Levis et al., 2019)

Self-care

- Self-referral for psychological therapy is available in most areas through NHS Talking Therapies services. These tend to offer a range of both group-based and individual interventions including cognitive behavioural therapy (CBT)
- Consider practical problem-solving, for example change of job – a clinician may help the person to navigate this but should avoid being directive
- Daily exercise, especially walking outdoors with a relative, friend or dog, is likely to help (Heissel et al., 2023)
- Try to resume activities previously enjoyed. The cycle of poor motivation leading to abandoning previously enjoyable activities, which then further compounds low mood and poor motivation, is not conducive to recovery
- Consider learning relaxation techniques. These may include mindfulness and meditation
- If not having enough restful sleep per night (they should be the judge of this), advise regarding 'sleep hygiene' measures (see later section on Insomnia)
- Ensure a regular intake of healthy food (omega-3 supplements have been suggested as a potential treatment for depression but high-quality real-world evidence is lacking)
- Avoid excessive caffeine
- If alcohol and substance misuse are contributing, self-refer to the appropriate service
- Self-help resources (see later section on Self-care Resources for Mental Health) – such as self-help CBT and mental wellbeing tips on the NHS website (www.nhs.uk/every-mind-matters/)

- Living Life to the Full (https://llttf.com/) is a free online self-help programme designed to help people with depression and anxiety. It teaches skills based on CBT
- Note that NICE specifically states not to recommend OTC St John's wort. Although there is reasonable evidence for its effectiveness, there is a lack of standardisation of products and a propensity for drug interactions
- Many Primary Care Networks (PCNs) have social prescribers; they can provide support with non-clinical issues such as debt, employment and housing, as well as opportunities for social connections and interactions (such as singing or gardening groups)

Action

Some actions will be universally applicable, whereas others will likely depend on the severity of depression. NICE recommends different approaches for people with less severe depression (PHQ-9 score <16) and more severe depression (PHQ-9 score ≥16).

For all

- Empathise and be positive about recovery
- If applicable, remind them that they have already learnt coping strategies that have previously helped them
- If taking regular medication, check side effects in the BNF. Benzodiazepines, steroids, simvastatin, opioids such as codeine, varenicline (Champix, used for smoking cessation), propranolol, anticonvulsants and hormonal medications (including contraceptives) are some of the drugs that may precipitate depression
- If experiencing work-related stress, would time off, limited duties or reduced hours help? Have they considered looking for a new job?
- The DVLA states that the person should notify them and should not drive if they have severe anxiety or depression with 'significant memory or concentration problems, agitation, behavioural disturbance or suicidal thoughts'
- Arrange a follow-up review after 2–4 weeks with a suitably competent and experienced practitioner. This should be earlier if any of the following: the person is aged <25, has more severe depression, postnatal depression or suicidal ideation

If less severe depression (PHQ-9 score <16)

- NICE does not recommend routinely offering an antidepressant medication as first-line treatment, but this can be used if the person wishes. If this is the case, *refer to an experienced colleague*
- Although it is recommended that the treatment choice should be matched to clinical needs and preferences, NICE has described a hierarchy of treatment options: counselling is far down the list, along with antidepressant medication; psychological therapies such as CBT or behavioural activation are positioned with greater preference
- In practice, it is not necessary to have a detailed understanding of the different types of talking therapy available locally, although awareness of local waiting times can be helpful. The role of the primary care practitioner is not to help choose the most appropriate talking therapy but to direct to the NHS Talking Therapies service (through referral or self-referral) so that a specialist practitioner can have this discussion

If more severe depression (PHQ-9 score ≥16)

- NICE describes a different hierarchy of treatment options for severe depression, although the choice should still be matched with clinical needs and the person's preferences. The preferred option is individual CBT with an antidepressant. Positioned lower in order of preference is individual CBT without an antidepressant, followed by individual behavioural activation and antidepressant medication alone
- In practice, antidepressants are suitable for use first-line (particularly in combination with a referral/self-referral to an appropriate service for psychological support)
- If the person wants to start an antidepressant, *refer to an experienced colleague* for initiation of a selective serotonin reuptake inhibitor (SSRI) or serotonin and norepinephrine reuptake inhibitor (SNRI)
  - Note that most antidepressants require 2–4 weeks before positive effects are seen
  - They are not addictive, but withdrawal symptoms are common if they are not appropriately weaned off; some antidepressants are more prone to causing these than others (e.g., stopping fluoxetine has a low risk of withdrawal due to both the drug and its active metabolites having long half-lives)
  - Safety-netting advice about side effects and potential for increased suicidal ideation, particularly in the first few weeks of treatment, is important

MHe

- Psychological therapies would usually be accessed through the local NHS Talking Therapies service (which offers self-referral). Particularly if motivation is impaired, it may be better to send a referral rather than relying on self-referral (but obtain consent first)
- Local NHS Talking Therapies services may be distinct from locally-commissioned specialist mental health services and do not usually accept referrals (or self-referral) for people whom they consider to be too high risk or whose needs are too complex (e.g., those with active suicidal ideation). If so, a referral to specialist mental health services may be necessary instead
- Occasionally, neither NHS Talking Therapies services nor specialist mental health services consider that a person is appropriate for them (being too high risk/complex for the former and insufficiently high risk/complex for the latter); the Community Mental Health Framework in England now seeks to address this. If the situation arises, *refer to an experienced colleague*

 RED FLAGS

- Recent childbirth (*suspect postnatal depression; consider using Edinburgh Postnatal Depression Scale and refer to experienced colleague. Specialist support may also be available through the local Health Visitor Team*)
- If suicidal thoughts are expressed, an urgent risk assessment should be made by an experienced colleague on whether to offer an immediate referral to a Crisis Team/A&E:
  - Active suicidal ideation (thoughts about harming oneself) suggests higher risk than passive suicidal ideation (thoughts of life not being worth living), particularly if associated with plans for how it would be done
  - If the person declines referral and is considered to have mental capacity, *the experienced colleague should give contact details of the local Urgent Mental Health Helpline (111, option 2) and the Samaritans (currently 116 123, www.samaritans.org) and arrange appropriate follow-up*

References

Apaydin, E.A., Maher, A.R., Shanman, R., et al. 2016. A systematic review of St. John's wort for major depressive disorder. *Syst Rev*; 5(1):148. https://doi.org/10.1186/s13643-016-0325-2 *St John's wort monotherapy for mild and moderate depression is superior to placebo in improving depression symptoms and not significantly different from antidepressant medication. However, evidence of heterogeneity and a lack of research on severe depression reduce the quality of the evidence. There is also a risk of drug interactions.*

Appleton, K.M., Voyias, P.D., Sallis, H.M., et al. 2021. Omega-3 fatty acids for depression in adults. *Cochrane Database Syst Rev*; 11:CD004692. https://doi.org/10.1002/14651858.CD004692.pub5 *This Cochrane review concluded that more evidence is required before omega-3 fatty acids can be recommended to help treat depression.*

Driver and Vehicle Licensing Agency (DVLA). 2022. Assessing fitness to drive – a guide for medical professionals. https://assets.publishing.service.gov.uk/government/uploads/system/uploads/attachment_data/file/1084397/assessing-fitness-to-drive-may-2022.pdf

Hartman, T.O., van Rijswijk, E., van Ravesteijn, H., et al. 2008. Mental health problems and the presentation of minor illnesses: data from a 30-year follow-up in general practice. *Eur J Gen Pract*; 14(Supp. 1):38–43. https://doi.org/10.1080/13814780802436150 *An interesting study looking at presentation rates for minor illness and association with depression and anxiety.*

Heissel, A., Heinen, D., Brokmeier L.L., et al. 2023. Exercise as medicine for depressive symptoms? A systematic review and meta-analysis with meta-regression. *Br J Sports Med*; 57:1049–1057. http://dx.doi.org/10.1136/bjsports-2022-106282 *Exercise is efficacious in treating depression and depressive symptom.*

Levis, B., Benedetti, A., and Thombs, B.D. 2019. Accuracy of Patient Health Questionnaire-9 (PHQ-9) for screening to detect major depression: individual participant data meta-analysis. *BMJ*; 365:l1476. https://doi.org/10.1136/bmj.l1476

Mental Health Foundation. 2023. www.mentalhealth.org.uk/

NHS England. 2019. The Community Mental Health Framework for adults and older adults. www.england.nhs.uk/wp-content/uploads/2019/09/community-mental-health-framework-for-adults-and-older-adults.pdf

NHS England. 2023. Adult and older adult mental health. www.england.nhs.uk/mental-health/adults/

NICE. 2022. NG222. Depression in adults: treatment and management. www.nice.org.uk/guidance/NG222

World Health Organization. 2023. Tackling adverse childhood experiences; state of the art and options for action. www.ljmu.ac.uk/-/media/phi-reports/pdf/2023-01-state-of-the-art-report-eng.pdf

ANXIETY

There is often significant overlap between anxiety and depression. However, some people can have marked symptoms of anxiety without other mood disturbance. Be mindful of the possibility of anxiety in people who attend frequently with physical symptoms such as insomnia, headaches, aches and pains, gastrointestinal symptoms or palpitations. Note that anxiety also frequently co-exists with physical health conditions and can exacerbate the experience and impact of associated symptoms (e.g., shortness of breath in COPD).

Similar to its recommendation for screening for depression, NICE suggests considering the first two questions from the validated Generalized Anxiety Disorder (GAD-7) questionnaire to identify possible anxiety disorders. This involves enquiring about how often the person has been bothered by 'feeling nervous, anxious or on edge' and 'not being able to stop or control worrying' within the last 2 weeks, with each question scoring 0 for not at all, 1 for several days, 2 for more than half the days, 3 for nearly every day. A cut-off of ≥3 has been shown to have good sensitivity and specificity for anxiety disorders (particularly generalised anxiety); if this threshold is met, NICE recommends that more detailed assessment should then follow.

Some people with anxiety may not report worry or psychological distress, instead presenting solely with physical symptoms. If suspecting anxiety, then continue to assess them as below, but it is usually a good idea to explore and assess their physical symptoms first (or at least concurrently). Attributing experienced physical symptoms to anxiety without properly assessing those symptoms, whatever their underlying cause, is unlikely to help and may make matters worse. Before requesting investigations, it is helpful to make clear that you expect the results to be normal. Otherwise the wait for results may also exacerbate anxiety.

History

Remember to use active, empathetic listening. Disclosing anxiety and phobias (which are often irrational in nature) can be much more difficult for people than talking about physical symptoms – be careful not to appear to pass any judgement or to trivialise the problem.

- Why have they come? Why today?
- How long has it been a problem?
- What, if anything, do they tend to worry about?
- Recent problems: at work, at home, with family or partner, financial
- Symptoms: feeling on edge or restless, dizziness, tiredness, palpitations, dry mouth, muscle tension, headaches, sweating, weight loss, urinary frequency, sleep disturbance, difficulty concentrating, irritability
- How is it affecting them? Has it impacted their family life, social activities or work?
- Is there co-existent depression? Ask about suicidal ideation (see earlier section on Depression and Red Flags box)
- Panic attacks
- Previous mental health problems and how they resolved them
- Potentially causative medication (e.g., levothyroxine [usually only if dose is excessive], decongestants, salbutamol, theophylline, corticosteroids)
- Caffeine, alcohol, recreational drugs

Examination

- Observe body language and look for tremor
- Consider checking heart rate

Tests

- Consider thyroid function tests, if not recently done
- Consider asking the person to complete the GAD-7 questionnaire to gauge severity of anxiety symptoms and monitor impact of any intervention (https://patient.info/doctor/generalised-anxiety-disorder-assessment-gad-7)

Self-care

- Self-referral for psychological therapy is available through NHS Talking Therapies services. These tend to offer a range of both group-based and individual interventions including CBT
- Consider practical problem-solving, for example a change of job

MHe

- Daily exercise, especially walking outdoors with a relative, friend or dog, can help
- Relaxation exercises or training (e.g., hypnotherapy) can be helpful; also yoga, tai chi, mindfulness, meditation, reading and listening to relaxing music
- Reduce or stop intake of caffeine, alcohol and recreational drugs
- Recommend self-help books and websites (see section at the end of this chapter)
- Living Life to the Full (https://llttf.com) is a free online self-help programme designed to help people with depression and anxiety. It teaches skills based on CBT
- Many PCNs have social prescribers; they can provide support with non-clinical issues such as debt, employment and housing, as well as opportunities for social connections and interactions (e.g., singing or gardening groups)

Action

- Empathise and be positive about recovery
- If panic attacks are reported, strongly reassure that these will not cause physical harm such as a heart attack
- If experiencing work-related stress, would time off, limited duties or reduced hours help? Have they considered looking for a new job?
- Recommend restorative sleep techniques (see later section on Insomnia)
- Remind the person of any previously learnt coping strategies that have helped them
- NICE recommends a stepped-approach to psychological therapy – usually the NHS Talking Therapies service will go through the details of available options and step up to offer more intensive interventions as necessary. It can be accessed through self-referral or direct referral from a healthcare practitioner
- If the person wants to start medication, *refer to experienced colleague* for initiation of an SSRI
- Do not routinely prescribe benzodiazepines for anxiety. They are addictive and will not be helpful in the long term. The possible exception is for short-term use (e.g., for up to 2 weeks) in a crisis or if there are severe symptoms and the person is planning to start an SSRI (which may worsen symptoms initially). If such a prescription might be appropriate, *refer to an experienced colleague*

RED FLAGS

- Chest pains on exertion (*suggests ischaemic heart disease; refer to experienced colleague*)
- Weight loss, heat intolerance, tachycardia (*suggests hyperthyroidism; check thyroid function blood test urgently*)
- Episodic pattern to symptoms, accompanied by high BP, headaches, palpitations (*may need assessment for rare adrenaline-secreting tumour [phaeochromocytoma]; refer to experienced colleague*)

Reference

Haftgoli, N., Favrat, B., Verdon, F., et al. 2010. Patients presenting with somatic complaints in general practice: depression, anxiety and somatoform disorders are frequent and associated with psychosocial stressors. *BMC Fam Pract*; 11(1):67. https://doi.org/10.1186/1471-2296-11-67 *A study looking at the presentation of mental health conditions with physical symptoms.*

NICE. 2020a. CG113. Generalised anxiety disorder in adults: management in primary, secondary and community care. www.nice.org.uk/guidance/cg113

NICE. 2020b. CG123. Common mental health problems: identification and pathways to care. www.nice.org.uk/guidance/cg123

NICE CKS. 2023. Generalized anxiety disorder. https://cks.nice.org.uk/topics/generalized-anxiety-disorder/

Romanazzo, S., Mansueto, G., and Cosci, F. 2022. Anxiety in the medically ill: a systematic review of the literature. *Front Psychiatry*; 13:873126. https://doi.org/10.3389/fpsyt.2022.873126 *A review looking at co-existent anxiety in people with physical health conditions.*

Sapra, A., Bhandari, P., Sharma, S., et al. 2020. Using Generalized Anxiety Disorder-2 (GAD-2) and GAD-7 in a primary care setting. *Cureus*; 12(5). https://doi:10.7759/cureus.8224 *Details the sensitivity and specificity for the screening and assessment questions suggested by NICE.*

HYPERVENTILATION

Over-breathing lowers the blood carbon dioxide level. This reduces the transfer of oxygen to the brain, which may cause dizziness, headache or fainting, and disturbs blood chemistry making it more alkaline and lower in free ionised potassium and calcium, in turn leading to paraesthesia (tingling or 'pins and needles') and muscle spasms.

History

- Episodes of being 'unable to take a deep enough breath'
- Absence of other respiratory symptoms, e.g., cough
- Previous episodes
- Precipitating psychosocial stress
- Chest discomfort
- Tingling around mouth, hands and feet
- In severe cases, spasm of hands and feet (tetany)
- Agoraphobia and panic disorder (up to 50% hyperventilate)
- Asthma (up to 30% hyperventilate)

Examination (to exclude respiratory disease)

- Observe respiration – often irregular or sighing, using upper chest muscles
- Note the ratio of inspiration time to expiration time:
  - In normal breathing, it is usually about 1:2
  - In asthma, expiration may be prolonged and through pursed lips
  - In hyperventilation, inspiration may be more energetic and expiration is not prolonged
- Examine chest:
  - Check percussion and that breath sounds are equal on both sides (to exclude pneumothorax)
  - Check for wheeze (suggests asthma)
- Record peak flow – should be normal (if low, see section on Asthma in Chapter 3)

Test

- Pulse oximetry to demonstrate to the person that their oxygen level is normal, i.e., $\geq 95\%$ (in hyperventilation, the level may actually be higher than normal for them, at 99%–100%)

Action

- Explain the problem
- If relevant to concerns, reassure that tingling in arms and hands is not a symptom of a heart attack
- If acute, ask them to breathe slowly in and out of a paper bag, or put their hands on their head to splint the upper chest
- Show them how to breathe using the diaphragm
- Suggest yoga (breathing exercises and relaxation are both likely to be helpful)
- Relaxation exercises/hypnotherapy may lower the underlying emotional arousal

References

Ito, H., Yokoyama, I., Iida, H., et al. 2000. Regional differences in cerebral vascular response to $PaCO_2$ changes in humans measured by positron emission tomography. *J Cereb Blood Flow Metab*; 20(8):1264–70. https://doi.org/10.1097/00004647-200008000-00011 *Evidence that low carbon dioxide levels reduce oxygen uptake by the brain.*

Patient.info. 2021. Hyperventilation. https://patient.info/doctor/hyperventilation

MHe

INSOMNIA

Insomnia is common and subjective. Some people feel rested with 5 hours of sleep a night, whereas others need 9 hours or more. The amount of sleep required tends to lessen with age and with lower activity levels. A 'good night's sleep' is not the same for everyone.

Despite popular perception, there is no compelling evidence to suggest that people who feel rested after naturally sleeping for relatively short periods (e.g., 5 hours), without having been prematurely woken, should be advised to sleep more. Though observational studies have shown around 7 hours of sleep to be associated with better cognition and mental health in people of middle to older age, this does not yet represent a target that all should aspire to; there is no evidence that outcomes improve for naturally shorter sleepers by prolonging sleep or for naturally longer sleepers through curtailment.

Almost everyone can have periods of insomnia at some stage. Tiredness is often considered the enemy, but building up a healthy level of tiredness over the course of a day can promote better sleep at night. The approach to managing insomnia largely relates to how long it has been a problem. A diagnosis of insomnia is dependent not only on sleep difficulties despite adequate opportunities for sleep, but also requires there to be resultant impairment to daytime functioning.

History

- What is their concern about their sleep pattern?
- When did the problem start and what was happening to them at that time?
- What is the sleep problem?
    - Difficulty falling asleep
    - Recurrent waking during the night
    - Early morning waking, feeling unrefreshed
- How is it affecting them? How is their daytime functioning impaired?
- Do they take daytime naps?
- Is the bedroom comfortable, quiet and dark?
- What is done to try to 'wind down' before sleep? (Do they watch television, browse the Internet, check social media, send text messages, read a book?)
- Any symptoms of depression (see earlier section)
- General health
- Potentially causative medication (see next section)
- Caffeine, nicotine, alcohol, recreational drugs
- Occupation – for example shift work, high-stress environment
- Their expectations – explore their ideas. What do they feel keeps them awake? Why are they coming to see you now? What help are they expecting?
- 🚩 Snoring with gasping or restlessness during the night (particularly applicable if overweight; may be reported by their partner/family)
- 🚩 Shortness of breath when lying down

Consider causes

- Physical: pain, discomfort, itching, shortness of breath, nocturia, indigestion/gastro-oesophageal reflux, tinnitus
- Pathological: sleep apnoea, restless legs syndrome, heart failure, nocturia
- Physiological: shift work, jet lag, pregnancy, irregular meals, low light levels while awake, bright artificial light in the evening (blue light is particularly implicated in circadian regulation, hence the 'night modes' now seen on electronic devices to reduce exposure in the evening)
- Psychological: emotional upsets, worries, bereavement
- Psychiatric: especially depression, anxiety and hypomania
- Pharmacological: are they taking medications which can disturb sleep, e.g., SSRIs, bupropion, lamotrigine, propranolol, corticosteroids (especially if not taken in the morning), salbutamol, theophylline, pseudoephedrine or laxatives, or taking excessive caffeinated drinks, alcohol, recreational drugs or nicotine
- Social: new baby, enuretic child, partner who has nocturia or who snores, noisy neighbours

Examination

- Look for agitation, depressed affect, 'washed-out' appearance
- Are they living with obesity? (Associated with obstructive sleep apnoea)
- If shortness of breath when lying down, check heart rate, BP, oxygen saturations and examine chest (fine crackles at lung bases suggest heart failure)

Self-care

- The website https://sleepeducation.org has useful self-care advice; people may also find it useful to complete the sleep diary there under 'Resources'
- Try to keep to regular times for going to bed and waking up
- There is only a certain amount of sleep an individual needs in 24 hours. If wanting to sleep more at night, avoid napping during the day
- Don't lie in after a poor night's sleep. Allow the tiredness to be used as 'fuel' for the next night's sleep and to help establish a routine
- Regular exercise is helpful, but avoid in the evening
- Don't drive if you feel sleepy
- OTC remedies are not recommended. Nytol contains a sedative antihistamine that may be temporarily effective but often causes morning drowsiness. Nytol Herbal contains valerian; this is unlikely to be harmful but lacks high-quality evidence for effectiveness
- Before going to bed:
  - Try not to eat a large, heavy meal late at night
  - Avoid caffeine, nicotine and alcohol within 6 hours of going to bed. Consider giving up caffeine altogether
  - Limit exposure to bright light in the evenings
  - A bedtime ritual (e.g., warm bath, milky drink) may help
  - Try to relax before going to bed. Relaxation exercises or training (e.g., hypnotherapy) can be helpful; also consider yoga, tai chi, meditation, reading and listening to relaxing music
  - Stop using electronic devices at least 30 minutes before bedtime
- After going to bed:
  - Keep the bedroom quiet, dark and at a comfortable temperature (usually cooler than other rooms)
  - Only use the bedroom for sleep and sex. Banish the television, laptop computer and smartphone
  - Don't keep checking the time throughout the night. Reading a book and watching the page numbers steadily rise can be just as frustrating
  - Don't lie in bed awake for more than roughly 20 minutes – it is better to get up and do something productive and then go back to bed when you feel sleepy

Action

- If resulting from work-related stress, would time off, limited duties, different shifts or reduced hours help? Have they considered looking for a new job?
- Consider adjusting the timing of medications if these are suspected to be affecting sleep
- The person must inform the DVLA if they have 'excessive sleepiness due to a medical condition' (this includes if obstructive sleep apnoea is suspected)
- For insomnia lasting ≥3 months, or lasting <3 months with daytime impairment causing significant distress and low likelihood of resolving soon, NICE recommends offering CBT for insomnia. This may be available online in your area or accessible through your local Talking Therapies service (which allows self-referral)

Prescription

- Hypnotic drugs such as zopiclone[PBCI] may cause addiction, daytime drowsiness, unsteadiness (with a risk of falls for frail or elderly people) and rebound insomnia on stopping. They are best avoided if possible

MHe

- Zopiclone[PBCI] (alongside other 'z-drugs') has a superior effect on sleep architecture compared with benzodiazepines such as temazepam[PBCI] and is therefore generally preferred as a hypnotic. However, it is more likely to cause driving impairment the next morning in older people (based on 7.5 mg of zopiclone vs. 20 mg of temazepam) (Leufkens and Vermeeren, 2009)
- Evidence suggests that the negative impact of these drugs increases with longer duration of use, while their benefits tend to decrease over time
- It may be reasonable to prescribe a short course (no more than 7 tablets) of zopiclone[PBCI] (7.5 mg in most adults and 3.75 mg in older people) in the following circumstances:
  - For insomnia lasting <3 months, if sleep hygiene measures have failed, daytime impairment is causing significant distress and there is a high likelihood of the insomnia resolving soon (e.g., there is a time-limited stressor)
  - For insomnia lasting ≥3 months, if there is an acute exacerbation (as a temporary adjunct to CBT)
- These can be used on alternate nights for a maximum of 14 days. Warn that they may impair driving the next morning and that alcohol should be avoided when they are used
- If prescribed, make clear that it is a one-off prescription. Long-term hypnotic treatment should not be prescribed
- Modified-release melatonin[PB] is licensed for use in people aged ≥55. It is non-addictive and acts on the circadian rhythm. Setting expectations is important; it is unlikely to have the same short-term effectiveness as hypnotic drugs and may take some weeks to 'reset the sleep cycle'. After an initial 3-week course, it can be continued for a further 10 weeks if there has been a positive response
- Daridorexant[PBCI] is a recently approved treatment for long-term insomnia. It may be offered if symptoms are present ≥3 nights a week for ≥3 months and CBT for insomnia is ineffective/unsuitable/not available. The BNF advises caution in the elderly and in people with depression or mental health problems, particularly if there is suicidal ideation, as these symptoms may be worsened. Treatment should be for as short a duration as possible and reviewed within 3 months

RED FLAGS

- Obese and reporting snoring and excessive tiredness (*may need assessment for sleep apnoea; refer to experienced colleague*)
- Difficulty sleeping due to shortness of breath when lying down (*possible heart failure; refer to experienced colleague*)

References

DeCrescenzo, F., D'Alò, G.L., Ostinelli, E.G., et al. 2022. Comparative effects of pharmacological interventions for the acute and long-term management of insomnia disorder in adults: a systematic review and network meta-analysis. *Lancet*; 400(10347):170–84. https://doi.org/10.1016/S0140-6736(22)00878-9 *A review of the efficacy and adverse event rates for commonly used medicines for treating insomnia.*

Driver and Vehicle Licensing Agency (DVLA). 2022. Assessing fitness to drive – a guide for medical professionals. https://assets.publishing.service.gov.uk/government/uploads/system/uploads/attachment_data/file/1084397/assessing-fitness-to-drive-may-2022.pdf

Espie, C.A., Kyle, S.D., Williams, C., et al. 2012. A randomized, placebo-controlled trial of online cognitive behavioral therapy for chronic insomnia disorder delivered via an automated media-rich web application. *Sleep*; 35(6):769–81. https://doi.org/10.5665/sleep.1872

Hemmeter, U., Müller, M., Bischof, R., et al. 2000. Effect of zopiclone and temazepam on sleep EEG parameters, psychomotor and memory functions in healthy elderly volunteers. *Psychopharmacology*; 147(4):384–96. https://doi.org/10.1007/s002130050007

Leufkens, T.R.M., and Vermeeren, A. 2009. Highway driving in the elderly the morning after bedtime use of hypnotics: a comparison between temazepam 20 mg, zopiclone 7.5 mg, and placebo. *J Clin Psychopharmacol*; 29(5). https://doi.org/10.1097/JCP.0b013e3181b57f43

Li, Y., Sahakian, B.J., Kang, J., et al. 2022. The brain structure and genetic mechanisms underlying the nonlinear association between sleep duration, cognition and mental health. *Nature Aging*; 2(5):425–37. *Characterised the association between duration of sleep and outcomes relating to mental health and cognition, but is observational evidence only.*

Mets, M.A., Volkerts, E.R., Olivier, B., et al. 2010. Effect of hypnotic drugs on body balance and standing steadiness. *Sleep Med Rev*; 14(4):259–67. https://doi.org/10.1016/j.smrv.2009.10.008

NICE. CKS. 2022. Insomnia. https://cks.nice.org.uk/topics/insomnia/

Rudisill, T.M., Zhu, M., Kelley, G.A., et al. 2016. Medication use and the risk of motor vehicle collisions among licensed drivers: a systematic review. *Accid Anal Prev*; 96:255–70. https://doi.org/10.1016/j.aap.2016.08.001

Scharner, V., Hasieber, L., Sönnichsen, A., et al. 2022. Efficacy and safety of Z-substances in the management of insomnia in older adults: a systematic review for the development of recommendations to reduce potentially inappropriate prescribing. *BMC Geriatr*; 22(1):87. https://doi.org/10.1186/s12877-022-02757-6

Shinjyo, N., Waddell, G., and Green, J. 2020. Valerian root in treating sleep problems and associated disorders-a systematic review and meta-analysis. *J Evid Based Integr Med*; 25:2515690X20967323. https://doi.org/10.1177/2515690X20967323 *The evidence is not of high quality and there seem to be differences between preparations. However, no serious side effects were reported.*

West, K.E., Jablonski, M.R., Warfield, B., et al. 2010. Blue light from light-emitting diodes elicits a dose-dependent suppression of melatonin in humans. *J Appl Physiol*; 110(3):619–26. https://doi.org/10.1152/japplphysiol.01413.2009

SELF-CARE RESOURCES FOR MENTAL HEALTH

Books

Your local library may have a 'Books on Prescription' scheme with recommended titles and online resources.

- Bradley, D., and Thomas, M. 2011. *Hyperventilation Syndrome: Breathing Pattern Disorders and How to Overcome Them*. Kyle Books. ISBN-13: 978-0857830296
- Griffin, J., and Tyrell, I. 2004. *How to Lift Depression Fast*. HG Publishing. ISBN-13: 978-1899398416
- Griffin, J., and Tyrell, I. 2006. *How to Master Anxiety: All You Need to Know to Overcome Stress, Panic Attacks, Trauma, Phobias, Obsessions and More*. HG Publishing. ISBN-13 978-1899398812
- Johnstone, M. 2007. *I Had a Black Dog*. Robinson Publishing. ISBN-13: 978-184529589. *A cartoon book – a picture is worth a thousand words*
- Singer, M. 2007. *Untethered Soul: The Journey Beyond Yourself*. NH Publications. ISBN: 978-1-57224-537-2
- Skynner, R., and Cleese, J. 1993. *Families and How to Survive Them*. Cedar Books. ISBN-13: 978-0749314101. *For those struggling with family dynamics*

Apps

Phone apps for mindfulness and breathing techniques may be helpful, for example Headspace and Breathe2Relax. They do not require a large time commitment and are free or low-cost. Your area may also have locally-commissioned apps/digital services available.

Websites

- Living Life to the Full: www.llttf.com *Free online CBT and other useful resources*
- Human Givens Institute: www.hgi.org.uk *Explanation of how unmet emotional needs can cause many mental health problems*
- Royal College of Psychiatrists: www.rcpsych.ac.uk/mental-health *Information leaflets in a range of languages*
- Mind: www.mind.org.uk *Many useful resources including access to free, moderated online peer support*
- NHS England – Every Mind Matters: www.nhs.uk/every-mind-matters *Includes tips and CBT-based resources for self-help*

Agencies

- Relate, for relationship difficulties: www.relate.org.uk, 0300 100 1234 (go to the website to find contact details for the nearest service)
- Drinkaware: www.drinkaware.co.uk
- Drinkline – National Alcohol Helpline: 0300 123 1110
- NHS Alcohol Support: www.nhs.uk/live-well/alcohol-advice/alcohol-support/
- Citizens' Advice (particularly helpful for debt or benefit problems): www.citizensadvice.org.uk
- National Debtline offers free, confidential and independent help over the phone (0808 808 4000) or via webchat for people in England, Scotland and Wales. You can also download sample letters from their website: www.nationaldebtline.org

MHe

- Civil Legal Advice (CLA). If you qualify for legal aid and live in England or Wales, CLA can provide free help or legal advice over the phone about debt, housing, employment, education, welfare benefits and tax credits: 0345 345 4345, www.gov.uk/civil-legal-advice
- Mind offers information and support for living with mental health problems. Infoline on 0300 123 3393, www.mind.org.uk
- Samaritans, a listening ear for all types of problems. Call 116 123, www.samaritans.org
- BBC Action Line – a gateway to a wide variety of support services: www.bbc.co.uk/actionline/
- Cruse, for bereavement: 0808 808 1677, www.cruse.org.uk
- National Domestic Abuse Helpline: 0808 2000 247 (24 hours), www.nationaldahelpline.org.uk
- Campaign Against Living Miserably (CALM), charity dedicated to preventing male suicide: 0800 58 58 58 (5 p.m.–12 a.m. every day), www.thecalmzone.net
- Health Visitor (for parents of children – age range seen varies by region, will always include <5 years, but may extend up to 19 years)
- NHS Services and support for parents: www.nhs.uk/conditions/baby/support-and-services/services-and-support-for-parents/ e.g., Sure Start children's centres provide family health and support services, early learning and full-day or temporary care for children from birth to 5 years

CHAPTER 12

Musculoskeletal/injuries

MANAGING ACUTE PAIN

OTC analgesics

People often talk about 'painkillers' but this term is unhelpful because it instils the idea that analgesics will completely relieve pain, whereas a partial reduction, perhaps around 50%, is more realistic. 'Pain relief' is a much better term.

Guidance from NHS England in 2018 stated that analgesics which are available OTC should not be prescribed for self-limiting musculoskeletal pain. Indeed, if the person pays prescription charges, ibuprofen[P] and paracetamol are considerably cheaper if bought OTC. They may be used together up to their maximum daily doses although, curiously, the low-dose combination of paracetamol 500 mg plus ibuprofen 200 mg provides results that are almost as good as the higher doses, so perhaps this should be our first suggestion for acute pain (Table 12.1).

Table 12.1 Comparison of single-dose pain relief (in a post-surgical context)

Medication (dose in mg)	NNT for at least 50% pain relief
Ibuprofen (acid) 200	2.9
Ibuprofen (acid) 400	2.5
Ibuprofen fast acting* 200	2.1
Ibuprofen fast acting* 400	2.1
Diclofenac sodium 50	6.6
Naproxen 500	2.7
Ibuprofen 200 + paracetamol 500	**1.6**
Ibuprofen 400 + paracetamol 1000	**1.5**
Paracetamol 500	3.5
Paracetamol 1000	3.2
Paracetamol 1000 + codeine 60	2.2
Ibuprofen 400 + codeine 60	2.2
Codeine 60	12

Source: Moore et al., 2015a.
Lower number needed to treat (NNT) = more effective pain relief.
* 'Fast acting' refers to particular compounds of ibuprofen: lysine, arginine or sodium. These are available OTC or on prescription, but are significantly more expensive than standard ibuprofen (ibuprofen acid).

Paracetamol alone has no benefit over placebo in back pain or osteoarthritis (da Costa et al., 2017). Combination analgesics containing codeine are available OTC in the UK, although banned in many other countries, but to obtain additional analgesia from codeine[PBC], most people need to take at least 25 mg per dose, and many common combinations contain suboptimal doses. It should also be noted that there is considerable individual variation in the response to opioids, as well as to non-steroidal anti-inflammatory drugs (NSAIDs).

Taking analgesics with food substantially reduces their efficacy. Despite the commonly recommended advice to take analgesics with food, evidence is lacking that this reduces adverse effects. Nor is there any evidence that rapidly dissolving formulations such as 'melts' are more effective or faster acting than ordinary tablets, but some compounds of ibuprofen (e.g., lysine, arginine or sodium) are more rapidly absorbed into the bloodstream than others.

There has been outcry surrounding the branding of some OTC medications, which may suggest targeted action against a particular cause of pain – that is, tension headache, period pain, migraine and back pain. Other than topical administration, there is no way of targeting the action of analgesics. Indeed, this type of branding can potentially be dangerous, with people inadvertently overdosing through taking the same analgesic compound (but branded differently) repeatedly in order to manage, for example, their period pain, tension headache and back pain. An advert in the UK for Nurofen Joint and Back was banned in 2016 for suggesting targeted pain relief, while in Australia, the manufacturer of Nurofen was fined AUD\$6 million in late 2016 for misleading consumers.

NSAIDs

NSAIDS have analgesic, antipyretic and, at higher doses, anti-inflammatory actions. They impair prostaglandin production by inhibiting the cyclo-oxygenase (COX) enzyme; inhibition of COX-2 is considered to be responsible for the anti-inflammatory action while inhibition of COX-1 is implicated in gastrointestinal toxicity.

NSAIDs may be divided into standard NSAIDs (such as ibuprofen and naproxen, which act on COX-1 and COX-2) and coxibs (such as etoricoxib, which inhibits COX-2 preferentially). All NSAIDs carry a risk of GI bleeds, which is much higher in the elderly, although it is lower for coxibs. Despite the common advice (and labeling instructions specified in the BNF) to take NSAIDs with food to mitigate GI risk, this is unlikely to have much benefit given that risk is largely related to blood levels of the NSAID rather than local effects on the GI mucosa (Moore et al., 2015b).

In the majority of situations in primary care which would benefit from using an anti-inflammatory, using a standard NSAID is most likely to be appropriate, although a coxib (alongside a proton pump inhibitor [PPI, e.g., omeprazole[Q], 20 mg daily in adults]) may be preferred for those at high risk of GI bleed (see Table 12.2).

Table 12.2 Common conditions/risks which may preclude the use of standard NSAIDs or coxibs

	Standard NSAID	Coxib
Uncontrolled hypertension	Caution, seek advice	Do not use
Mild heart failure	Caution, seek advice	Do not use
Severe heart failure	Do not use	Do not use
Other cardiovascular disease	Do not use	Do not use
High risk of GI bleed	Do not use	Caution, seek advice, add PPI
Chronic kidney disease (eGFR <30)	Do not use	Do not use

NSAIDs also substantially increase the risk of cardiovascular disease; this risk is higher for coxibs. Before recommending or prescribing an NSAID (whether a standard NSAID or a coxib), you should consider any contraindications, drug interactions, medical history, GI and cardiovascular risk, and any monitoring requirements. The lowest effective dose for the shortest possible time should be used.

- Do not use NSAIDs if:
  - Relevant allergy
  - Current/previous peptic ulcer or GI bleed
  - Kidney disease (eGFR <30)
  - Liver failure
  - Severe heart failure
  - Chickenpox or shingles (Mikaeloff et al., 2008)
  - Cardiovascular disease (Bally et al., 2017)
  - Pregnancy or trying to conceive (Salman et al., 2015)
- Also take caution if using NSAIDs if:
  - High risk for VTE (e.g., previous DVT, taking COC, immobilisation) or cardiovascular disease (e.g., uncontrolled hypertension, diabetes, heavy smoker); avoid diclofenac, high-dose ibuprofen or coxibs
  - Inflammatory bowel disease
  - Within 48 hours of a fracture, sprain or (possibly) operation (Schug, 2021; Wheatley et al., 2019)
  - Asthma – although most people with asthma can take NSAIDs without a problem. Ask whether they have ever taken one and, if so, what happened (Kanabar et al., 2007)
  - Breastfeeding (naproxen[PBCI] is best avoided; if an NSAID is required, ibuprofen[P] is preferable)
  - Increased risk of GI ulceration/bleed (see Box 12.1)
- If one NSAID is ineffective, it is worth trying another, as there is considerable individual variation in response

BOX 12.1 CONSIDERING RISK OF GI ADVERSE EVENTS WITH NSAID USE – INCLUDING WHEN TO CO-PRESCRIBE PPI

- The following are risk factors for GI ulceration/bleed with NSAIDs:
  - Prolonged requirement for NSAIDs
  - Age ≥65 (GI bleed risk with NSAIDs doubles with every decade above 55 years [Petersen et al., 2014])
  - Using other medications which increase the risk of GI adverse events; anticoagulants (e.g., warfarin, apixaban), antiplatelets (e.g., aspirin, clopidogrel), corticosteroids, SSRIs (e.g., fluoxetine, sertraline)
  - Significant comorbidity, such as liver or kidney disease, diabetes, or hypertension
  - Heavy smoker
  - Excessive alcohol intake
  - Low platelet count or coagulation defect
  - Previous adverse reaction to NSAIDs
  - High dose of NSAID would be indicated
- High risk of GI bleed is defined as having ≥3 risk factors; if present, avoid standard NSAIDs. If essential and not otherwise unsuitable, an experienced colleague may cautiously use a coxib with PPI
- Moderate risk is defined as having 1–2 risk factors; if present and NSAIDs not otherwise unsuitable, co-prescribe PPI with standard NSAID (or use a coxib if appropriate)

Gabapentinoids

The gabapentinoid group consists of gabapentin[PCI] and pregabalin[PBCI]. They may be used in neuropathic pain, such as post-herpetic neuralgia (nerve pain after shingles). Although commonly used in other situations, such as low back pain or sciatica, they are not recommended and should be avoided here as there is evidence of harm and no overall evidence of benefit.

Their use had been increasing until 2019, potentially driven by a desire to avoid prescribing opioids. In 2019, they were reclassified as Class C drugs in the UK due to an increase in the number of deaths caused by misuse and addiction. The risk factors for gabapentinoid abuse are largely the same as for opiates: a history of abuse, comorbid psychiatric condition and young age. Studies show gabapentinoid misuse to be higher in people with opioid use disorders; pregabalin is thought to enhance the effects of opiates and reduce withdrawal symptoms. Concern has been expressed over the increasing use of gabapentinoids, mainly when prescribed alongside opioids or benzodiazepines, due to a synergy of central depressant effects (Hofmann and Besson, 2021).

Opioids

Opioids relieve pain by acting on endorphin receptors in the central nervous system (CNS) rather than tackling the cause of the pain; they have no anti-inflammatory action. Short-term use for musculoskeletal conditions may be needed if other analgesics fail to relieve pain, but, beyond a 2-week course, dependency is a major risk and non-pharmacological treatments provide a far better option. In contrast to NSAIDs (where if a person does not respond well to one, it is useful to try an alternative), the variation in response to opioids is more often related to genetic variations in the enzymes that metabolise opioids, rather than which opioid is used. The same dose of one opioid may give widely different therapeutic and adverse effects for different individuals. This is particularly true of tramadol (Leppert and Mikolajczak, 2011), which is one reason why the National Minor Illness Centre (NMIC) does not encourage its use.

Codeine[PBC] is the most frequently prescribed opioid in the UK; 1-2% of the population are ultra-fast metabolisers, converting up to 50% of a dose of codeine to morphine, in contrast with a more usual rate of 10% conversion. In some ethnic groups (e.g., people of North African, Ethiopian or Arab ethnic origin), up to 28% may be ultra-fast metabolisers (Dean and Kane, 2021). Ultra-fast metabolisers will gain more analgesic effect but also have more side effects; if the person is breastfeeding, a higher amount of morphine can be passed via the milk to the baby.

Previously the MHRA has advised against the use of codeine[PBC] by breastfeeding mothers, but a large population study from Canada showed no increase in baby deaths or hospital admissions. However, other adverse effects such as drowsiness and poor feeding were not studied (Zipursky et al., 2023). The UK's Specialist Pharmacy Service (SPS) recommends that codeine should not be taken by breastfeeding mothers, recommending dihydrocodeine instead

MSK

(SPS, 2023a), although both drugs are metabolised by the same enzyme. Based on the pharmacology, morphine would be a safer option (SPS, 2023b) because the received dose is predictable, in contrast to codeine, which metabolises to varying morphine levels depending on enzyme activity.

Children are very susceptible to the adverse effects of morphine, so codeine[PBC] is contraindicated for all children aged <12 years and not needed for any minor illness for those aged <18. If required as a short course for adults, prescribe codeine separately from other analgesics such as paracetamol to allow flexibility in the dose and choice. When the pain is more severe, the person can take both drugs, and when pain starts to improve, the dose of codeine can be reduced first. As constipation is almost inevitable with opioid use, always advise also taking a stimulant laxative (see section on Constipation in Chapter 9).

MANAGING CHRONIC PAIN

- Defined as pain that persists or recurs for ≥3 months
- This may be primary (no obvious cause) or secondary (known underlying condition, e.g., osteoarthritis). Primary chronic pain may be described as 'functional'; although it can be felt in a specific part of the body (i.e., back, pelvis, abdomen), it may be a problem with the pain system itself, rather than pathology in the area in which the pain is experienced
- In 2021, NICE published NG193, a guideline on chronic pain. Although this guides the **assessment** of primary and secondary chronic pain in people aged ≥16, the recommendations on **management** relate only to primary chronic pain (i.e., pain with no clear underlying cause, or pain [or its impact] that is out of proportion to any observable injury or disease). It is important to appreciate this, to avoid a common misconception that the guideline refers to all chronic pain conditions

Pharmacological management of primary chronic pain

- The NICE guideline advises that paracetamol, NSAIDs, benzodiazepines, gabapentinoids or opioids should not be used to manage primary chronic pain
- Antidepressants can be considered for primary chronic pain even in the absence of a diagnosis of depression, as they may target an abnormally heightened sensitivity to pain and thereby help with quality of life, pain, sleep and psychological distress. This is an *unlicensed indication*

Non-pharmacological management of chronic primary pain

- Offer a person-centred assessment of how the pain affects their life and vice versa, including the impact on day-to-day activities, work, sleep, mental health and social factors such as employment, housing and income. Explore their understanding of the cause of their pain and their expectations of how it might change in the future
- Explain that symptoms may fluctuate over time
- Explore the person's expectations and explain that, even if their pain does not fully resolve, they can still have a good quality of life
- There are various approaches/treatments which can help:
  - Keeping active, including supervised group exercise programmes
  - Acceptance and commitment therapy (ACT)/CBT; these may be available through local pain clinics
  - Acupuncture
  - Ultrasound therapy or transcutaneous electrical nerve stimulation (TENS) (although not recommended by NICE due to limited evidence of benefit, the risks of such treatments are very low). TENS machines can be bought for around £30; note that use is not advised in people with epilepsy, a pacemaker or in early pregnancy
  - Self-help resources such as the Pain Toolkit (www.paintoolkit.org)

References

Bally, M., Dendukuri, N., Rich, B., et al. 2017. Risk of acute myocardial infarction with NSAIDs in real world use: Bayesian meta-analysis of individual patient data. *BMJ*; 357:j1909. https://doi.org/10.1136/bmj.j1909 *This huge observational study found that all NSAIDs were associated with an increased risk of acute myocardial infarction of up to 50%, greatest during the first month of NSAID use and with higher doses. For this reason, NMIC believes that NSAIDs are contraindicated in all people with cardiovascular disease despite the European Medicines Agency statement: www.ema.europa.eu/en/medicines/human/referrals/ibuprofen-dexibuprofen-containing-medicines*

da Costa, B.R., Reichenbach, S., Keller, N., et al. 2017. Effectiveness of non-steroidal anti-inflammatory drugs for the treatment of pain in knee and hip osteoarthritis: a network meta-analysis. *Lancet*; 390(10090):e21–33. http://dx.doi.org/10.1016/S0140-6736(17)31744-0 *The authors see no role for single-agent paracetamol for the treatment of people with osteoarthritis, irrespective of dose.*

Dean, L., and Kane, M. 2021. Codeine therapy and CYP2D6 genotype. BTI – medical genetics summaries. *Medical Genetics Summaries*. www.ncbi.nlm.nih.gov/books/NBK100662/ *The hepatic CYP2D6 enzyme metabolises a quarter of all prescribed drugs, including codeine. Genetic variation in the efficiency of this process is very large.*

Faculty of Pain Medicine. 2021. Core standards for Pain Management Services in the UK. https://fpm.ac.uk/standards-guidelines/core-standards

Hofmann, M., and Besson, M. 2021. Gabapentinoids: the rise of a new misuse epidemics?. *Psychiatry Res*; 305:114193. https://doi.org/10.1016/j.psychres.2021.114193 *Gabapentinoids increase the risks associated with opioids or other sedatives, due to a synergy of central depressant effects.*

Kanabar, D., Dale, S., and Rawat, M. 2007. A review of ibuprofen and acetaminophen use in febrile children and the occurrence of asthma-related symptoms. *Clin Ther*; 29(12):2716–23. https://doi.org/10.1016/j.clinthera.2007.12.021 *This literature review found a low risk for asthma-related morbidity associated with ibuprofen use in children and a possible protective and therapeutic effect compared with paracetamol.*

Leppert, W., and Mikolajczak, P. 2011. Analgesic effects and assays of controlled-release tramadol and o-desmethyltramadol in cancer patients with pain. *Curr Pharm Biotechnol*; 12(2):306–12. https://doi.org/10.2174/138920111794295738 *The blood level of tramadol cannot be predicted by the dose. If there is no suitable alternative, start at a low dose and titrate carefully.*

Mathieson, S., Lin, C-W.C., Underwood, M., et al. 2020. Pregabalin and gabapentin for pain. *BMJ*; 369:m1315. https://doi.org/10.1136/bmj.m1315 *A useful summary.*

Meaidi, A., Mascolo, A., Sessa, M., et al. 2023. Venous thromboembolism with use of hormonal contraception and non-steroidal anti-inflammatory drugs: nationwide cohort study. BMJ, 382;e074450. https://doi.org/10.1136/bmj-2022-074450 *The rate of extra VTE events associated with NSAID use is significantly greater if combined hormonal contraception is being used.*

MHRA Drug Safety Update. 2013. Codeine for analgesia: restricted use in children because of reports of morphine toxicity. www.gov.uk/drug-safety-update/codeine-for-analgesia-restricted-use-in-children-because-of-reports-of-morphine-toxicity

MHRA Drug Safety Update. 2017. Gabapentin (Neurontin): risk of severe respiratory depression. www.gov.uk/drug-safety-update/gabapentin-neurontin-risk-of-severe-respiratory-depression#reminder-of-risk-with-concomitant-use-of-opioids

Mikaeloff, Y., Kezouh, A., and Suissa, S. 2008. Nonsteroidal anti-inflammatory drug use and the risk of severe skin and soft tissue complications in patients with varicella or zoster disease. *Br J Clin Pharmacol*; 65(2):203–9. https://doi.org/10.1111/j.1365-2125.2007.02997.x *Use of NSAIDs is associated with an elevated risk of severe skin and soft-tissue complications of varicella*

Moore, R.A., Derry, S., Straube, S., et al. 2014. Faster, higher, stronger? Evidence for formulation and efficacy for ibuprofen in acute pain. *Pain*; 155(1):14–21. https://doi.org/10.1016/j.pain.2013.08.013 *Interesting reference suggesting that ibuprofen arginine, lysine and sodium salts are more effective than standard ibuprofen.*

Moore, R.A., Derry, S., Aldington, D., et al. 2015a. Single dose oral analgesics for acute postoperative pain in adults – an overview of Cochrane reviews. *Cochrane Database Syst Rev*; 9:CD008659. https://doi.org/10.1002/14651858.CD008659.pub3 *For single-dose pain relief after surgery.*

Moore, R.A., Derry, S., Wiffen, P.J., et al. 2015b. Effects of food on pharmacokinetics of immediate release oral formulations of aspirin, dipyrone, paracetamol and NSAIDs – a systematic review. *Br J Clin Pharmacol*; 80(3):381–8. https://doi.org/10.1111/bcp.12628 *There is evidence that high, early plasma concentrations produce better early pain relief, better overall pain relief, longer-lasting pain relief and lower rates of re-medication. Taking analgesics with food may make them less effective, resulting in greater population exposure. It may be time to rethink research priorities and advice to professionals and the public.*

NICE. 2020. NG59. Low back pain and sciatica in over 16s: assessment and management. www.nice.org.uk/guidance/NG59

NICE. 2021. NG193. Chronic pain (primary and secondary) in over 16s: assessment of all chronic pain and management of chronic primary pain. www.nice.org.uk/guidance/ng193

NICE CKS. 2020. NSAIDs – prescribing issues. https://cks.nice.org.uk/topics/nsaids-prescribing-issues/

Petersen, J., Hallas, J., de Muckadell, O.B., et al. 2014. A model to assess the risk for ASA/NSAID-related ulcer bleeding for the individual patient based on the number of risk factors. *Gastroenterology*; 146(5):S-319. https://doi.org/10.1111/bcpt.13370 *Doubling of NSAID GI bleed risk with every decade of age.*

Salman, S., Sherif, B., and Al-Zohyri, A., 2015. Effects of some non steroidal anti-inflammatory drugs on ovulation in women with mild musculoskeletal pain. *Ann Rheum Dis* 74:117–18. *There was significant inhibition of ovulation in 39 people treated with diclofenac, naproxen and etoricoxib.*

Schug, S.A., 2021. Do NSAIDs really interfere with healing after surgery? *J Clin Med*, 10(11):2359. https://doi.org/10.3390/jcm10112359 *There are few human RCTs on this important topic.*

SPS (Specialist Pharmacy Service). 2023a. Using codeine, dihydrocodeine or tramadol during breastfeeding. www.sps.nhs.uk/articles/using-codeine-dihydrocodeine-or-tramadol-during-breastfeeding/

SPS. 2023b. Using strong opioid analgesics during breastfeeding. www.sps.nhs.uk/articles/using-strong-opioid-analgesics-during-breastfeeding/

MSK

Wheatley, B.M., Nappo, K.E., Christensen, D.L., et al. 2019. Effect of NSAIDs on bone healing rates: a meta-analysis. *J Am Acad Orthop Surg*; 27(7):e330–e336. https://doi.org/10.5435/JAAOS-D-17-00727 *NSAIDs double the rate of non-healing of fractures (except in children).*

Zipursky, J.S., Gomes, T., Everett, K., et al. 2023. Maternal opioid treatment after delivery and risk of adverse infant outcomes: population based cohort study. *BMJ*; 380:e074005. https://doi.org/10.1136/bmj-2022-074005 *The authors say that their large study suggests no association between maternal opioid prescription after delivery and adverse infant outcomes, including death. But the only other adverse outcome that they considered was hospital admission.*

NECK PAIN

This common symptom is usually caused by muscular pain or occasionally by lymph node enlargement. Meningitis is extremely rare in UK primary care and would typically feature additional symptoms such as fever or altered mental state; however concern about meningitis may be a driver for the consultation.

History

- What is worrying them? (May be concerned about meningitis)
- Onset: gradual/sudden/upon waking
- Duration
- Any injury (e.g., whiplash)
- Site of pain
- Fever
- Sore throat
- Occupation (e.g., checkout/keyboard operator)
- 🏴 Rheumatoid or inflammatory arthritis
- 🏴 Neurological symptoms
- 🏴 History of cancer

Examination

- Range of movement
- Location of pain (muscle or vertebra)
- If infection suspected:
    - Temperature, heart rate and respiratory rate
    - CRT in children aged <12 years/BP in adults and older children
    - Cervical lymph nodes
    - Neck stiffness (can a child kiss their knees?)

Self-care

- If relevant to concerns, appropriately reassure about meningitis
- Explain that neck pain is common and likely to resolve in 3–4 weeks
- Continue normal activity as much as possible
- Cervical collars are not recommended
- Sleep with one firm pillow
- Try to maintain good posture
- Consider workstation assessment
- Do not drive if neck movements are restricted
- Analgesia with ibuprofen[P] or paracetamol
- If pain is muscular, try topical diclofenac emulgel 2.32%[PC]

RED FLAGS

- Neurological symptoms (*possible prolapsed cervical disc/myelopathy; refer to experienced colleague*)
- Evidence of infection and neck stiffness (*possible meningitis; give IV/IM benzylpenicillin and admit very urgently under Medical/Paediatrics*) (the absence of a rash does not exclude meningitis)
- Sudden-onset severe headache with neck stiffness (*possible subarachnoid haemorrhage; send very urgently to hospital*)
- Rheumatoid or inflammatory arthritis (*may affect the atlantoaxial joint, making it unstable; send urgently to A&E if any limb weakness or numbness; otherwise refer urgently to Rheumatology*)
- Osteoporosis with severe pain over a vertebra, relieved by lying down and with tenderness on examination (*possible spinal wedge fracture; refer to experienced colleague*)
- History of cancer with localised vertebral tenderness (*possible metastatic deposit; discuss urgently with Oncology*)

References

Derry, S., Wiffen, P.J., Kalso, E.A., et al. 2017. Topical analgesics for acute and chronic pain in adults – an overview of Cochrane Reviews. *Cochrane Database Syst Rev*; 5:CD008609. https://doi.org/10.1002/14651858.CD008609.pub2 *There is good evidence that topical NSAIDs are useful in acute pain conditions such as sprains or strains. Different formulations varied in effectiveness; the best was diclofenac emulgel (NNT 1.8).*

Maloney, J., Pew, S., Wie, C., et al. 2021. Comprehensive review of topical analgesics for chronic pain. *Curr Pain Headache Rep*; 25:1–8. https://doi.org/10.1007/s11916-020-00923-2 *There is evidence to support the use of topical NSAIDs, high-concentration topical capsaicin and topical lidocaine for various painful conditions.*

NICE CKS. 2023. Neck pain – non-specific. https://cks.nice.org.uk/topics/neck-pain-non-specific/

BACK PAIN

Most back pain is muscular; the differential diagnosis includes sciatica (about 10% of cases, due to irritation or compression of a nerve root) and rarer conditions such as spinal cord compression, spinal fracture, metastases, infection and spondyloarthritis. However, 'sciatica' is a much misused term; unless the person's symptoms are experienced below the knee, sciatic nerve irritation is unlikely.

History

- What is worrying them? (Often prolonged debility)
- Onset: gradual/sudden/while lifting
- Duration
- Any previous episodes
- Site – make sure it really is in the back, not the kidney, lung or hip
- Radiation to leg – especially below the knee
- Numbness/tingling of each leg
- Weakness in any area, particularly movements of each leg
- Occupation
- Psychosocial stress
- Where are they sleeping (e.g., bed, sofa or floor)?
- What has been tried already and what was the response?
- ⚑ Bilateral leg pain
- ⚑ Loss of bladder or bowel control
- ⚑ Disturbed sensation in perineum (wiping after going to the toilet may feel different/numb)
- ⚑ Abdominal pain/coldness/cyanosis of legs
- ⚑ Fever
- ⚑ Weight loss/malaise

MSK

🏴 Osteoporosis

🏴 History of cancer/TB

🏴 Immunosuppressed

🏴 Person who injects drugs

Examination

- Ask them to point out the site of pain and then palpate the area. Is it over muscle or bone?
- Spinal tenderness/scoliosis/abnormal shape
- Spasm of paraspinal muscles
- Can they walk on tiptoe and on their heels?

Tests

- Most back pain is muscular and no current scan can pinpoint this
- Imaging tests are generally not necessary or helpful in primary care. People who expect an x-ray should be gently told that it is very unlikely to be of help in finding the cause of their pain (unless a bone issue such as a fracture is suspected), and the dose of radiation required is 120 times that of a chest x-ray
- MRI scans are not recommended by NICE (2020) unless the person is considering surgery, there are rapidly evolving neurological symptoms, or red flag pathology is suspected. Lumbar MRI scans have a high proportion of false-positives (Wnuk et al., 2018)

Action

- Reassure them that most back pain, even with sciatica, is not serious and will get better without treatment. Pain does not equal damage
- Explain that psychosocial stress causes muscular tension and can contribute to pain; relaxation or meditation may help
- Reducing movement may delay recovery, so encourage gentle mobilisation (activity within the limits of pain as soon as possible)
- For acute back pain, regular analgesics (e.g., ibuprofen[P] OTC) are recommended because they help the person to keep mobile. Paracetamol OTC may be used in addition (but is ineffective for low back pain on its own)
- Give exercise leaflet, e.g., from Versus Arthritis (www.versusarthritis.org – though explain that this does not mean that their back pain is caused by arthritis; note that Versus Arthritis has many other excellent resources)
- If their mattress is >10 years old, advise them to consider buying a replacement
- They may find it helpful to carefully apply heat to the area
- Manual therapies such as spinal manipulation or massage are available privately (or through insurance schemes). NICE recommends that they should be used only in conjunction with an exercise regime
- TENS is not recommended by NICE guidance due to limited evidence of benefit but, given its relative safety, may be worth trying. Its use is not advised in people with epilepsy, a pacemaker or in early pregnancy. Machines can be bought for around £30
- Emotional health plays a major part in the resolution of back pain; it is important that clinicians convey a positive attitude from the beginning. The STarT Back tool (https://startback.hfac.keele.ac.uk/) may be used to identify people who are at high risk of persistent symptoms – if so, *refer to Musculoskeletal Service*
- Consider early referral to your local musculoskeletal service for people with risk factors for developing chronic back pain, e.g., obesity, physical inactivity, mental health problems
- At the time of writing, NICE had issued draft guidance that some apps may be an additional option for the treatment for non-specific low back pain, while more evidence is generated on their clinical and cost-effectiveness. Check if any such options are available in your area and how they may be accessed
- See earlier section on Managing Chronic Pain if appropriate

Prescription

- If ibuprofen[P] OTC has been ineffective, consider naproxen[PBCI] (500 mg initial dose followed by 250 mg every 6–8 hours as required)

- Codeine[PBC] may be prescribed separately from paracetamol as codeine phosphate[PBC] tablets (adult dose: initially 30 mg every 4 hours as required, increasing to 60 mg if necessary; maximum dose 240 mg per 24 hours) if necessary for acute pain. This is likely to cause constipation, which may be difficult to manage when the person has back pain, so always offer a stimulant laxative (see section on Constipation in Chapter 9). Opioids should not be used for chronic low back pain

- NICE recommends that gabapentinoids should not be offered for sciatica due to evidence of causing harm, alongside an overall lack of evidence of benefit

- There is continuing debate over the utility of muscle relaxants such as diazepam for managing muscle spasm in acute low back pain. Although CKS does not recommend their use, a recent Cochrane review (Cashin et al., 2023) has shown some benefit of such muscle relaxants for pain relief and improving physical function in this context. Pragmatically, they can be useful in people with muscle spasm, but must only be used short term as they are highly addictive and can have problematic side effects. The adult dose of diazepam[PBC] is 2–15 mg daily in divided doses

RED FLAGS

- Progressively worsening symptoms (*may need investigation; refer to experienced colleague*)
- Any of the following: numbness/tingling in perianal area, bladder or bowel dysfunction, bilateral leg pain/weakness/numbness (*possible cauda equina syndrome; send urgently to hospital with referral to Orthopaedics*)
- Sudden-onset severe back and abdominal pain, with discoloration of legs or stiffness (*possible dissection of aortic aneurysm; send very urgently to hospital*)
- Sudden-onset severe headache with back stiffness (*possible subarachnoid haemorrhage; send very urgently to hospital*)
- History of cancer with localised vertebral tenderness (*possible metastatic deposit; discuss urgently with Oncology*)
- Any of the following: thoracic pain, weight loss, severe pain that remains when supine, night pain that disturbs sleep or pain aggravated by straining (*possible metastatic cancer; refer to experienced colleague*)
- Pain with standing or walking eased by sitting or bending forwards (*suggestive of lumbar spinal stenosis; refer to experienced colleague*)
- Osteoporosis with severe pain over a vertebra, relieved by lying down and with tenderness on examination (*possible spinal wedge fracture; refer to experienced colleague*)
- New onset in person aged ≥50 (*higher risk of osteoporotic fracture or cancer; refer to experienced colleague*)
- Aged <50 with morning stiffness and fatigue (*possible ankylosing spondylitis; refer urgently to Rheumatology*)
- Fever and malaise, especially in people with immunosuppression, people who inject drugs or people with tuberculosis (*possible spinal infection; send urgently to hospital with referral to Orthopaedics*)

MSK

References

Cashin, A.G., Wand, B.M., O'Connell, N.E., et al. 2023. Pharmacological treatments for low back pain in adults: an overview of Cochrane Reviews. *Cochrane Database Syst Rev*; 4:CD013815. https://doi.org/10.1002/14651858.CD013815.pub2 *An overview of the evidence for various classes of medicines in managing low back pain, including muscle relaxants.*

Keele University. STarT Back Tool. https://startback.hfac.keele.ac.uk/

Mathieson, S., Maher, C.G., McLachlan, A.J., et al. 2017. Trial of pregabalin for acute and chronic sciatica. *N Engl J Med*; 376(12):1111–20. https://doi.org/10.1056/NEJMoa1614292 *Treatment with pregabalin did not significantly reduce the intensity of leg pain associated with sciatica and did not significantly improve other outcomes.*

NICE. 2020. NG59. Low back pain and sciatica in over 16s: assessment and management. www.nice.org.uk/guidance/NG59

Wnuk, N.M., Alkasab, T.K., and Rosenthal, D.I. 2018. Magnetic resonance imaging of the lumbar spine: determining clinical impact and potential harm from overuse. *Spine J*; 18(9):1653–8. https://doi.org/10.1016/j.spinee.2018.04.005 *Of over 5000 lumbar MRI scans, the false-positive rate was 81%.*

SPRAINS AND STRAINS

A sprain is an overstretch or tear of a ligament; a strain is an overstretch or tear of a muscle.

History

- How and when did it happen?
- Severity of impact
- Location of any pain and what makes it worse
- Timing of pain (delayed pain and swelling suggest soft-tissue injury)
- Relevant medical and drug history, particularly osteoporosis and anticoagulants
- 🚩 Functional loss (e.g., weakness)
- 🚩 Instability or 'giving way'
- 🚩 Neurological symptoms
- 🚩 Any safeguarding concerns

Examination

- Swelling (note that this takes time to develop – in primary care, people may present early)
- Assess possibility of fracture/dislocation (see Box 12.2):
  - Degree of bruising (again, takes time to develop)
  - Any deformity
  - Bony tenderness
  - Ability to weight bear, if relevant
  - Restriction of movement. If passive movements are pain-free, then fracture is unlikely
- Assess circulation (warmth/pulses/capillary refill) and sensation distal to injury
- If stressing/pushing on a ligament reproduces the pain, then this is likely to be the location of injury
- If a joint feels unstable (e.g., moves out of alignment when examined) then there is likely to be a ligament tear

Self-care

- Follow **PEACE** in the first few days after injury and then **LOVE** thereafter (Dubois and Esculier, 2019):
  - **P**rotect from further injury and avoid exacerbating activities for a few days
  - **E**levation above the level of the heart as often as possible
  - **A**void NSAIDs and ice
  - **C**ompression (e.g., with Tubigrip) may relieve symptoms of joint injuries
  - **E**ducation on allowing the body to heal itself and avoiding unnecessary investigations

and

  - **L**oad the injured site in accordance with improvements in the level of pain
  - **O**ptimism is important for supporting recovery – the injury is very likely to improve
  - **V**ascularisation (get blood pumping with pain-free activity to help tissue repair)
  - **E**xercise to restore mobility, strength and functioning
- Note that CKS still recommends the acronyms PRICE and HARM, but NMIC prefers the above due to the emphasis on longer-term recovery, education and positive thinking. Additionally, some elements of PRICE, such as applying ice, are not supported by good evidence (Halabchi and Hassabi, 2020)
- Take paracetamol or use topical diclofenac emulgel[PC] for pain relief, but oral NSAIDs are not recommended in the first 48 hours because they may delay the healing process; inflammation plays an important part in healing. NSAIDs are no more effective than paracetamol after sprains (Jones et al., 2020)
- Opioids do not appear to be more effective in acute sprains and fractures than the combination of paracetamol and ibuprofen (at least at the doses conventionally used)

BOX 12.2 INDICATIONS FOR X-RAY AFTER ACUTE INJURY (IF NOT OBVIOUS FRACTURE)

- Ankle: pain over the malleolus AND any of the following:
  - Inability to take four weight-bearing steps (transferring weight twice onto each leg)
  - Bone tenderness along the distal 6 cm of the posterior edge of the fibula or tip of the lateral malleolus
  - Bone tenderness along the distal 6 cm of the posterior edge of the tibia or tip of the medial malleolus

- Foot: pain in the midfoot zone AND any of the following:
  - Inability to take four weight-bearing steps (transferring weight twice onto each leg)
  - Bone tenderness at base of the fifth metatarsal
  - Bone tenderness of the navicular bone (distal to the medial malleolus)

- Knee: any of the following:
  - Inability to take four weight-bearing steps (transferring weight twice onto each leg)
  - Age ≥55
  - Tenderness at the head of fibula
  - Isolated tenderness of patella
  - Inability to flex knee to 90 degrees

- Wrist:
  - Pain or tenderness over the scaphoid bone

Diagrams available online:
www.mdcalc.com/calc/1670/ottawa-ankle-rule
www.mdcalc.com/calc/368/ottawa-knee-rule

 RED FLAGS

Send urgently to hospital (Paediatrics/Orthopaedics/A&E) if:
- Safeguarding concerns; any injury in a non-mobile child is suspicious (*call ahead and highlight your concerns about possible non-accidental injury with the Paediatric team before the child arrives at hospital*)
- Swelling of a joint and known bleeding disorder (*possible haemarthrosis – bleeding into a joint which is typically very painful with rapid swelling*)
- Penetrating injury to joint and/or fever with hot, red and swollen joint (*high risk of septic arthritis*)
- Deformity/instability/inability to perform certain movements (*suspected dislocation, complete muscle tear or complete tendon rupture*)
- Possible damage to nerves (e.g., loss of sensation distal to injury) or circulation (e.g., prolonged cap refill/cool to touch distal to injury)
- Inability to take four weight-bearing steps (*possible fracture*)
- Other suspicion of possible fracture (see Box 12.2)

MSK

References

Chang, A.K., Bijur, P.E., Esses, D., et al. 2017. Effect of a single dose of oral opioid and nonopioid analgesics on acute extremity pain in the emergency department: a randomized clinical trial. *JAMA*; 318(17):1661–7. https://doi.org/10.1001/jama.2017.16190 *In this RCT of people with limb pain following injury, there was little difference in the effects of various combinations of analgesics.*

Derry, S., Wiffen, P.J., Kalso, E.A., et al. 2017. Topical analgesics for acute and chronic pain in adults – an overview of Cochrane Reviews. *Cochrane Database Syst Rev*; 5:CD008609. https://doi.org/10.1002/14651858.CD008609.pub2 *There was good evidence that topical NSAIDs are useful in acute pain conditions such as sprains or strains. Different formulations varied in effectiveness; the best was diclofenac emulgel (NNT 1.8).*

Dubois, B., and Esculier, J-F. 2019. Soft-tissue injuries simply need PEACE and LOVE. *Br J Sports Med*; 54(2):72–3. https://doi.org/10.1136/bjsports-2019-101253 *Advocating new acronyms to replace RICE/PRICE/POLICE with the addition of education and encouraging optimism.*

Halabchi, F., and Hassabi, M. 2020. Acute ankle sprain in athletes: clinical aspects and algorithmic approach. *World J Orthop*; 11(12):534–58. https://doi.org/10.5312/wjo.v11.i12.534 *Highlighting the lack of evidence for various aspects of management of ankle sprains, including applying ice.*

Jones, P., Lamdin, R., and Dalziel, S.R. 2020. Oral non-steroidal anti-inflammatory drugs versus other oral analgesic agents for acute soft tissue injury. *Cochrane Database Syst Rev*; 8:CD007789. https://doi.org/10.1002/14651858.CD007789.pub3 *Compared with paracetamol, oral NSAIDs make no difference to pain after sprains. Inflammation is integral to the healing process; by reducing inflammation, healing may be impaired. NSAIDs delay, but do not reduce, the inflammatory response to injury.*

NICE CKS. 2020. Sprains and strains. https://cks.nice.org.uk/topics/sprains-strains/

Vuurberg, G., Hoorntje, A., Wink, L.M., et al. 2018. Diagnosis, treatment and prevention of ankle sprains: update of an evidence-based clinical guideline. *Br J Sports Med*; 52(15):956. http://dx.doi.org/10.1136/bjsports-2017-098106 *NSAIDs may be used to reduce pain and swelling after ankle sprains, but usage is not without complications and NSAIDs may suppress the natural healing process.*

JOINT PAINS

Arthralgia is common; people may be concerned that they have developed rheumatoid arthritis (RA). Here is a brief overview:

- **Shoulder pain**: younger adults may suffer from dislocations or disorders of the acromioclavicular joint. In people aged 30–60, pain is most likely to be rotator cuff-related, although 'frozen shoulder' also increases in prevalence between ages 50–60, particularly in people with diabetes. Once aged >60, osteoarthritis becomes more likely

- **Elbow pain** in an adult is most likely to be tennis elbow (lateral epicondylitis)

- **Knee pain** in adolescents may be due to Osgood–Schlatter disease, an inflammation at the site where the patellar tendon attaches to the tibia. In young adults, patellofemoral pain syndrome (pain at the front of the knee on exercise or when sitting for too long) is common. In older adults, suspect osteoarthritis; if the history is suggestive and the person is aged ≥45, there is no need for an x-ray to confirm the diagnosis

- **Hip pain** in older people is most likely to be due to osteoarthritis or greater trochanteric pain syndrome. Beware hip pain and limp in children; this needs urgent orthopaedic assessment (slipped femoral epiphysis, Perthes' disease)

- **Thumb and finger pain** is usually due to osteoarthritis

- **Toe pain** is usually caused by gout if it occurs episodically or osteoarthritis if more continuous in an older person

Osteoarthritis is a common joint disorder that mostly affects the knees, hips and small joints of the hands. It is much more common with increasing age but may also affect people in their 40s. The joints are painful when used, with pain generally worse after activity or at the end of the day. There may be crepitus or restriction of movement but morning stiffness should generally last <30 minutes. Diagnosis can usually be made clinically without the need for imaging, with tests such as x-rays not always correlating with clinical severity and generally only useful if surgery is being considered.

The concept of 'wear and tear' for osteoarthritis has been recently superseded by 'tear, flare and repair' to allude to the imbalance between damage and repair to joint tissue. Injury can result in flares with some inflammation; NSAIDs can therefore be helpful, as can steroid injections in the short term (see earlier section on NSAIDs and their risks; also note that steroid injections have been associated with potential for long-term harm to the joint).

NICE recommends that the core treatments are therapeutic exercise and weight management if appropriate (particularly for osteoarthritis affecting the knees or hips), along with information and support. For lower limb osteoarthritis, walking aids can also be useful. Referral for surgical management may be necessary if symptoms are substantially affecting quality of life and other approaches have been insufficiently effective.

RA and other causes of inflammatory arthritis are, as the term suggests, characterised by inflammation of the joints. RA usually starts with the small joints of the hands and the feet. It affects 1% of the population and is more common in women in their 40s and 50s. The key features are swelling, heat and pain in the affected joints, often with stiffness after inactivity. Morning stiffness lasting ≥30 minutes is suggestive; symptoms are usually symmetrical.

There are other causes of inflammatory arthritis including systemic lupus erythematosus, psoriatic arthritis and ankylosing spondylitis; it is not essential for a practitioner in primary care to work out which one might be present. Instead, anyone with suspected inflammatory arthritis should be *referred urgently to Rheumatology*. Blood tests (e.g., CRP, rheumatoid factor, anti-cyclic citrullinated peptide [anti-CCP]) can be requested to accompany the referral but cannot make or exclude a diagnosis on their own, so normal results should not dissuade you from referral. Prompt diagnosis and treatment of these conditions can help avoid permanent joint damage and disability.

References

Birrell, F., and Johnson, A. 2022. The tear, flare, and repair model of osteoarthritis. *BMJ*; 377:o1028. https://doi.org/10.1136/bmj.o1028

Gray, M., Wallace, A., and Aldridge, S. 2016. Assessment of shoulder pain for non-specialists. *BMJ*; 355:i5783. https://doi.org/10.1136/bmj.i5783

NICE. 2022. NG226. Osteoarthritis in over 16s: diagnosis and management. www.nice.org.uk/guidance/NG226

Speers, C.J., and Bhogal, G.S. 2017. Greater trochanteric pain syndrome: a review of diagnosis and management in general practice. *Br J Gen Pract*; 67(663):479–80. https://doi.org/10.3399/bjgp17X693041

GOUT

This disorder of purine metabolism is more common in men aged 30–60. Due to high levels of uric acid in the blood, crystals form in the cooler areas of the body, typically the first metatarsophalangeal joint (at the base of the great toe) but also in tophi (swellings often found on the elbow or pinna).

History

- Location of pain
- Speed of onset (often rapid, within 24 hours)
- Previous episodes and response to treatment
- Alcohol intake
- Diet – particularly offal, game, oily fish, seafood and meat/yeast extracts (Bovril or Marmite)
- Medication – aspirin, diuretics
- ⚑ Fever/malaise (*possible septic arthritis*)

Examination

- Temperature, heart rate and respiratory rate (fever, rapid heart or respiratory rate suggest possible septic arthritis)
- The joint is swollen, hot, red and painful on passive movement with gout. It may affect any joint, though usually on the lower limb, and is often asymmetrical. Over time, attacks of gout can involve multiple joints at once
- Tophi may be seen – firm white nodules on pinnae, elbows, fingers, toes or knees. Usually occur when gout is long standing

Tests

- Serum uric acid measurement may help the diagnosis, but:
  - Should be delayed until at least 4 weeks after the attack
  - False-positives and false-negatives are common
- If the diagnosis is uncertain, consider testing CRP, ESR, rheumatoid factor and anti-nuclear antibodies

Self-care

- Rest and elevate the limb
- Use an ice pack, for example frozen peas wrapped in a towel
- Drink plenty of water
- Reduce alcohol intake – particularly beer and spirits
- Reduce consumption of sugars, especially fructose
- The evidence base for dietary interventions is poor, but guidelines suggest that people should reduce their consumption of food high in purines, e.g., liver, kidneys, game, oily fish, yeast/meat extracts and shellfish
- A diet sheet is available from the UK Gout Society (note that this recommends vitamin C supplements, though the evidence is not convincing [Brzezińska et al., 2021]) – see www.ukgoutsociety.org/docs/goutsociety-allaboutgoutanddiet-0113.pdf

MSK

Action

- First-line treatment is naproxen[PBCI] (for adults, initially 750 mg, then 250 mg every 8 hours until 1–2 days after the attack has passed). When assessing the suitability of naproxen, note that people with gout are also at increased risk of cardiovascular disease

- If an NSAID is not suitable for the person, prescribe colchicine[PCI] (for adults, 500 micrograms 2–4 times a day until symptoms are relieved, maximum 6 mg per course; do not repeat course within 3 days). An unfortunate side effect of colchicine is diarrhoea; this is not ideal when mobilising is painful, although the risk is low within the maximum of 6 mg per course

- If neither an NSAID or colchicine can be used, an alternative is prednisolone[PI] (for adults, 30 mg daily for 5 days)

- Intra-articular corticosteroid injections can be used if oral treatment is unsuitable or ineffective

- People with multiple or troublesome flares of gout, tophi or particular risk factors for recurrence of gout (e.g., CKD with eGFR <60, diuretic therapy) should be offered prophylaxis with allopurinol[PCI]; NICE also recommend discussing the option of prophylaxis with everyone else with gout. Allopurinol takes 2–3 months to work, during which time an NSAID or colchicine should be co-prescribed, and urate levels should be monitored

- Offer a cardiovascular risk assessment. If the person is taking prophylactic aspirin, they should be offered an alternative. Thiazide diuretics such as bendroflumethiazide and indapamide also increase the risk of gout and should be reviewed

RED FLAG

- Pain, heat and swelling in a single joint associated with fever or malaise (*suspect septic arthritis; send urgently to hospital with referral to Orthopaedics*)

References

Brzezińska, O., Styrzyński, F., Makowska, J., et al. 2021. Role of vitamin c in prophylaxis and treatment of gout—a literature review. *Nutrients*; 13(2):701. https://doi.org/10.3390/nu13020701 *The results do not clearly define the benefits of a high daily intake of vitamin C in preventing the development and recurrence of gout.*

Jamnik, J., Rehman, S., Blanco Mejia, S., et al. 2016. Fructose intake and risk of gout and hyperuricemia: a systematic review and meta-analysis of prospective cohort studies. *BMJ Open*; 6(10):e013191. https://doi.org/10.1136/bmjopen-2016-013191 *Fructose consumption was associated with an increased risk (62%) of developing gout in predominantly white health professionals.*

Neilson, J., Bonnon, A., Dickson, A., et al. 2022. Gout: diagnosis and management—summary of NICE guidance. *BMJ*; 378:o1754. https://doi.org/10.1136/bmj.o1754

NICE. 2022. NG219. Gout: diagnosis and management. www.nice.org.uk/guidance/ng219/chapter/Recommendations

NICE CKS. 2022. Gout. https://cks.nice.org.uk/topics/gout/

ROAD TRAFFIC COLLISION

Be aware that people may present for a range of reasons other than concern over their symptoms; they may think it important that they attend to justify a future claim for compensation, or may have been advised to be 'checked over' by the police or an insurance company. The first doctor to provide emergency treatment after a road traffic accident is entitled to charge a fee of £21.30 if the care occurs outside an NHS hospital: see www.bma.org.uk/pay-and-contracts/fees/fees-for-doctors-services/fees-for-emergency-treatment-in-a-road-traffic-accident

History

- Date and time of the collision
- Were they the driver or passenger/pedestrian/cyclist?
- Details of the collision – how did it happen, were they moving or stationary?
- Direction of impact
- If in a car, whether a seat belt was worn, whether there was a head rest and if airbags were activated
- Descriptions of the injuries: pain, stiffness, bruising, exacerbating movements
- If neck pain, was it immediate with restricted movement (more concerning) or delayed?
- Psychological effects: shaking, insomnia, nightmares, fear of driving, flashbacks
- Time off work/school

🏴 Any loss of function (e.g., weakness)

🏴 Instability or 'giving way'

🏴 Disturbance of bladder/bowel function or perianal numbness

Examination

- Appropriate to affected area
- Extent of grazing and bruising – measure these
- Movement of affected limbs – check for any limitation of range
- Check how far they can move their neck (ask them to try putting their chin to their chest, looking up at the ceiling, looking over each shoulder and tilting their head to each shoulder)
- Assess possibility of fracture/dislocation (see Box 12.2 for indications for x-ray)

Action

- Give treatment and advice dependent on, and appropriate to, the injuries
- Sketch areas of grazing and bruising, or recommend they take photos
- Often the main purpose of the person's visit is to document the injuries for a possible future compensation claim. Record the details carefully

RED FLAGS

- Any suspicion of fracture or dislocation (see Box 12.2) (*immobilise affected area and send urgently to hospital with referral to Orthopaedics*)
- Inability to laterally rotate the neck more than 45 degrees (*needs x-ray of cervical spine; consider immobilisation and send urgently to A&E*)
- Suspicion of spinal cord or cauda equina compromise, including any of the following: weakness in limbs, loss of sensation, disturbance of bladder or bowel function, perianal numbness (*send urgently to hospital with referral to Orthopaedics*)

References

British Medical Association. 2021. Fees for emergency treatment in a road traffic accident. www.bma.org.uk/pay-and-contracts/fees/fees-for-doctors-services/fees-for-emergency-treatment-in-a-road-traffic-accident

Michaleff, Z.A., Maher, C.G., Verhagen, A.P., et al. 2012. Accuracy of the Canadian C-spine rule and NEXUS to screen for clinically important cervical spine injury in patients following blunt trauma: a systematic review. *CMAJ*; 184(16):E867. https://doi.org/10.1503/cmaj.120675

NICE. 2016. NG41. Spinal injury: assessment and initial management. www.nice.org.uk/guidance/ng41

HEAD INJURY

A crucial element of the initial assessment of acute head injury in primary care is considering whether the person should be sent to hospital. NICE recently published detailed guidance on this.

History

- How did it happen?
- How long ago?

🏴 Recent intake of alcohol or recreational drugs

🏴 Persistent headache since injury

🏴 Any loss of consciousness

🏴 Vomiting since injury – particularly worrying if worsening

🏴 Confusion, amnesia, drowsiness

🏴 Convulsions

🏴 Neurological disturbance (e.g., numbness, weakness, double vision)

MSK

🚩 Blood or clear fluid from ear or nose

🚩 Bleeding disorder or taking anticoagulants/antiplatelets (except aspirin monotherapy)

🚩 Previous brain surgery

🚩 Any safeguarding concerns

Examination

- Examine site of injury, look for and measure any bruising or swelling
- Check pupils:

    🚩 Are they unequal?

    🚩 Are they not reacting normally or equally to light?

🚩 Confused/drowsy (assess using the Glasgow Coma Scale – anything below the maximum score (i.e., scoring <15) is abnormal [see Box 12.3])

🚩 Bruising around the eyes or behind the ears (signs of a skull fracture)

🚩 Bulging fontanelle (check for this in children aged <2 years)

🚩 Any impairment to moving all limbs properly with normal and equal power

---

BOX 12.3 GLASGOW COMA SCALE (GCS) FOR ADULTS AND VERBAL CHILDREN

Best eye response:

- Eyes open spontaneously – score 4
- Eyes open in response to voice – score 3
- Eyes open in response to painful stimuli – score 2
- Does not open eyes – score 1

Best verbal response:

- Orientated and converses normally – score 5
- Confused and disorientated – score 4
- Inappropriate words – score 3
- Incomprehensible sounds – score 2
- Makes no sounds – score 1

Best motor response:

- Obeys simple commands – score 6
- Localises painful stimuli – score 5
- Flexion or withdrawal in response to painful stimuli – score 4
- Abnormal flexion in response to painful stimuli – score 3
- Extension in response to painful stimuli – score 2
- Makes no movement in response to pain – score 1

Self-care for adults

- Should be monitored by another responsible person for 24 hours after the injury
- Rest as much as possible
- Take paracetamol, if needed, for headache. Avoid ibuprofen (increased bleeding risk)
- If appropriate, inform employer about head injury and consider graded return to work
- Until completely recovered, avoid:
    - Being alone or out of telephone contact
    - Alcohol or sedative medicines
    - Contact sports
    - Driving or operating machinery
- Safety-netting is essential – see next section

Advice to parents about caring for children

- Offer paracetamol if required for headache. Avoid ibuprofen (increased bleeding risk)
- Offer only light meals for 1 or 2 days
- Until completely recovered, avoid:
  - Leaving the child alone. Check them every couple of hours while they are asleep (but do allow them to sleep)
  - Overexcitement
  - Contact sports and rough play
- If appropriate, inform teacher that child has had a head injury and consider graded return to school
- Safety-netting is essential – see next section

Safety-netting advice

- Go to A&E immediately if person:
  - Becomes drowsy or confused
  - Leaks fluid from ear or nose
  - Develops bruising behind the ears
  - Develops problems with sight, understanding, memory or speech
  - Develops loss of balance or weakness in arms or legs
  - Has worsening headache
  - Vomits
  - In children – has persistent crying, altered behaviour or is irritable
  - In children – concern from parent(s)/family

RED FLAGS

Send urgently to A&E or appropriate specialty if:

- High-energy impact to head, e.g., fall from a height of ≥1 metre (roughly the height of a supermarket trolley handle) or ≥5 stairs
- GCS <15 (i.e., any impairment)
- Any history of loss of consciousness
- Amnesia
- Confusion, irritability or altered behaviour
- Weakness or numbness in any limbs, visual disturbance, loss of balance
- Convulsions or any other neurological disturbance
- Vomiting (use clinical judgement in children aged ≤12 years, e.g., if there is a cause for the vomiting other than the head injury)
- Persistent/worsening headache
- Bleeding disorder or taking anticoagulant/antiplatelet (except aspirin monotherapy)
- Previous brain surgery
- Intoxication (alcohol or recreational drugs)
- Suspected skull fracture (*suggested by periorbital bruising without local injury, deafness, clear cerebrospinal fluid from ear or nose, bleeding from ear, bruising behind ear*)
- Pupils unequal or non-reactive
- Suspicion of a non-accidental injury (*e.g., non-mobile child, inadequate explanation, delayed presentation, other injuries, previous safeguarding concerns – call ahead to Paediatric team to inform them of your concerns before the child arrives at hospital*)
- Bulging fontanelle, indicating raised intracranial pressure (*the anterior fontanelle has generally closed by 2 years of age*)
- Bruise, swelling or laceration of >5cm on the head of a child aged <1 year
- No responsible adult is able to stay with the person for the first 24 hours after the injury, even if none of the other criteria above is met

MSK

Reference

NICE. 2023. NG232. Head injury: assessment and early management. www.nice.org.uk/guidance/ng232

BURNS AND SCALDS

A burn is caused by heat, friction, electricity, chemical solids or radiation, whereas a scald is caused by hot liquid, chemical fluids or steam. Superficial burns or partial-thickness burns covering <5% of the body are classed as minor burns.

History

- Parts and extent of body affected
- Cause of burn/scald
- How it occurred and duration of contact
- What has been done so far?
- Is it painful? (Full-thickness burns are not painful)
- 🚩 Any safeguarding concerns

Examination

- Check temperature, heart rate and respiratory rate – is there evidence of sepsis?
- Extent of burn – how many palm prints of the person is the size of the burn? (Each palm print is estimated to be around 1% of the body surface area)
- Depth of burn is assessed through colour change/vesicles/capillary refill (tested using sterile cotton bud or swab)
  - Superficial epidermal burns are red but not blistered. Capillary refill: blanches and refills rapidly
  - Superficial dermal (partial-thickness) burns are pale pink with blistering. Capillary refill: blanches and refills slowly
  - Deep dermal (partial-thickness) burns are blotchy and red with possible blistering. Capillary refill: does not blanch
  - Full-thickness burns look leathery or waxy. The skin may be white, brown or black with no blisters. Capillary refill: does not blanch
- In dark skin, superficial or partial thickness burns may not appear red
- Evidence of possible inhalation injury (burnt nasal hairs, carbon in sputum)

Self-care

- Ensure safety (e.g., from flames, chemicals or electricity)
- Irrigate the burn as soon as possible by immersing the area in cool running water for at least 20 minutes. Do not use iced water
- Keep warm to avoid hypothermia if cooling large areas
- If swollen, elevate the affected limb
- Take paracetamol for pain relief
- Apply emollients two to three times daily
- Avoid sun exposure to the affected area
- If being referred to hospital (see next section), cover the burn with cling film, but do not wrap it all around the limb. Use a clean, clear plastic bag for hands or feet

Action

- Ensure that the area has been adequately irrigated as above
- Consider aspirating any vesicles/bullae that are likely to burst; otherwise leave them intact
- If blistered, cover with a non-adherent dressing (e.g., paraffin gauze – Jelonet) then a dressing pad and bandage
- Check whether tetanus prophylaxis is indicated. If the person has not received an adequate priming course of tetanus vaccine (at least 3 doses) or their immunisation status is uncertain, then an immediate dose of tetanus

vaccine would be indicated (potentially with other measures in addition, depending on the specifics of the burn). The guidance is complex; a useful summary can be found at https://assets.publishing.service.gov.uk/media/5de1352340f0b650c194cb2c/Tetanus_quick_guide_poster.pdf

- Review after 48 hours as burn depth may increase over time and/or infection may develop
- Safety-netting: advise to seek urgent attention if they develop signs or symptoms of infection, such as increased pain, odour, exudate, fever or redness

RED FLAGS

- *Admit urgently under Medical/Paediatrics/Plastic Surgery if:*
  - Signs of infection/sepsis/systemically unwell
  - Safeguarding concerns (call ahead to inform team of concerns before child's arrival)
  - Deep dermal or full-thickness burn
  - Burn goes completely around the body or a limb
  - Area larger than two palm prints in a child aged <16 years
  - Area larger than three palm prints in an adult
  - Involving the face, hands, feet, perineum, genitalia or any flexure
  - Any electrical, cold or chemical burn
  - Any inhalation injury

- *Consider admitting urgently under Medical/Paediatrics/Plastic Surgery if:*
  - Superficial dermal burn
  - Child aged <5 years
  - Adult aged >60
  - Comorbidities/immunosuppressed/pregnant
  - Social reasons, pain control or if dressings difficult to manage

- If a burn has not healed after 2 weeks, *refer to a specialist burn unit*

References

Griffin, B.R., Frear, C.C., Babl, F., et al. 2020. Cool running water first aid decreases skin grafting requirements in pediatric burns: a cohort study of two thousand four hundred ninety-five children. *Ann Emerg Med*; 75(1):75–85. https://doi.org/10.1016/j.annemergmed.2019.06.028 *In this cohort study of 2500 children, the odds of skin grafting were decreased among children who had 20 minutes of cold running water (odds ratio 0.6).*

NICE CKS. 2023. Burns and scalds. https://cks.nice.org.uk/topics/burns-scalds/

Norman, G., Christie, J., Liu, Z., et al. 2017. Antiseptics for burns. *Cochrane Database Syst Rev*; 7:CD011821. https://doi.org/10.1002/14651858.CD011821.pub2 *This review found that it was uncertain whether antiseptics were associated with any difference in healing, infections or other outcomes.*

SUNBURN

History

- Intensity and duration of exposure
- Sunscreen usage
- Fluid intake and urine output
- 🚩 Any safeguarding concerns *(contact safeguarding lead or admit urgently under Medical/Paediatrics)*

Examination

- Temperature
- Extent of burn
- Redness
- Blistering
- Skin loss

MSK

Self-care

- Cool the skin by having a cool shower or bath; do not apply ice
- Drink plenty of cool fluids
- Avoid alcohol
- Apply emollient or aloe vera gel (only to intact skin)
- Leave blisters intact if possible
- Apply non-adherent dressings, for example Jelonet, to blisters or areas of skin loss

Caution

- If temperature is elevated, assess level of hydration, and treat for heatstroke with rest, fluids and cooling

References

Genuino, G.A.S., Baluyut-Angeles, K.V., Espiritu, A.P.T., et al. 2014. Topical petrolatum gel alone versus topical silver sulfadiazine with standard gauze dressings for the treatment of superficial partial thickness burns in adults: a randomized controlled trial. *Burns*; 40(7):1267–73. https://doi.org/10.1016/j.burns.2014.07.024 *Petrolatum gel without top dressings may be at least as effective as silver sulfadiazine gauze dressings in the treatment of minor superficial partial-thickness burns in adults.*

Tidy, C. 2022. Sunburn. Patient professional article. https://patient.info/doctor/sunburn

BITES – ANIMAL AND HUMAN

History

- Which part of the body?
- How did it happen? What animal? (Note that the answer may not be truthful, particularly if a human bite)
- Date/time of bite
- Was the skin broken? Did it bleed?
- Any contamination
- Did it happen abroad?
- 🚩 Immunosuppressed
- 🚩 Severe liver disease
- 🚩 Structural heart disease (e.g., prosthetic valve)
- 🚩 Prosthetic joint
- 🚩 Any safeguarding concerns

Examination

- Temperature, heart rate and respiratory rate
- Look for cellulitis – is the surrounding area hot, red or tender?
- Is there discharge or signs of bleeding from the wound?
- How deep is the wound? – This may be difficult to assess in puncture wounds, so err on the side of caution
- Any teeth or foreign bodies in the wound?

Tests

- Consider wound swab

Self-care

- Check for signs of infection and, if these develop, seek help immediately
- If bite on limb then elevate the affected limb

Action

- If fresh wound, irrigate well with water

- If possible, remove any foreign bodies or debris from the wound
- Any wound that needs debridement or closure will likely require attendance at A&E. However, note that it is not usual practice to surgically close bites
- Consider need for vaccination against:
  - Tetanus (e.g., due to exposure to soil; but tetanus prophylaxis in people who have received an adequate priming course of vaccination (at least 3 doses) is not generally needed for bites from domestic pets (UKHSA, 2023). A useful summary of the guidance can be found at https://assets.publishing.service.gov.uk/media/5de1352340f0b650c194cb2c/Tetanus_quick_guide_poster.pdf
  - Hepatitis B (if bitten by a human; although note that the biter is likely to be at greater risk of contracting a blood-borne virus from the incident than the person who was bitten)
- Consider post-exposure prophylaxis against rabies and HIV
- Consider antibiotic only if the bite has broken the skin (Table 12.3)

Table 12.3 Indications for antibiotic treatment following a bite that has broken the skin

Type of bite	If bite has broken the skin but not drawn blood	If bite has broken the skin and drawn blood
Human	Consider antibiotic if high risk	Offer antibiotic
Cat	Consider antibiotic if wound could be deep	Offer antibiotic
Dog or other traditional pet	Do not offer antibiotic	Offer antibiotic if high-risk bite. Consider if high-risk site or person

High-risk situations:
- **Bite** (deep, contaminated, from an unusual animal or acquired under water)
- **Site** (hands, feet, face, genitals, over joints or cartilage)
- **Person** (immunosuppressed, severe liver disease, structural heart disease, prosthetic valve or joint, baby or frail)

Antibiotic choice in adults

- Co-amoxiclav, 500/125 mg three times daily for adults: 3 days for prophylaxis (no signs of infection), or 5 days for treatment
- If allergic to penicillin:
  - Doxycycline[PBC], 200 mg on first day, then 100–200 mg daily, plus metronidazole[Q], 400 mg three times daily for adults: 3 days for prophylaxis (no signs of infection), or 5 days for treatment
  - Review in 1–2 days, as not all pathogens are covered by the alternatives to penicillin

RED FLAGS

- Safeguarding concerns, for example human or dog bite to a child (*contact safeguarding lead or admit urgently under Medical/Paediatrics if significant concern [call ahead if doing so]*)
- Risk of rabies, for example bat bite (*phone Rabies and Immunoglobulin Service at UK Health Security Agency on 0330 128 1020*)
- Risk of hepatitis B or HIV (*seek specialist advice or send urgently to A&E*)
- *Send urgently to A&E or relevant specialty if*:
  - Penetrating wound affecting deeper structures
  - Bites to poorly vascularised areas, for example ear or nose
  - Facial wounds (unless very minor) or scalp bite in a child
  - Suspected foreign body in wound or in need of closure
  - Severe cellulitis/infected wounds not responding to treatment/systemically unwell
  - High-risk group: immunosuppressed, severe liver disease, structural heart disease, prosthetic valve or joint

MSK

References

NICE. 2020. NG184. Human and animal bites: antimicrobial prescribing. www.nice.org.uk/guidance/ng184

UK Health Security Agency. 2023. Guidance on the management of suspected tetanus cases and on the assessment and management of tetanus prone wounds. www.gov.uk/government/publications/tetanus-advice-for-health-professionals
Although smaller bites from domestic pets are generally puncture injuries, animal saliva should not contain tetanus spores unless the animal has been rooting in soil or lives in an agricultural setting.

INSECT BITES AND STINGS

There is a temptation to overtreat insect bites or stings with antibiotics because the appearance of the normal inflammatory response to the sting toxin may look like an infection. In fact, it is uncommon for insect bites in the UK to become infected. If the bite was sustained abroad, record the details carefully in case the person presents later with symptoms that could be a disease from the bite, such as malaria or leishmaniasis.

History

- Site
- Time of bite/sting
- Nature of insect (if known)
- Itching
- Generalised rash
- 🚩 Breathing difficulty
- 🚩 Swelling of the mouth, tongue or throat
- 🚩 Severely immunosuppressed (*increased risk of infection*)
- 🚩 Previous systemic allergic reaction to same type of bite

Examination

- Temperature, heart rate and respiratory rate
- Size of reaction
- Evidence of lymphangitis or cellulitis
- Is sting still in situ (rare)

Self-care

- Wash area with soap and water and apply ice pack to reduce swelling (except for jellyfish stings, which should be washed in vinegar and have heat applied for 40 minutes)
- If the site is itchy:
  - Try not to scratch (to reduce the risk of infection); rub or slap the area instead. Consider brushing with a clean paintbrush to manage itching without damaging the skin
  - Take an oral antihistamine, for example loratadine[PB] (10 mg once daily for adults), although note that there is uncertainty about their effectiveness in this context (NICE, 2020)
  - If still itching, consider adding oral chlorphenamine[PBI] (4 mg for adults) at night, if sedation tolerated
  - Topical antihistamines have poor absorption so are unlikely to be effective
  - Piezo-electric devices may reduce itching; they are available OTC for around £7
- Safety-netting advice, including to seek help if any of the following:
  - Breathing difficulty (*requires urgent attention*)
  - Fever or signs of infection
  - Rash develops after tick bite (could be Lyme disease; see Box 12.4)

Action

- If stinger still in place, remove it as soon as possible by scraping with a scalpel blade, not tweezers
- Remove ticks as soon as possible. Specialist tick removers are available; otherwise, tweezers may be used (do not twist the tick during removal). Heat, Vaseline and alcohol are not recommended. Warn about signs of Lyme disease (Box 12.4)
- Timing is the best guide to distinguish the expected normal inflammatory response/allergy from infection. Allergic reactions usually occur within the first 24 hours, although a large local reaction may peak at 48 hours (Pesek and Lockey, 2013). Signs of infection usually develop after 24 hours, with increasing redness, tenderness and swelling; other signs of infection may include:
  - Fever
  - Pus
  - Lymphangitis (tracking)
- People at risk of severe reaction or infection may need admission; see Red Flags box

Prescription

- If infection is suspected, treat with flucloxacillin (500 mg four times daily for adults for 5–7 days) or, if allergic to penicillin, clarithromycin[PIQ] (500 mg twice daily for adults for 5–7 days). A delayed prescription may be appropriate
- Consider a few days' course of oral prednisolone[PI] (40 mg once daily for adults) if severe local reaction not responding adequately to oral antihistamine and there is no suspicion of infection

RED FLAGS

- Anaphylaxis (features include swelling of lips or tongue or throat, breathing difficulty, feeling faint; see section in Chapter 8) (*get help and administer IM adrenaline; send very urgently to hospital*)
- Consider *seeking specialist advice* or *admitting urgently under Medical/Paediatrics* if:
  - Systemically unwell
  - Severely immunosuppressed and symptoms/signs of an infection
  - Previous systemic allergic reaction to the same type of bite or sting
  - Bite or sting is in the mouth or throat, or around the eyes
  - Caused by an unusual or exotic insect
  - Fever or persisting lesions associated with a bite or sting that occurred while travelling abroad

RED FLAG CONDITION

BOX 12.4 LYME DISEASE

A bacterial infection carried by deer ticks. Cases occur mainly in forested areas, especially the New Forest. The risk is low if the tick has been attached for <24 hours, but people do not always notice the tick. In the UK, post-exposure prophylaxis is not recommended for tick bites.

A round red area develops around the site of the bite, typically 1–4 weeks later, and then spreads to become >5 cm (usually), with central clearing. It may be painful or itchy, and the person may feel unwell with flu-like symptoms.

Laboratory tests are available but are not necessary if the classical rash is present. If diagnosis is likely, treat adults with doxycycline[PBC], 100 mg twice daily for 21 days. There is a risk of long-term health problems if untreated.

MSK

References

Doyle, T., Headlam, J., Wilcox, C., et al. 2017. Evaluation of *Cyanea capillata* sting management protocols using ex vivo and in vitro envenomation models. *Toxins*; 9:215. https://doi.org/10.3390/toxins9070215 *After a sting by a lion's mane jellyfish (the most common UK type), washing in vinegar and applying a hot pack for 40 minutes was the most effective treatment.*

NICE. 2018. NG95. Lyme disease. www.nice.org.uk/guidance/ng95

NICE. 2020. NG182. Insect bites and stings: antimicrobial prescribing. www.nice.org.uk/guidance/ng182

NICE CKS. 2021. Insect bites and stings. https://cks.nice.org.uk/topics/insect-bites-stings/

Pesek, R.D., and Lockey, R.F. 2013. Management of insect sting hypersensitivity: an update. *Allergy Asthma Immunol Res*; 5(3):129–37. https://doi.org/10.4168%2Faair.2013.5.3.129 *Large local reactions usually peak at about 48 hours and then may take a week to resolve.*

CUTS/WOUNDS

Assess the risk of infection (e.g., contamination, comorbidities, immunosuppression) and check for signs of sepsis, if relevant.

History

- Wound location
- How did it occur?
- How long ago did it happen?
- Any contamination
- 🚩 Immunosuppression and/or diabetes
- 🚩 Any safeguarding concerns

Examination

- Check temperature, heart rate and respiratory rate
- Is there evidence of infection?
- Wound length
- Wound margins – are they jagged?
- Is there any contamination?
- Is the appearance consistent with the reported history?
- If on limb, check for normal range of movements near wound site and distally (assessing for possible tendon damage)
- Are there any healed scars? (Multiple injuries are less likely to be accidental)

Self-care

- Disinfect the skin with antiseptic, but try not to get it into the wound
- Take paracetamol for pain relief
- Seek help if increasing pain/redness/swelling or fever/malaise

Action

- Irrigate with sodium chloride 0.9% solution or cool water
- Remove any foreign bodies, under local anaesthetic if necessary
- Assess risk of infection – high risk would be wound contamination or >1 of the following (although use your clinical judgement):
  - Age ≥65
  - Wound length >5 cm
  - Jagged wound margin
  - Immunosuppression and/or diabetes
- If infected, take a swab and prescribe flucloxacillin (500 mg four times daily for adults for 5–7 days) or, if allergic to penicillin, clarithromycin[PIQ] (500 mg twice daily for adults for 5–7 days). If wound contaminated with high-risk material, use co-amoxiclav instead (500/125 mg three times daily for adults for 5–7 days)
- For infected wounds after surgery, take a swab and contact the responsible surgeon (ideally before prescribing, although this may not be practical)
- If high risk but no features of current infection, consider prophylactic antibiotic

- Check whether tetanus prophylaxis is indicated. If the person has not received an adequate priming course of tetanus vaccine (at least 3 doses) or their immunisation status is uncertain, then an immediate dose of tetanus vaccine would be indicated (potentially with other measures in addition, depending on the specifics of the wound). The guidance is complex; a useful summary can be found at https://assets.publishing.service.gov.uk/media/5de1352340f0b650c194cb2c/Tetanus_quick_guide_poster.pdf
- Dress with a clear vapour-permeable dressing; use an absorbent pad if exudate is present
- Consider closure only if no signs of infection and low risk:
  - Tissue glue, self-adhesive strips or both can be used to close wounds ≤5 cm where the edges can be easily pulled together. This is not practical near the eye (where glue could seriously damage the surface), for areas that cannot be covered by a dressing to stop them getting wet (where adhesives will fail) or on a joint (unless it is going to be immobilised for at least 5 days)
  - Suturing: for wounds not suitable for closure with glue or self-adhesive strips (see above)
  - Strips/sutures can be removed after 3–5 days for head wounds, 10–14 days for wounds over joints and 7–10 days for other sites
- If wound not closed initially due to infection/high risk, review in 3–5 days to see if wound can be closed

 RED FLAGS

- *Admit urgently under Medical/Paediatrics/Orthopaedics/Plastic Surgery if any:*
  - Signs of sepsis
  - Damage to bone, artery, nerve or tendon
  - Facial laceration
  - Signs of infection of the hand, face or near a joint
- *Safeguarding concerns (contact safeguarding lead or admit urgently under Medical/Paediatrics if significant concern [call ahead if doing so])*
- *Suspected self-inflicted injury (refer to experienced colleague)*

References

Aresti, N., Kassam, J., Bartlett, D., et al. 2017. Primary care management of postoperative shoulder, hip, and knee arthroplasty. *BMJ*; 359:j4431. https://doi.org/10.1136/bmj.j4431 *Do not treat suspected wound infections empirically with antibiotics without advice from the operating surgeon, as it may diminish the ability to later isolate an organism to treat.*

Hagiga, A., Arif, T., Gultiaeva, M., et al. 2021. ProTetanus – a rapid tetanus antibody status test for the assessment of tetanus-prone wounds. *Plast Surg Nurs*; 41(4):181. https://doi.org/10.1097/PSN.0000000000000390 *Incorporating this test may improve safety, reduce unnecessary interventions and reduce costs.*

NICE CKS. 2022. Lacerations. https://cks.nice.org.uk/topics/lacerations/

Health Security Agency. 2023. Guidance on the management of suspected tetanus cases and on the assessment and management of tetanus prone wounds. https://www.gov.uk/government/publications/tetanus-advice-for-health-professionals/guidance-on-the-management-of-suspected-tetanus-cases-and-the-assessment-and-management-of-tetanus-prone-wounds

MSK

CHAPTER 13

Management of minor illness

EVIDENCE-BASED PRACTICE

Evidence-based practice is 'integrating the best available research evidence with clinical expertise and the patients' unique values and circumstances' (Straus et al., 2010). There has been a quiet revolution going on over the past 20 years. Access to high-quality, clinical information has never been so good. The speed at which you can find the answer to a question is now so fast that searches can be done during a consultation if necessary.

Clear presentation of evidence is far more than making it look pretty; it saves lives. At its core, the power of evidence-based practice is about getting knowledge from research into practice to make a real difference to patients and outcomes. Original research is essential, but getting the benefit for people is a vital next step. Evidence-based practice has a few hazards and traps for the unwary, for example confusing quantity of evidence with certainty, or statistical significance ('p-values') with clinically meaningful impact. The references below give an overview of what evidence-based practice can do and what it can't do.

It is helpful for all clinicians working in primary care to be consistent and evidence based in managing minor illness. Where differences in practice are apparent, you should be able to access up-to-date, high-quality research evidence to aid discussion and help you to reach agreement. Critical analysis of published research has become highly complex and very time-consuming; thankfully, there are now several agencies such as the National Institute for Health and Care Excellence (NICE), the Scottish Intercollegiate Guidelines Network (SIGN) and Cochrane that analyse the evidence on our behalf and provide easy access to this information online. The Trip database helpfully ranks high-quality evidence over lower-quality, even though that may be in greater quantity.

Although reviewers explore possible flaws in the published papers, there are several factors that inherently bias the whole process of evaluating evidence. They include the following:

- Old drugs may appear inadequately researched compared with new ones
- Large samples are needed to reliably compare one intervention with another, but this can obscure the benefit or harm to a smaller group of people, with a particular characteristic, who form just part of that larger group
- Participants in research trials are often highly selected; they may be healthier and younger than those typically seen in practice, or have just the one disease requiring a treatment being researched, whereas, in reality, people often have several diseases and may be taking many drugs
- In addition to environmental differences, there are some physiological differences between different populations (hence variations in protocols for the control of hypertension, for example). The population evaluated in a trial may not reflect the individual in front of you
- Trials on new medicines are too short to pick up long-term side effects – this must come later from monitoring
- When real outcomes are too infrequent to be examined, surrogate measures are used (e.g., serum lipids as opposed to death from heart attack), but these may not truly reflect the important outcome of interest
- Few trials examine the whole person: an antihypertensive may reduce the risk of stroke, but did it cause more falls or road traffic accidents due to faintness?
- The rigorous standards and large sample sizes that are now expected in clinical trials lead to very high costs, which make it difficult to attract funding other than from pharmaceutical companies with a high turnover
- Funded research is more likely to favour a sponsor's product
- Negative results are less likely to be published
- Little research is conducted in primary care but that is where most people are assessed and treated
- Therapies that do not employ the same disease categories as Western medicine are difficult to research using randomised controlled trials (e.g., traditional Chinese medicine is aimed at balancing energy flow to correct disharmony; people with similar illnesses but different 'patterns', as identified through pulse and tongue findings, would be managed differently from each other under this approach)
- Many established therapies do not have a good evidence base because it would be unethical to withhold them for trial purposes. 'No evidence of effectiveness' is not the same as 'evidence of non-effectiveness'

Min

What we call 'evidence' is an artificial construction, a modern concept that should not be confused with truth. Patients will have a very different perspective from clinicians on what factors would persuade them to try a new therapy. Bearing these limitations in mind, it is important to recognise that guidance needs to be placed in the context of an individual's situation. The more experienced you become, the more confidence you will have to deviate from standard advice and target treatment to the needs of an individual; it is important that your reasons are documented.

We recommend the following resources:

- NICE: www.nice.org.uk *World-renowned clinical guidelines. Text and visual summaries give an overview and direct you to where to find more detail if you need it*
- NICE CKS: https://cks.nice.org.uk *Although under the NICE umbrella, CKS is an independent organisation which provides an interpretation of NICE and other evidence-based guidance presented in a way that is fast to navigate*
- SIGN: www.sign.ac.uk *Clinical guidelines for Scotland. These high-quality guidelines sometimes differ in their recommendations from those of NICE; the date of publication is helpful in assessing which is more likely to be based on up-to-date evidence*
- NICE OpenAthens: https://openathens.nice.org.uk/Hub *A portal to a variety of evidence sources. An Athens password is needed; those working in the NHS can obtain this by registering on the site*
- Cochrane Library: www.cochranelibrary.com *A huge database of systematic reviews*
- Trip (Turning Research into Practice) database: www.tripdatabase.com *User-friendly, huge database that shows the quality or type of evidence found from a search and displays evidence after just a few clicks. The normal version is powerful and free; there is also a pro version with more features for a low annual fee for individuals, but check first if your organisation already has paid for access*

HOLISTIC CARE

It is apparent from reading the other chapters of this book that the previous optimism of Western medicine about the eradication of infectious diseases through antibiotics has not been fulfilled. The more that we research these drugs, the more evidence we find that their benefits in most cases of minor illness are marginal, yet little evidence exists to support alternative treatments (including traditional self-care advice about rest and fluids); nor is such evidence likely to be provided because funding for research into minor illness and the relief of self-limiting symptoms is scarce.

You may feel that this lack of evidence-based treatments leaves you in an awkward position; someone is coming to you for help and you have little to offer. Your priority must be to establish that there is no indication of serious disease and, if so, to reassure the person accordingly and give appropriate safety-netting. It is important to be sensitive to their ideas, concerns and expectations, or 'agenda'. They may have attended in order to legitimise their illness to an employer or at the insistence of a relative. Stress can also arise from their own sense that they should not 'give in' to feeling unwell; it can be helpful to give them 'permission' to be ill and remind them that they are human and not a robot. Social factors, such as an impending holiday or examination, are often of far greater importance to people than any medical issues, and inevitably influence their assessment of the relative risks and benefits of any treatment. People often attend for reassurance and do not necessarily want advice on managing their illness. Furthermore, offering unsolicited medical advice and treatment as opposed to self-care, though well-meaning, may inadvertently encourage them to come back the next time they have the same self-limiting symptoms, which is wasteful for the health service and creates a culture of dependency.

In Western medicine, the 'placebo effect' is often regarded as a nuisance that interferes with the evaluation of the 'real' effects of a treatment in clinical trials, yet the placebo effect is itself very real and enhances the intrinsic healing ability of the body (curiously this may happen even if people are aware that they are taking a placebo – seen in so-called 'open-label placebo' trials). You can harness this effect very easily by establishing a good relationship, being positive and emphasising that a good recovery is likely.

The placebo effect of any treatment that you suggest will be enhanced by the fact that you have recommended it. If you recommend a treatment that does not have a good evidence base, you need to use your clinical judgement as to how to share this information (which will inevitably reduce the effectiveness). It is also clearly inappropriate to recommend such a treatment if there is a risk that it may do harm. More often though, there is little risk of harm and some of the limited evidence available shows possible benefit, such as suggesting pelargonium for acute cough, valerian for insomnia or adequate hydration to avoid headaches. Advising people about self-care does more than reducing the impact of minor illnesses: it empowers them and gives them more confidence so they can manage a wider range of future symptoms without reliance on health services.

References

Blease, C.R., Bernstein, M.H., and Locher, C. 2020. Open-label placebo clinical trials: is it the rationale, the interaction or the pill? *BMJ Evid Based Med*; 25(5):159–165. https://doi.org/10.1136/bmjebm-2019-111209 *A new programme of research in placebo studies indicates that it may be possible to harness placebo effects in clinical practice via ethical, non-deceptively prescribed 'open-label placebos'.*

Gabbay, J., and le May, A. 2016. Mindlines: making sense of evidence in practice. *BJGP*; 66(649):402–3. https://doi.org/10.3399/bjgp16X686221 *'Coffee-room chat may impact on evidence-based practice at least as much as all those guidelines'.*

Greenhalgh, T., Howick, J., and Maskrey, N. 2014. Evidence based medicine: a movement in crisis? *BMJ*; 348:g3725. https://doi.org/10.1136/bmj.g3725 *A critique of evidence-based medicine.*

Haynes, R.B., Devereaux, P.J., and Guyatt, G.H. 2002. Clinical expertise in the era of evidence-based medicine and patient choice. *Evid Based Med*; 7(2):36. https://doi.org/10.1136/ebm.7.2.36 *The nature and scope of clinical expertise must expand to balance and integrate the traditional focus of assessing the person's state with the pertinent research evidence and the person's preferences and actions.*

Jefferson, T., and Jørgensen, L. 2018. Redefining the 'E' in EBM. *BMJ Evid Based Med*; 23:46–7. https://doi.org/10.1136/bmjebm-2018-110918 *An editorial about the difficulty in clearly defining what we mean by evidence. 'By the law of Garbage In Garbage Out, whatever we produce in our reviews will be systematically assembled and synthesised garbage with a nice Cochrane logo on it'.*

Resnick, B. 2017. The weird power of the placebo effect, explained. *Vox*. www.vox.com/science-and-health/2017/7/7/15792188/placebo-effect-explained *A very clear explanation of the complex mechanisms though which placebos work and the new ways of using them. 'Placebo is … the water that medicine swims in'.*

Straus, S.E., Glasziou, P., Richardson, W.S., et al. 2010. *Evidence-based Medicine: How to Practice and Teach It*, 4th edition. Churchill Livingstone Elsevier. ISBN-13: 978-0702031274.

MAKING A DIAGNOSIS

The skills needed to make a diagnosis take time to acquire. Experienced clinicians employ a range of skills to assess the description of symptoms and then combine this with knowledge of the probability of various diagnoses to arrive at the most likely one. The front runner in this skillset is *active listening*. The diagnostic power of someone struggling to find the right words to describe a classic symptom is far greater than a yes/no answer to a question asked by a clinician. How do you know if you are listening well? If you find yourself asking something that has already been said, or that can be inferred from what the person has said already, then you are missing things.

Nuances and precision matter. For example, someone with a localised chest pain says, 'I was lying on my side on the sofa watching TV and then as I got up the pain suddenly came on.' They mean the pain started precisely at the moment they got up, not before, not after, making a diagnosis of a pulled muscle more likely than a coincident heart attack or pulmonary embolus. Not a diagnosis in full yet, just an indicator adding weight to a musculoskeletal cause rather than alternatives. As the conversation proceeds, indicators accumulate and when the majority point to a particular cause, a diagnosis can be made.

Beware of descriptions of a symptom that sound so classic they would fit well on a Wikipedia page or come straight out of NHS Health A to Z. Indeed, that could be where they have come from, driven by health anxiety about a particular diagnosis. Instead of just chasing other features of such a diagnosis, which may encourage responses suggested from the same source, seek the opposite; ask a question that will not normally form part of the diagnosis. For example, if someone says, 'I have crushing central chest pain that radiates to my left arm and up into my jaw', ask about non-cardiac features. 'OK. What happens when you lift your left arm?'

'Oh that makes it much worse.' Gradually, you can steer the conversation back to their main concern and cover some diagnostically important areas in a different frame of context. 'Anything else make it worse?'

'Lifting my right arm up also seems to – though not as much.'

'How about your legs?'

'They're fine. Doesn't make any difference to the chest pain.'

'Walking's OK?'

'Yep.'

'Going up stairs?'

'No problem.'

Min

The next skill in the set is a combination of clinical knowledge, particularly anatomy and common sense. Fear not, you don't need a detailed knowledge of human anatomy to reach useful conclusions. My recent experience of observing a consultation by a GP trainee serves as a good example. Trying to be supportive, I asked the junior doctor why angina is not normally tender, i.e., pressing on the chest doesn't make the pain worse, as was being described. Alas the trainee was visibly perplexed by this apparently simple question. Now, there are lots of possible physiological and psychological answers to the question, but to keep things simple we rely on the anatomical fact that there are ribs in the way. Pressing on the outside of the chest is not going to result in pressure on the heart.

You may find it surprising that anatomy and other clinical insights plus a little logic can have such an impact on diagnosis and further management in a wide range of cases. Practise the technique and your diagnostic ability will take a leap forwards. Take otitis media, for example. Here the clinical insight is that it is an infection of the middle ear which lies beyond the tympanic membrane. Therefore, taking a swab is unhelpful if there is no perforation because the bacteria would have to cross an intact tympanic membrane. Perforation would reduce auditory acuity, so if the hearing is unaffected, then taking a swab would be unlikely to be helpful and topical antibiotics would not reach the site of the infection. For the minority of cases of otitis media where an antibiotic was indicated, it would have to be oral.

If a specific symptom would make a diagnosis because that symptom has great diagnostic power, there is a temptation to simply ask whether or not it is present. The drawback is that by suggesting it, you bias the answer towards affirmative. Far better to try to reframe the context so, if present, the symptom would be mentioned. 'Don't lead the witness!' One technique for doing this is approximation, whereby a direct question is used that includes a crucial alteration, akin to a 'deliberate mistake'. For example, you become concerned that the 72-year-old person with you is describing a severe headache that might be caused by giant cell arteritis. Rather than asking outright about temporal tenderness (think of that as a last resort), instead ask 'What happens if you press on the centre of your forehead?' If the response is a curious expression and a self-test with the reply, 'Doesn't make much difference, but it hurts real bad when I press on the left side here…' with a demonstration of a hand going to the affected temple, then you have enough for your diagnosis to move on to examination, tests and urgent treatment.

A *working diagnosis* often starts at a very early stage – even when you are reviewing the person's notes before calling them into the room. It may be changed by your observation of their behaviour and appearance in the waiting room or how they walk through a corridor, then change again with their first sentence. Information that is volunteered spontaneously is much more likely to be relevant than that acquired by asking direct questions. This 'working diagnosis' process is usually efficient, but it has some pitfalls; jumping to the wrong conclusion is the most obvious. In order to reduce this risk, it is wise to ask yourself three questions:

- Is there anything that does not fit with this diagnosis?
- What other diagnoses are possible?
- Am I confident that the management of this situation is within my boundaries of expertise and clinical practice?

Sometimes a working diagnosis is so important that it can demand a shortcut to the outcome to bypass the delay of all the usual next steps. For example, if a remote consultation identifies someone who collapsed with a thunderclap headache, the diagnosis of a subarachnoid haemorrhage needs urgent confirmation or exclusion. Immediate transfer to hospital is essential, as imaging of the head or lumbar puncture will not be available elsewhere.

It is also worth noting that the most likely diagnosis is not always the most important. A hoarse voice lasting 3 weeks in a 45-year-old is probably not due to cancer, but cancer remains the most important potential diagnosis to consider. Indeed, the thresholds for referral for suspected cancer are not set at when the diagnosis is more likely than not. Rather, the bar is generally set at a risk of around 3%. This may sound low but, framed a different way, equates to approximately 1 in 33 people with that risk actually having cancer; meaning that if you saw 17 such people and did not refer them, you would be more likely than not to have missed a cancer diagnosis.

REMOTE ASSESSMENT

Early in the COVID-19 pandemic, Matt Hancock, the then UK Secretary of State for Health and Social Care, announced that all GP consultations should be remote by default. In response, the Royal College of General Practitioners expressed concern, and by the following year national newspapers were running a campaign that some called 'The new face-to-face revolution'. In fact, face-to-face consulting had never gone away, but the pandemic did make primary care practitioners reconsider who needs to be seen and who can be safely managed remotely by telephone, video, online or via a third party. The proportion of GP appointments which are face-to-face was 76% in April 2019, before the pandemic, and 62% in April 2023, but the total number of appointments per month increased by 8% in this period (The Health Foundation, 2023). These figures hide a large variation between practices.

Often the decision to see someone face-to-face (rather than conduct a consultation entirely remotely) is based on practical aspects, for example when a parent is vague about their child's symptoms and it would be better to hear them directly from the child. There are also the added benefits of being able to observe their behaviour and interact with them in a softer way than via a video link. In contrast, a child with recent-onset earache without discharge who is otherwise healthy and behaving normally can safely be managed remotely.

Note, however, that the reasoning behind that safety relies on medical knowledge that seeing the child is unlikely to change the diagnosis or treatment, an insight that may not be appreciated by the parent who is expecting their child to be seen and examined. The same principle applies to adults. Whilst you can be confident in a diagnosis of shingles by taking a good history over the phone, it may be hard for someone with a physical sign as obvious as a rash to accept that examining it is unnecessary. Box 13.1 gives medical and patient reasons why a person may be better seen face-to-face than assessed remotely, but bear in mind that whilst there may be a good medical rationale for safe remote assessment, patient factors may override this and make a face-to-face consultation more helpful from a social or psychological point of view.

BOX 13.1 WHO NEEDS A FACE-TO-FACE ASSESSMENT?

Medical reasons:

- Examination may help make a diagnosis that is not apparent from the history alone (*ask yourself – 'Will examination findings change my management?'*)
- When this cannot be done via a video link (*e.g., too small or indistinct, tissue warmth or tenderness, texture, signs of dehydration, auscultation, awkward site such as the inner ear, intimate examinations, and clinical measurement such as urine dipstick*)
- The story is far from clear (*observing body language may help and this is far easier with the wide field of view in a face-to-face contact. More reliance on examination may be needed for diagnosis. Acute confusion may be part of the illness*)
- Babies and infants too young to describe symptoms (*some common conditions, such as nappy rash, do not need face-to-face assessment, but for systemic illnesses the absence of a first-hand history makes examination more necessary*)
- Repeat presentations of persistent or worsening symptoms (*was the original diagnosis correct? If it was made remotely, could a physical sign have been missed?*)
- Safeguarding concerns
- Clinician unease (*trust your intuition – if it feels insecure, see the person face-to-face*)

Patient reasons:

- Reassurance needed (*for patients, parents or carers – health anxiety is a major factor*)
- To encourage appropriate treatment (*e.g., antibiotic not needed OR essential*)
- Loneliness or isolation (*being ill on your own is frightening and even a video link provides little comfort compared with seeing a friendly clinician*)
- Rare consulters or those with a high threshold to seek help (*e.g., a farmer at harvest time*)

Through the National Minor Illness Centre's courses, we have encountered some confusion amongst attendees about whether it is appropriate for an independent prescriber to prescribe for someone following a remote consultation. There is nothing in the regulations to prevent this; the Competency Framework for all Prescribers from the Royal Pharmaceutical Society (RPS, 2021) requires that the prescriber 'Identifies and minimises potential risks associated with prescribing via remote methods'. In other words, you need to be satisfied that the prescription is needed and appropriate and that risks, such as allergies, interactions or adverse reactions, are considered in the context of the past medical history and balanced against the potential benefit.

The Nursing & Midwifery Council (NMC) website gives the 10 key principles agreed by a collaboration of professional bodies to safeguard people accessing healthcare remotely (NMC, 2019). A face-to-face consultation or physical examination may be helpful to establish a diagnosis, but is not mandatory. An example of a diagnosis when a remote consultation would provide adequate assessment is uncomplicated cystitis, which can be diagnosed and treated based on a good history.

Min

References

NMC. 2019. High level principles for good practice in remote consultations and prescribing. www.nmc.org.uk/globalassets/sitedocuments/other-publications/high-level-principles-for-remote-prescribing-.pdf

RPS. 2021. A competency framework for all prescribers. www.rpharms.com/resources/frameworks/prescribers-competency-framework

The Health Foundation. 2023. General practice tracker. www.health.org.uk/news-and-comment/charts-and-infographics/general-practice-tracker#:~:text=Since%20then%2C%20it%20has%20broadly,staff%20were%20face%20to%20face

SAFETY-NETTING

There are two aspects to safety-netting at the end of a consultation: positive and negative. Positive safety-netting describes what is expected to happen, how symptoms should resolve over a specified time and how to manage them in the meantime. It is usually followed by advice that if this doesn't happen, or if a new symptom arises, then further medical advice should be sought. Negative safety-netting warns of what to look out for, in this particular situation, as signs of more serious illness (the original diagnosis may have been wrong or incomplete). This is best done as specifically as possible, because vague advice about seeking further medical advice '*if symptoms get worse*' may be too open to interpretation. Table 13.1 gives features of the two aspects.

Table 13.1 Safety-netting

Negative	Positive
–	+
Can be concerning for the patient	Reassuring, supportive
Discourages self-care	Encourages self-care
Specific	Less specific about the risks
Will not reduce the risk from worsening scenarios not mentioned	Helps to reduce the risks linked to new or unanticipated symptoms
Anxiety may be transferred from clinician to patient	Informative and empowering

Whilst negative safety-netting is common, used in isolation it may miss a worsening situation not mentioned. For example, a couple bring their young son for an assessment resulting in a diagnosis of a simple cold. The clinician is confident in the diagnosis but warns of major issues: that should the child stop breathing, have a convulsion or turn blue, the parents should call an ambulance. This leaves the parents concerned that the diagnosis may be insecure, but they are further reassured by the clinician and take their child home. Later in the night, after his anxiety about the child has been raised, the father checks on his son and notices that, although asleep, he is breathing very quickly. He calls his partner and she reassures him, 'No, at the surgery they said if he *stops breathing or goes blue* we have to dial 999. Well clearly, he isn't stopping, is he? And he's pink. So it's OK.'

Increased respiratory rate was not specifically included in the safety-netting, but we cannot cover every adverse possibility. The clinician would be very concerned if they knew the child had developed tachypnoea, which is not a feature of an upper respiratory infection and raises the likelihood of pneumonia. In contrast, positive safety-netting is more about empowering people/parents to raise their concerns if something unexpected happens, which does not form part of the natural progress as described. Practically, often a combination of the positive aspects and a few important negative aspects works well. Maybe a form of words like 'Ask for advice if you are getting worse, or if new symptoms develop that concern you. Keep an eye out for...' (mention only things which relate to the context of the problem).

Reference

Edwards, P.J., Silverston, P., Sprackman, J., et al. 2022. Safety-netting in the consultation. *BMJ*; 378:e069094. https://doi.org/10.1136/bmj-2021-069094

ARE THERE ANY PEOPLE OR CONDITIONS THAT YOU SHOULD NOT SEE?

Clinicians come to manage minor illness from a wide range of backgrounds, so it is not possible to make blanket recommendations. It is more efficient for you to exclude people with issues that you are unable to resolve, such as someone requesting a second or third opinion for a complex chronic problem. Paediatricians sometimes recommend that only clinicians with a paediatric qualification should see children; this is simply impractical and would exclude many GPs.

It is sometimes also suggested that only those with an obstetric or midwifery qualification should see pregnant women. This would be potentially dangerous, resulting in 'de-skilled' clinicians failing to consider the possibility of pregnancy in someone who is perhaps unaware. The Royal College of Nursing (RCN) provides the following guidance for independent prescribers: '*A useful distinction may be whether the "condition" is related to the pregnancy or not; even then we would recommend consideration of the possible impact on pregnancy and consult appropriately*'.

If there are several clinicians within an organisation who see people with minor illness and they all have different exclusions, it becomes a logistical nightmare to book someone with the appropriate clinician.

References

BNF. Prescribing in pregnancy. https://bnf.nice.org.uk/medicines-guidance/prescribing-in-pregnancy/

RCN. 2021. Advanced level nursing practice and care of pregnant and postnatal women. www.rcn.org.uk/Professional-Development/publications/rcn-care-of-pregnant-and-postnatal-women-uk-pub-009-756

CHILDREN

The examination of children requires a child-friendly environment and special skills; see the *Spotting the Sick Child* website.

- Bring your face to their level
- Keeping your voice soft, try to include them in the history-taking where appropriate and explain what you want to do on examination, but do not explicitly ask their permission. The parent/guardian has already given their implied consent
- Talk about something of interest to them
- Distraction, e.g., by a bubble machine or phone video, may be helpful
- Encourage parent to cuddle them
- Non-threatening examination first – for example hands
- Then chest, in case the child cries later
- With an anxious or uncooperative child, it may help for the parent to hold them facing their chest while you listen to their back. If they resist being undressed, first listen to the chest through thin clothes, then lift the clothing and listen again
- If the child is crying by then, listen carefully during inspiration
- Leave throat until last, and examine only if necessary
- Firm hold is needed for ear examination to avoid hurting the child if they wriggle

If the child becomes distressed during examination, abandon the attempt. For a minor illness, it is not appropriate to cause psychological trauma, hoping to improve the accuracy of your diagnosis. Explain this to the parents, with appropriate safety-netting.

All clinicians working with children should be aware of current advice on safeguarding children and should have undergone training to Level 3. This can be accessed through your local Safeguarding Children Partnership and may be available online.

References

BNF. Prescribing in children. https://bnf.nice.org.uk/medicines-guidance/prescribing-in-children/

HM Government. 2018. Working together to safeguard children. www.gov.uk/government/publications/working-together-to-safeguard-children--2 *Statutory guidance on inter-agency working to safeguard and promote the welfare of children.*

Spotting the sick child editorial team. 2020. Spotting the sick child. https://spottingthesickchild.com *An excellent free resource with many learning materials on the signs and symptoms of serious illness in children.*

Min

INFECTIONS

The traditional Western explanation of the infectious process portrays the human body as a sterile environment that has been invaded by a hostile organism. Our scientists' efforts have been concentrated on finding newer and better chemical weapons to defeat these enemy forces. However, the spread of antibiotic resistance is one of the biggest threats to global health. Our ability to develop new antibiotics is limited; all antibiotics in our formulary were developed more than 40 years ago.

We are beginning to see that this war-like model is fundamentally flawed. The human body is more like an ecosystem, supporting a myriad of other organisms far greater in number than the cells in our body. Some of them are essential for our survival and exist with us in symbiosis, such as the intestinal bacteria that manufacture vitamin K. Broad-spectrum antibiotics dramatically alter our internal flora, leading to side effects such as diarrhoea and vaginal thrush.

Many of the organisms that can cause infections are also normal inhabitants of the healthy human body (commensals) (see Table 13.2). The process that causes them to become pathogenic is not well understood, but it often seems to be initiated by a fall in the vigilance of the immune system rather than a change in the organism itself. The immune system has intricate links with all other systems of the body, is in communication with the gut bacteria, and is susceptible to the effects of nutrition and psychosocial stress. It follows from this that the maintenance of a healthy body and mind is important, both in reducing the chances of developing an infection and in aiding recovery. It also seems logical that medicines that interfere with the natural defences of the body (e.g., antipyretic, antiemetic and anti-inflammatory drugs) should be used with caution.

Table 13.2 Some of the bacteria that cause common infections and the antibiotics most frequently used against them

Organism	Commensal	Diseases	Antibiotic susceptibility
Streptococcus	Throat	Pharyngitis, otitis media, pneumonia, meningitis, cellulitis	**Phenoxymethylpenicillin**, amoxicillin, clarithromycin[PIQ]
Staphylococcus	Nose	Impetigo, boils, abscesses, cellulitis, pneumonia (typically after viral infection)	**Flucloxacillin**, co-amoxiclav, clarithromycin[PIQ]
Haemophilus influenzae	Upper respiratory tract	Otitis media, epiglottitis, meningitis, chest infections	**Amoxicillin** (83%), co-amoxiclav, clarithromycin[PIQ], doxycycline[PBC]
Escherichia coli	Intestine	UTI, abscesses, gastroenteritis	**Nitrofurantoin***[PBC] (98%), trimethoprim[PI] (78%), cefalexin, pivmecillinam* (96%)

* Nitrofurantoin and pivmecillinam are suitable to treat lower UTI (cystitis) only, as blood levels are inadequate to treat pyelonephritis, abscesses or bacterial gastroenteritis.

References

Hullegie, S., Venekamp, R.P., van Dongen, T.M.A., et al. 2021. Prevalence and antimicrobial resistance of bacteria in children with acute otitis media and ear discharge: a systematic review. *Pediatr Infect Dis J*; 40(8):756–62. https://doi.org/10.1097/INF.0000000000003134

Office for Health Improvement & Disparities. 2022. AMR local indicators – produced by the UKHSA. https://fingertips.phe.org.uk/profile/amr-local-indicators *Local and national antibiotic resistance figures*.

Recurrent infections

Sometimes, someone presents with several different types of infection over a short period of time. Consider if they are in a high-risk group for infections (see Chapter 1). If there is no apparent reason for the recurrences, there may be an underlying problem (see Box 13.2).

BOX 13.2 HIDDEN CAUSES OF RECURRENT INFECTIONS

- Increased exposure to infections (*e.g., child starting school*)
- Psychosocial stress (*a potent immunosuppressant for viral infections*)
- White cell dysfunction (*e.g., leukaemia – check FBC and differential*)
- Undiagnosed diabetes (*check FPG or HbA1c; see Box 8.3*)
- Human immunodeficiency virus (*HIV; offer testing*)
- Immunoglobulin deficiency, in children and young people (*check immunoglobulin levels*)

References

Blaser, M.J. 2014. The microbiome revolution. *J Clin Invest*; 124(10):4162–5. https://doi.org/10.1172/JCI78366 *An overview of new approaches to the microorganisms that live in and on the human body. For the full story, see Blaser's book,* Missing Microbes: How the Overuse of Antibiotics Is Fueling Our Modern Plagues. Macmillan USA. ISBN-13: 978-1250069276.

Pedersen, A., Zachariae, R., and Bovbjerg, D.H. 2010. Influence of psychological stress on upper respiratory infection – a meta-analysis of prospective studies. *Psychosom Med*; 72(8):823–32. https://doi.org/10.1097/PSY.0b013e3181f1d003 *Meta-analysis found that psychological stress is associated with increased susceptibility to upper respiratory tract infection.*

Song, H., Fall, K., Fang, F., et al. 2019. Stress related disorders and subsequent risk of life-threatening infections: population based sibling controlled cohort study. *BMJ*; 367:l5784. https://doi.org/10.1136/bmj.l5784 *In the Swedish population, stress-related disorders were associated with a subsequent risk of life-threatening infections, after controlling for familial background and physical or psychiatric comorbidities.*

Spector, T. 2020. *Spoon-Fed – Why Almost Everything We've Been Told about Food Is Wrong.* London: Jonathan Cape. ISBN-13: 978-1787332294.

Thaiss, C.A., Zmora, N., Levy, M., et al. 2016. The microbiome and innate immunity. *Nature*; 535(7610):65–74. https://doi.org/10.1038/nature18847 *Presents the intestinal microbiome as a signalling hub that integrates environmental inputs, such as diet, with genetic and immune signals to affect the host's metabolism, immunity and response to infection.*

NOTIFIABLE DISEASES

Diseases that must be notified to the local Health Protection Team (HPT) include:

- Chickenpox (only NI)
- COVID-19
- Food poisoning (not S)/infectious bloody diarrhoea (only E & W)
- Invasive group A streptococcal disease (only E & W)
- Measles
- Monkeypox
- Mumps
- Rubella
- Scarlet fever (not S)
- Whooping cough

(E = England; NI = Northern Ireland; S = Scotland; W = Wales)

Full lists for each of the four UK countries and contact details of local HPTs are given on the websites below. This notification is statutory and does not require the person's consent. Warn them that they may be contacted by the local HPT, and explain that their role is to identify the source of infection and prevent its spread. If there are any implications for the community, for example suspected food poisoning in a chef or a rare infectious disease, notify the local Health Protection Team by telephone. Information about specific diseases is given in Table 13.3.

Resources for notifiable diseases

- England: www.gov.uk/guidance/notifiable-diseases-and-causative-organisms-how-to-report#list-of-notifiable-diseases
- Northern Ireland: www.niinfectioncontrolmanual.net/notifiable-diseases
- Scotland: www.legislation.gov.uk/asp/2008/5/schedule/1
- Wales is covered by the same UK Health Security Agency (UKHSA) regulations as England

Min

Table 13.3 Infectiousness and exclusion periods for various infectious diseases

Disease	Incubation period	Infective period	Exclusion from school/work	Action for contacts
Chickenpox	11–20 days	From onset of rash until all lesions are crusted about 5–7 days later	At least 5 days from onset of rash and until all lesions have crusted over	Refer babies <4 weeks old and non-immune, immunosuppressed or pregnant contacts
Conjunctivitis	1–3 days for viral, 5–12 for bacterial	While discharge present	None	None, but contact HPT if an outbreak or cluster occurs
COVID-19	2–14 days	5 days after test	5 days (or at least 3 days if age ≤18 years) after a positive COVID-19 test and no longer with high fever or feeling unwell	None
Cryptosporidium	2–10 days	From onset of diarrhoea until 2 weeks after it stops	Until 48 hours after last diarrhoea or vomiting episode. No swimming for 2 weeks after infection cleared	HPT will decide
Diarrhoea and vomiting	1 hour–14 days (depending on cause)	While diarrhoea lasts	Until 48 hours after last diarrhoea or vomiting episode	No exclusion unless particular cause, when HPT will decide
Glandular fever	4–7 weeks	Very variable, from 7 weeks before to 18 months after symptoms	None	None
Hand, foot and mouth disease	3–5 days	7 days	None	None, but contact HPT if a large number of children are affected
Head lice	7–10 days	As long as lice or live eggs are present	None	None
Impetigo	1–10 days	While purulent lesions persist	Until lesions crusted, or 48 hours after treatment started	None
Measles	1–3 weeks	From 4 days before onset of rash to 4 days after	4 days from onset of rash	Refer babies <1 year and non-immune, immunosuppressed or pregnant contacts
Mumps	12–25 days	From 2 days before onset of symptoms to 5 days after	5 days from onset of swelling	None
Parvovirus (slapped cheek)	14–21 days	Until 24 hours after fever goes	None	Refer pregnant contacts at <30 weeks' gestation
Pertussis (whooping cough)	5–21 days	Up to 3 weeks if untreated	Until 2 days after starting antibiotic, or 3 weeks after onset of symptoms if no antibiotic given	Consult HPT about contact tracing
Rubella (no confirmed case in UK since 2019)	12–23 days	From 7 days before onset of rash to 5–7 days after	5 days from onset of rash	Refer non-immune pregnant contacts at <20 weeks' gestation
Scabies	4–6 weeks	Until mites and eggs have been destroyed	Until first treatment done	Household and close contacts require treatment at the same time
Scarlet fever	12 hours–5 days	Up to 24 hours after antibiotic, but up to 3 weeks if treatment declined	24 hours after starting antibiotic treatment or, if treatment declined, excluded until resolution of symptoms	Contact HPT if more than one suspected case

(Continued)

Table 13.3 (*Continued*) Infectiousness and exclusion periods for various infectious diseases

Disease	Incubation period	Infective period	Exclusion from school/work	Action for contacts
Shingles	Not relevant	From onset of rash until all lesions are dry, but rare as a cause of chickenpox (may cause chickenpox only by direct contact)	None, provided lesions covered	Refer babies <4 weeks and non-immune, immunosuppressed or pregnant contacts if exposed to uncovered lesions
Threadworms	2–6 weeks	As long as eggs present	None	Treatment recommended for child and household
Tinea	4–14 days	While lesions are active	None	None
Verrucae (plantar warts)	1–24 months	As long as warts are present	None (but cover warts with waterproof plaster for swimming/barefoot sports)	None

References

European Centre for Disease Prevention and Control (ECDC). 2016. Systematic review on the incubation and infectiousness/shedding period of communicable diseases in children. www.ecdc.europa.eu/sites/default/files/media/en/publications/Publications/systematic-review-incubation-period-shedding-children.pdf *Discusses the variation in advice about incubation and infectiousness from different sources.*

General Medical Council. 2018. Confidentiality: good practice in handling patient information: disclosing information about serious communicable diseases. https://www.gmc-uk.org/professional-standards/professional-standards-for-doctors/confidentiality---disclosing-information-about-serious-communicable-diseases/disclosing-information-about-serious-communicable-diseases

HM Government: Health Protection. 2023. Infectious diseases: detailed information. www.gov.uk/topic/health-protection/infectious-diseases

Marin, M., Leung, J., Lopez, A.S., et al. 2021. Communicability of varicella before rash onset: a literature review. *Epidemiol Infect*; 149:e131. https://doi.org/10.1017/S0950268821001102 *Chickenpox transmission before rash onset seems unlikely, although the possibility of pre-rash, respiratory transmission cannot be entirely ruled out.*

UK Health Security Agency. 2022a. Pertussis: guidance, data and analysis. www.gov.uk/government/collections/pertussis-guidance-data-and-analysis

UK Health Security Agency. 2022b. Viral rash in pregnancy. www.gov.uk/government/publications/viral-rash-in-pregnancy#full-publication-update-history

UK Health Security Agency. 2023. Children and young people settings: tools and resources. Exclusion table. www.gov.uk/government/publications/health-protection-in-schools-and-other-childcare-facilities/children-and-young-people-settings-tools-and-resources#exclusion-table

CERTIFICATES

NHS certificates (fit notes, MED3s)

Since 1 July 2022, healthcare professionals who can now certify fit notes (in addition to doctors) are nurses, occupational therapists, pharmacists and physiotherapists. In April 2022, a new version of the fit note was introduced to replace the signature in ink with the name and profession of the issuer completed by computer systems in primary care.

- May be used to state that the person is unfit for any work
- Alternatively, the person may be certified fit for limited work:
  - Phased return
  - Altered hours
  - Amended duties
  - Workplace adaptations
  - Other (in 'Comments' box), for example time off to attend appointments
- You do not need to issue a fit note for the first 7 calendar days of a person's sickness absence. People can self-certify for this period. Employees who have been unwell for 4 or more consecutive days can claim Statutory Sick Pay by completing an SC2 form online (just type SC2 into a search engine)

Min

- Does not require face-to-face assessment
- May be completed after remote consultation
- May be based on a written report by another registered healthcare professional (e.g., computer entry by minor illness nurse or pharmacist, a discharge summary or electronic communication from an out-of-hours organisation)
- Choice of 'open' statements (this will be the case for...) and 'closed' statements (from... to...)
- Use closed statements for most minor illness:
  - If the period is <14 days, and
  - The person does not need to be reassessed
- In the first 6 months of a condition, a fit note can cover a maximum of 3 months. If a condition has lasted longer than 6 months, a fit note can be for any clinically appropriate period up to 'an indefinite period'
- Cannot be forward dated, although overlapping is permitted
- Closed statements can be backdated
- Employers must fill in the SSP1 form when an employee is not entitled to Statutory Sick Pay (SSP), or when their SSP is ending
- Those unable to claim SSP, such as self-employed people, may be eligible for Employment and Support Allowance or Universal Credit

Private certificates

These can be issued by GP practices at their discretion. There is a fee, which should be reclaimed from the employer. If requested by a third party, signed consent of the person would be required. There is no need to supply sick notes for children's exams.

References

British Medical Association. 2021. Medico-legal aspects of providing certificates. www.bma.org.uk/pay-and-contracts/fees/medico-legal-fees/medico-legal-aspects-of-providing-certificates

Citizens Advice. 2020. www.citizensadvice.org.uk/work/sick-leave-and-sick-pay/check-if-you-can-get-sick-pay/

HM Government Department for Work and Pensions. 2022. Fit note. www.gov.uk/government/collections/fit-note

HM Government. Employment and Support Allowance. www.gov.uk/employment-support-allowance

CHAPTER 14

Prescribing for minor illness

SCOPE

The range of medication to treat minor illness found in this manual comprises 150 commonly used medicines. Recommended indications and specific doses for those indications are given in the prescribing section of each condition described. Each drug also has an entry in the Prescribing Insights section of our website, for which you have 6 months' free access using the voucher inside the front cover. Information gathered there is either hard to find from standard reference sources, or needs careful interpretation. As an example, the entry for the antibiotic nitrofurantoin MR is shown in Figure 14.1. We use a wide range of information sources, but have limited the references for any drug to three, the first of which links directly to the drug's entry in the British National Formulary (BNF) or the British National Formulary for Children (BNFC), where you will find the current recommendations on dose.

Online resources

- BNF: bnf.nice.org.uk
- BNFC: bnfc.nice.org.uk
- NMIC: www.minorillness.co.uk/content/insights
- emc: www.medicines.org.uk
- Pregnancy – UKTIS: https://uktis.org
- Breastfeeding – LactMed: www.ncbi.nlm.nih.gov/books/NBK501922/
- QT interval – CredibleMeds: www.crediblemeds.org
- Sudden arrhythmic death – SADS: www.sads.org.uk

SAFE PRESCRIBING

To prescribe any medication safely, you need to be aware of its action, side effects, interactions and contraindications. Independent prescribers should be familiar with all these medicines already, but this range of knowledge alone is not enough to ensure safe practice. Understanding key concepts in pharmacology, the actions of common long-term drugs and how drugs interact is essential because so many people will be taking other medication. Furthermore, side effects of long-term medication are so common that about 1 in 30 consultations are because of medication-related symptoms masquerading as illness. Elderly people, who have the greatest burden of medication, are at greatest risk.

Above all, make sure the prescription specifies the drug you intended. Most prescriptions in primary care are generated using a computer. The difference in selecting from a menu between drugs with similarly spelt names can be as little as the gap between two adjacent keys on a keyboard. One of the most dangerous examples is selecting penicillamine when penicillin was intended. Such an inadvertent swap from an antibiotic to an immunosuppressant could be fatal. Computer systems help to reduce errors, for example by potentially alerting the practitioner when a 'high-risk drug' has been selected and requiring the selection of 'phenoxymethylpenicillin', not just 'penicillin'. But it is not just a problem of typing the wrong letters; the real risk is from confusion in the mind between similar-sounding drugs. It may seem that such a gross error is unlikely, but none of us is immune.

In 2004, the Royal College of General Practitioners, in collaboration with many other national professional healthcare organisations and universities, sent a newsletter on prescribing entitled 'In Safer Hands' to all 9265 GP practices in England and Wales at that time. The edition focused on different drugs with similar names. 'We have tried to make suggestions for redesigning systems to make medicines safer; however, as you will see, there is often no substitute for checking.' Next came a list of nine pairs of drugs most commonly confused with one another. Out of the 18 drug names, three were incorrectly spelt in the newsletter. This error rate of 1 in 6 is rather more than the average error rate on prescriptions in primary care of 1 in 20, as found in the PRACtICe Study (Avery et al., 2012).

As a final check before issuing a prescription, the acronym *DDPASS* can be used.

- the right Drug (*i.e., the one intended*)
- the right Dose (*the dose appropriate for the indication, age or weight, and any special adjustments*)

R_x

- Pregnant or breastfeeding?
- Allergic?
- Some other drug? (*Another medication that might interact*)
- System impairment? (*Kidney especially, liver, heart*)

When considering if someone is pregnant, bear in mind those hoping to become pregnant but who have not yet missed a period; breastfeeding mothers also need caution when prescribing.

Having the full general practice record on the computer system from which you are issuing a prescription helps (through the use of alerts), but this is not always available, particularly if you are working in a location other than the person's general practice. Even then, the records are not always complete, so it is good practice to always ask the person if they are allergic to the drug you are about to prescribe. Phrase the question to include the group of the drug. For example, someone may know they are allergic to penicillin but not realise that co-amoxiclav is also a form of penicillin. If you were prescribing naproxen, ask 'Are you allergic to any anti-inflammatory pain relievers, such as ibuprofen or naproxen?'

Always consider the possibility of an interaction with any other current medication. It would be impractical to expect that every possible interaction is checked manually. Experienced prescribers know which drugs out of several are likely to interact and check those. This is one reason why a broader knowledge of pharmacology, not just the drugs used for minor illness, is so important. Your computer system may help in this regard, although it is not always clear which of the many interactions that it may flag are clinically significant. The BNF has a very useful interactions section that can quickly check one drug for interactions with several others, and the App is even smarter by being able to cross-check for any interactions between any of the drugs entered into the search.

Some drugs are *contraindicated* (N.B. this means 'should not be used') or should be given at lower dosage for people with kidney, liver or heart failure. Information on this is given in the BNF in the individual drug entries and on our website for minor illness medication. If in doubt, ask an experienced prescriber.

If you do need to write a prescription by hand, be aware of some additional pitfalls. The prescription form has a box at the top where the number of days' treatment may be entered. This avoids the need to calculate quantities but is awkward to use. It cannot be used for variable-dose drugs, creams, lotions and so forth. Remember that the box is an instruction to the pharmacist as to how much to dispense, not a direction to the patient, so anything written there does not appear on the dispensed medication instructions unless repeated in the main body of the prescription. It is simpler, clearer and safer to specify an amount to be dispensed in the main text and leave the top box blank.

Clear, uncluttered prescriptions are safest. Try to avoid decimal points (e.g., 500 mg is preferable to 0.5 g), repeating words, using superfluous words (e.g., 'spoonful') or adding instructions that are on the medication label anyway. The wording of the cautionary and advisory label for any drug (e.g., 'Protect your skin from sunlight…' or 'Take with a full glass of water') can be found in the 'Medicinal forms' section of the drug's entry in the BNF. As the dispensing pharmacist adds any required label to the dispensed medication by default, there is no need to repeat it on a prescription. A different instruction can be added to a prescription if required, but it is best to avoid adding specific instructions when none is required, in case you inadvertently contradict the standard advice on how the medicine should be taken. It also saves your valuable clinical time.

PHARMACODYNAMICS

Take every opportunity to learn about the actions of the wide range of drugs people are commonly taking when they seek your help for a minor illness. One of the drugs they are already taking might be part of the problem (the majority of adverse reactions are an exaggeration of the known effect of the drug) or might affect the use of the normal choice of treatment for their current condition. If you are simply curious to discover how a particular drug works, check out its 'Pharmacodynamic properties' in section 5 of the drug's entry in emc (www.medicines.org.uk/emc).

To give an example as to why this is helpful and makes for far better prescribing: you see someone with wheezing who had asthma as a child but was infrequently troubled by it as an adult. You notice they are taking propranolol, which they started 2 weeks ago as prophylaxis against migraine. Knowing that the action of this drug is to block beta receptors to adrenaline, including those in the lungs, you appreciate that the wheezing may not be a recurrence of the asthma, but an adverse drug reaction, in that their natural adrenaline-type messenger molecules can no longer activate the receptors that would open up the airways. Instead of your focus being on prescribing a bronchodilator, it shifts to stopping the propranolol. Nevertheless, a prescription might still be needed to relieve the wheeze. Normally you might issue one for salbutamol, but your insight tells you that, as it mimics adrenaline, it too will be less effective than normal. Therefore, it might be better to use a different type of bronchodilator, one that does not rely on the adrenaline pathway, such as ipratropium bromide. Had this all been asthma, you might have considered if a corticosteroid was also indicated, but as the asthma seems to have been significant only in childhood, and the recent attack coincided with the propranolol, it is more likely to be caused by the medication than any inflammatory process. A steroid is therefore less likely to be needed, or to help.

PHARMACOKINETICS

Absorption

Not surprisingly, tablets and capsules are designed to dissolve very fast in the warm acid environment of the stomach. There is no need to prescribe liquid or dispersible forms of medication to speed up their absorption. Solid preparations are preferable to liquids, being chemically more stable and less expensive. Even in acute migraine, when the stomach may be immobile, the average difference in speed of absorption between tablets and liquid is only 10 minutes. Some tablets dissolve on the tongue (e.g., 'melts'), but the resulting liquid still needs to be swallowed. This is useful when ordinary tablets cannot be swallowed easily, for example when there is no ready access to water, but does not significantly increase the speed of onset. There are very few preparations designed to be absorbed directly into the circulation from the mouth; one example is buccal prochlorperazine.

Modified-release tablets are intended to dissolve slowly to give a prolonged effect or reduced side effects. Gastro-resistant or enteric coating is a way of protecting a drug from damage by gastric acid. The coating resists acid, but dissolves in the more alkaline small bowel, which is the main site of absorption of oral drugs. Note that the coating is required to protect the drug, and hardly ever is it helpful in protecting the stomach. Gastric side effects are usually due to the overall effect of a drug after it has been absorbed, so the route by which it is given is immaterial. An NSAID can cause a gastric bleed from its systemic action, whether it is given orally, rectally or by injection.

Gastro-resistant coating overcomes a problem but introduces new ones for the prescriber. For example, 70%–90% of a dose of erythromycin is destroyed by normal gastric acid (Boggiano and Gleeson, 1976). Now consider the doses of erythromycin recommended in the BNF for different ages, which are all four times daily: 2–7 years, 250 mg, doubled in more severe infection; 8–17 years, 250–500 mg, doubled in more severe infection; and adults, 250–500 mg, doubled in more severe infection. Can you see why the children's doses are so similar to the adult doses? There is a hidden assumption here that children will be prescribed a liquid form of the medicine, whereas adults are likely to have a gastro-resistant form that preserves the dose swallowed.

This has implications for prescribers. A child who objects to the taste of a liquid medicine might prefer a solid form, but the use of a gastro-resistant form can result in a considerable increase in the effective dose absorbed. A pregnant woman with pneumonia who is allergic to penicillin might be prescribed erythromycin as an alternative, but beware that if they find it difficult to swallow capsules or tablets, a switch to a liquid preparation could reduce the absorbed dose to a fraction of what was intended. Trying to compensate for this by prescribing a higher dose would be fraught with difficulty because the amount of acid present when any one dose is swallowed might vary.

If an entire tablet or capsule is protected from dissolving in gastric acid, then the onset of action following the dose is delayed until the intact tablet or capsule happens to be near the opening of the pylorus, allowing passage into the duodenum and then on to the small bowel, the main site of absorption. This gives rise to a variable delay in onset of action that could be many hours. Furthermore, if the gut is upset with vomiting or diarrhoea, the drug may not be absorbed at all. The reason is that the complete, undissolved tablet or capsule in the stomach is vulnerable to being vomited up in its entirety or being rushed through the gut without adequate time to be dissolved and absorbed. In contrast, uncoated (non-gastro-resistant) drugs will be quickly dissolved in the stomach contents, and although people may claim they 'vomit everything up', it is often only a proportion of the gastric liquid.

The conclusion for prescribers is to avoid gastro-resistant coating when possible. If there is no form listed in the BNF without such coating, such as for omeprazole, or if most preparations that are listed are coated, then it may be necessary, but if there are many forms listed without gastro-resistant coating (such as for prednisolone) or an alternative medication is available that is stable in acid (such as clarithromycin instead of erythromycin), then it is simpler and safer to use the uncoated option.

Elimination and half-life ($t_{1/2}$)

The speed at which a drug is eliminated from the body is usually proportional to the concentration of drug in the blood. Elimination is more rapid just after a dose has been absorbed, when the drug is present in high concentration, than later when it is present only in low concentration. Drugs that are eliminated in proportion to their concentration are said to have first-order kinetics, and they have a constant $t_{1/2}$. This is the time taken for the concentration of the drug to reduce to half of its starting level.

R_x

Drugs with more complex kinetics may not have a constant $t_{1/2}$, but if it varies within a reasonably narrow range, then an average can be taken for practical purposes. It is useful to know the $t_{1/2}$, even if it is only an approximation, to help to understand how long the action of a drug will last and when a further dose may be needed. This information may be found under 'Elimination' in the 'Pharmacokinetics properties' in section 5 of the drug's Summary of Product Characteristics (SmPC) in emc (www.medicines.org.uk/emc). $t_{1/2}$ varies widely: less than an hour for phenoxymethylpenicillin, around 3 days for azithromycin and over a decade for alendronic acid (used for treating osteoporosis). Although knowledge of $t_{1/2}$ is often helpful, some drugs have actions that last longer than the presence of the drug in the circulation, for example the antiplatelet action of aspirin.

For a few drugs, the elimination rate is constant because, even at low concentrations, the metabolism for deactivating or eliminating is saturated (i.e., working at full capacity). Any further rise in the concentration of the drug in the blood does not drive faster elimination, as the process simply cannot go any faster. The maximum rate of ethanol (alcohol) metabolism is about one unit (10 ml) per hour, whether a single glass or a whole bottle of wine has been consumed. Over time, regular consumption induces greater activity of the pathway to eliminate ethanol, until liver damage starts to impair the system.

UNWANTED EFFECTS OF DRUGS

Allergic reactions

Many reported allergies are just coincidences, for example the appearance of a viral rash just after starting a course of an antibiotic. Of the UK population, 5.6% are labelled as being allergic to penicillin; when tested, 95% of these labels are incorrect (Savic et al., 2022). However, any report of swelling of the tongue or face, or difficulty in breathing, must be taken seriously.

Allergic reactions are usually:

- Itchy
- Generalised
- Confluent (abnormal areas of skin merging into one another)
- Either immediate (within 1 hour – often a more serious reaction), occurring 6–10 days after the drug is taken for the first time, or about 3 days (sometimes later) after a subsequent exposure

If someone has a true allergy to one type of penicillin, *all* drugs of this class should be avoided. This does not apply if they experience non-allergic side effects, such as diarrhoea with co-amoxiclav; phenoxymethylpenicillin may not produce this side effect.

If penicillin is the first-line treatment but cannot be used because of a known penicillin allergy, the usual alternative is clarithromycin because it is a macrolide of very different structure to penicillin, yet its spectrum of activity is similar. However, this too may be undesirable in view of its drug interactions. Azithromycin helps to overcome this problem (it has fewer interactions by a different mechanism), but both drugs are not recommended in pregnancy or for people with a long QT interval. For further information, see the sections on Prescribing in Pregnancy, Breastfeeding and QT Interval see the relevant later section.

Cefalexin is an alternative that can be used in pregnancy and also for people sensitive to penicillin unless they have had an anaphylactic reaction to penicillin previously. If not pregnant, doxycycline may be a suitable alternative to penicillin depending on the indication.

Anaphylaxis

Every frontline clinician needs to know how to recognise anaphylaxis and give emergency treatment. Update courses are usually done annually, and guidance is available online (Resuscitation Council UK, 2021). It is not that uncommon. Expect one person a year to present to a general practice that happens to be nearby when the symptoms start, whilst the majority present to A&E. Although it can be life-threatening, most reactions do not result in severe outcomes (Anagnostou and Turner, 2019). Food is a common trigger in children, whereas drugs are much more common triggers in older people.

The key message regarding treatment is that the only drug acting quickly is intramuscular adrenaline. Make sure you know where it is kept and, if in doubt, give it. An antihistamine may be used, but its role is not in the primary resuscitation (an oral antihistamine may help if taken by the patient as soon as they realise they have been exposed to their allergen, *before* much histamine has been released). Corticosteroids (e.g., hydrocortisone) are no longer advised for the emergency treatment of anaphylaxis, being too slow to act (and rarely hydrocortisone can trigger a further allergic response). Intravenous fluids are recommended for refractory anaphylaxis, and need to be given early if hypotension or shock is present. Anaphylactic reactions should be reported to the UK Anaphylaxis Registry at the international site www.anaphylaxie.net (to register, email anaphylaxis.registry@ic.ac.uk).

Adverse drug reactions

Adverse drug reactions (ADRs), often referred to as 'side effects', are very common and becoming more so with increasing prescribing to prevent or control long-term conditions. A meta-analysis of hospital admissions between 1988 and 2015 showed that, for older people, 8.7% of hospital admissions resulted from an adverse reaction to medication (Oscanoa et al., 2017). We found no recent research into the impact of such reactions on primary care consultations, but our experience at the National Minor Illness Centre is that, in about 1 in 30 consultations, the presenting symptom is a result of an unwanted effect of medication. This equates to about one a day for a clinician in minor illness.

Thus, it is essential to consider acute symptoms in light of concurrent medication. If an ADR is suspected, the principle to follow is that it is far better to stop or change a medication that is causing problems than to start another to control the unwanted effects. However, this is not always possible. If you do not normally prescribe the medication in question, seek advice from a clinician who does.

It may help in structuring your thoughts about ADRs to divide them into different types (Box 14.1).

BOX 14.1 CLASSIFICATION OF ADVERSE DRUG REACTIONS

Two basic types:

> **A**ugmented (80%) (adverse amplified therapeutic effect – this type of effect is predictable from the intended action of the drug)
> **B**izarre (20%) (but how could I have known that would happen? – sometimes termed idiosyncratic)

These can be divided into:

> **C**ontinuous (occurs while the drug is being taken)
> **D**elayed (occurs sometime after starting the drug)
> **E**nd of use (starts after the drug has been discontinued)

One example of a drug that has the potential for an ADR in every one of these categories is prednisolone:

A It is an immunosuppressant and therefore it increases the risk of infection
B Psychotic symptoms can be triggered; nothing to do with the therapeutic intention
C Immunosuppression continues while the drug is being taken
D Skin atrophy occurs later only if the drug is continued
E Stopping suddenly after prolonged use could precipitate an adrenal crisis

Discussing 'side effects'

The debate over how much to say about side effects continues, with advocates at each end of the spectrum – from the view that one should say as little as possible for fear that otherwise the person might not take necessary treatment, to those who champion the notion that every possible side effect should be fully discussed. We must discount these extremes for what they are. The best way to encourage people to take treatment when they really do need it is to involve them in the decision. It helps to have a background of not prescribing unnecessary treatment for them in the past.

Always warn about important or common side effects, or any that are particularly relevant to them. Such a conversation may give you an insight into how much more information they would like to be given. Too little leaves them feeling uninformed and perhaps more vulnerable if problems do occur and too much may cause unnecessary concern and confusion. Imagine trying to discuss fully the possible side effects of trimethoprim with the parents of a 3-year-old child with a proven urinary tract infection, namely that the antibiotic might cause toxic epidermal necrolysis or aseptic meningitis. Such serious side effects are vanishingly rare, but from the parents' point of view, it is difficult to appreciate the balance between the tiny risk involved and the essential need for treatment. The information leaflets

R_x

that are provided with drugs may help by giving the frequency of side effects, separating common side effects that amount to no more than a nuisance from serious ones listed as very rare.

It is the middle road for us – somewhere between the two extremes. It depends on your consultation skills exactly how well you manage to inform the person about their proposed treatment. The aim is to give them any information that they either need or want. Always give instructions on how to take a medicine, even if it is on the prescription and will be duplicated on the label. If asked, 'Are there any side effects?', the answer should be along the lines of 'Yes, all drugs have side effects, including this one', followed by an invitation to the person to hear more about the specific side effects associated with the proposed treatment. Aim to cover everything they **need** to know and provide an easy opening for them to ask about anything they **want** to know as well.

The BNF provides lists of known adverse reactions, but for more information or frequencies, look up a drug's SmPC, section 4.8 'Undesirable effects' (www.medicines.org.uk/emc). For antibiotic treatment, a study on people in hospital concluded that one in five would experience at least one adverse reaction (Tamma et al., 2017). These were not all serious, but certainly an unwanted burden, with a fifth of them suffering for no benefit because they had conditions for which antibiotics were not indicated.

Any treatment has non-specific effects related to the perception of the therapy being administered. We are familiar with the placebo effect (a positive effect), but a negative context, including information about adverse effects, may lead to low expectations and poor outcomes, called the nocebo effect. Far less is known about the nocebo effect; clinical trials on these effects are generally considered unethical as they trigger negative outcomes and do not provide any benefit to the participants.

An example of this is the concern that statin therapy might cause muscle pain or weakness. A study showed that >90% of all reports of muscle symptoms by participants allocated statin treatment were not due to the statin, but rather to the nocebo effect, encouraged by drug labelling and misleading sources of information (Reith et al., 2022). Positive framing can help reduce the nocebo effect. For example, saying 'the great majority of people tolerate this treatment very well' is construed more positively than '5% of patients report…' (Planès et al., 2016).

Black triangle symbol ▼

This symbol means that there is limited experience of the use of this product, and the Medicines and Healthcare products Regulatory Agency (MHRA) requests that *all* suspected adverse reactions should be reported online at https://yellowcard.mhra.gov.uk or through the Yellow Card app. The report can be submitted by any health professional.

Adverse drug reactions presenting as symptoms of minor illness

Many drugs are used in primary care, and each one may have multiple adverse effects, so it is always worth considering if symptoms could be due to a drug rather than a new illness. Table 14.1 gives some of the more common ones. Unless you are an independent prescriber or have another specialist role, you may not be initiating these medications, but as a specialist in minor illness it is important to recognise symptoms that might result from the person's medication. Often the symptoms start shortly after initiating a medication or changing the dose, but remember that type D adverse reactions are delayed.

Table 14.1 Symptoms which may be adverse reactions to medication

Adverse reaction symptom	Causative medication
Abdominal pain	Mebendazole, PPIs (e.g., omeprazole)
Arthralgia (gout)	Thiazides (e.g., bendroflumethiazide), aspirin
Confusion (hypoglycaemia)	Oral hypoglycaemics (e.g., gliclazide), insulin
Confusion (elderly)	Anticholinergics*, benzodiazepines (e.g., diazepam)
Constipation	Opioids, PPIs, iron, cyclizine, amitriptyline
Cough	ACE inhibitors (e.g., lisinopril)
Diarrhoea	Metformin, broad-spectrum antibiotics, laxatives, PPIs, colchicine, orlistat
Drowsiness	Sedative antihistamines (e.g., chlorphenamine), some antidepressants (e.g., amitriptyline, mirtazapine), antiepileptics (e.g., carbamazepine, gabapentin, pregabalin, topiramate), opioids, benzodiazepines

(Continued)

Table 14.1 (*Continued*) Symptoms which may be adverse reactions to medication

Adverse reaction symptom	Causative medication
Dyspepsia	NSAIDs including aspirin, bisphosphonates (e.g., alendronic acid), corticosteroids (e.g., prednisolone)
Eye pain (glaucoma)	Anticholinergics*, prednisolone
Fever	Vaccines (particularly meningitis B)
Flushing	Tamoxifen, calcium channel blockers (CCBs, e.g., amlodipine), nitrates (e.g., isosorbide mononitrate)
Headache	Analgesia overuse/withdrawal (particularly codeine), CCBs, nitrates, PPIs, initial few weeks of SSRI (e.g., fluoxetine)
Light-headedness	Antihypertensives (e.g., doxazosin), diuretics (e.g., furosemide), sudden withdrawal of prednisolone
Myalgia	Statins (e.g., atorvastatin) – *but rarer than people think*
Nausea/vomiting	Colchicine, opioids, PPIs, metronidazole, nitrofurantoin, erythromycin, initial few weeks of SSRI (e.g., fluoxetine), some antidiabetic drugs (e.g., semaglutide, dulaglutide)
Petechiae	Antiplatelet drugs (e.g., aspirin), anticoagulants (e.g., warfarin, apixaban), corticosteroids
Photosensitive skin	Tetracyclines (e.g., doxycycline)
Rash	Many drugs (e.g., penicillin, allopurinol)
Sore mouth (oral thrush)	Corticosteroid inhalers
Sore throat (urgent FBC needed)	Carbimazole, propylthiouracil, immunosuppressants
Swollen ankles	CCBs (e.g., amlodipine), corticosteroids (e.g., prednisolone)
Tremor/cramp/muscular spasm	Metoclopramide, prochlorperazine
Urinary frequency	Diuretics, SGLT2 inhibitors (e.g., dapagliflozin)
Urinary retention	Anticholinergics*
Wheezing	Beta blockers (e.g., propranolol), NSAIDs

* Anticholinergic drugs have inhibitory action on acetyl choline receptors; this may be the intended target of a medication (e.g., ipratropium/tiotropium inhaler, solifenacin) or an unwanted side effect (e.g., **chlorphenamine**, amitriptyline, paroxetine). See Ghossein et al. (2023) for more information.

QT interval

A long interval between the Q and T waves on an electrocardiogram (ECG) indicates an increased risk of cardiac arrhythmias that can cause sudden death. People who inherit this characteristic must avoid all drugs that prolong the interval; they are usually well informed and aware of potential risk.

Anyone with a family history of unexplained sudden death should have an ECG, but if this has not been done before they need a medication, it would be wise to assume that they might have an inherited long QT interval and avoid any drug that prolongs it. Those who acquire a long QT interval by taking a drug that prolongs it need to avoid taking a second drug that also prolongs the interval and would thereby increase the risk. In this case, the responsibility for this rests with the prescriber because most people are completely unaware that they may be taking a drug that affects the QT interval. Full information on which drugs prolong the QT interval can be found at the sudden arrhythmic death syndrome (SADS) website (www.sads.org.uk) or the American site CredibleMeds (www.crediblemeds.org).

Table 14.2 provides a list of medications commonly prescribed in primary care or available OTC in the United Kingdom that are known to affect the QT interval. Not all carry the same risk. The drugs in bold type are associated with higher risk. You will spot several that are used in minor illness.

R_x

Table 14.2 Common drugs that affect the QT interval (bold type indicates high risk)

Anti-arrhythmic	**Sotalol**
Anti-cancer	Tamoxifen
Anti-emetic	**Domperidone**, metoclopramide, **ondansetron**, prochlorperazine
Anti-fungal	**Fluconazole**, itraconazole, ketoconazole
Anti-hypertensive	Bendroflumethiazide, indapamide (by causing hypokalaemia)
Anti-migraine	Naratriptan, sumatriptan, zolmitriptan
Asthma inhalers	Salbutamol, salmeterol, terbutaline
Gastrointestinal	Esomeprazole, lansoprazole, loperamide, omeprazole
Macrolides	**Azithromycin, clarithromycin, erythromycin**
Mental health	**Amitriptyline, chlorpromazine, citalopram, escitalopram**, fluoxetine, **haloperidol**, hydroxyzine, lithium, paroxetine, quetiapine, risperidone, sertraline, trazodone, venlafaxine
Quinolones	**Ciprofloxacin, levofloxacin**, ofloxacin
Urological	Solifenacin, tolterodine
OTC	Nytol Original and One-a-Night (diphenhydramine), Sudafed (pseudoephedrine), many cold remedies
Others	Furosemide, metronidazole, quinine

Interactions

A simple theoretical model, based purely on probability, shows that if the chance of an interaction between any two drugs is 1%, the chance of an interaction occurring when someone is taking 12 drugs is about 50%. Further prescribing will clearly increase this risk. Fortunately, many interactions are not serious; the prime aim is to avoid those that are. Warnings from clinical computer systems are helpful, but if you find that your attention to such alerts wanes because of their frequency, consider changing the user settings to alert you only to higher-priority issues.

Table 14.3 shows some examples of relevance to the management of minor illness.

Table 14.3 Examples of long-term medications that interact with acute medications (bold type indicates high risk)

Long-term medication	Interacting acute medication for minor illness
Aspirin	**NSAIDs** – *increased risk of gastrointestinal haemorrhage and reduced cardiovascular protection*
Amiodarone	Colchicine – *increased toxicity*
Ciclosporin	Azithromycin, clarithromycin, fluconazole, itraconazole – *increased ciclosporin level* Colchicine – *increased toxicity* NSAIDs, trimethoprim – *increased renal toxicity*
Digoxin	Colchicine – *increased toxicity*
Lithium	**NSAIDs** – *increased lithium level*
Methotrexate	**Trimethoprim** – ***serious dual interference with folate metabolism*** NSAIDs – *increased methotrexate level*
Statin	Clarithromycin, fluconazole – *increased statin level and risk of rhabdomyolysis*
Theophylline	Clarithromycin, fluconazole, itraconazole, colchicine – *increased theophylline level*
Ticagrelor	Clarithromycin – *increased ticagrelor level*
Warfarin	**NSAIDs** – *enhanced anticoagulation and risk of gastrointestinal haemorrhage* Antibiotics (particularly clarithromycin and erythromycin), fluconazole, itraconazole, **topical miconazole** – *enhanced anticoagulation*

Table 14.3 gives just a few examples of the many interactions that can occur, but take another look and see if you can spot a few themes (NSAIDs, colchicine, clarithromycin and fluconazole are a good starting point). Rather than trying to remember all the different interactions, it is more practical to have a high index of suspicion for certain types of drug and check for possible interactions using the BNF or the computer system (Box 14.2).

BOX 14.2 FACTORS THAT INCREASE THE RISK OF A SIGNIFICANT DRUG INTERACTION

- Drugs that **share** an effect – e.g., aspirin and warfarin can both cause GI bleeding
- Drugs that have **opposite** effects – e.g., salbutamol will not be so effective if the person is taking propranolol
- A drug that affects the **liver** metabolism of other drugs – e.g., clarithromycin or fluconazole inhibits liver metabolism whereas carbamazepine or prednisolone may enhance it
- A drug that affects **kidney** function and the excretion of other drugs – e.g., NSAIDs
- A drug that needs careful adjustment of dose or **monitoring** – e.g., digoxin, methotrexate, lithium

Drugs that take a long time to be eliminated from the body (e.g., amiodarone, azithromycin, fluoxetine) can interact with other drugs several days or even weeks after they have been discontinued. You can suspect that a drug may have a long half-life if it is administered once a day or less often. This is not always the case, but it is useful as an alert; the actual half-life can then be checked in the SmPC (www.medicines.org.uk).

Be wary of drugs that require careful dose adjustment (e.g., warfarin, ciclosporin, antiepileptics), as small effects from another drug on the metabolism can decrease the drug's effectiveness or increase its toxicity. A clue to recognising these drugs is that the blood levels are often monitored. People who are stabilised on very small doses may be at greater risk of a significant interaction.

None of the antibiotics recommended in this book interacts with oral contraceptives. In fact, the only antibiotics that do interact are the few that enhance liver metabolism, such as some used to treat tuberculosis (Faculty of Sexual and Reproductive Healthcare Clinical Effectiveness Unit, 2022). There is no need to advise women taking antibiotics for minor illness to change their normal pill routine.

Not all interactions are from prescribed medication. St John's wort affects the metabolism of many other drugs, as does grapefruit juice. Cranberry juice increases the effect of warfarin, and alcohol interacts with metronidazole.

PRESCRIBING FOR SPECIAL GROUPS

Children

Children are not just small adults; their chemistry is still developing and they may metabolise drugs differently. Some drugs that are safe for use by adults cannot be taken by children because of the risk of a side effect that affects only children – for example, aspirin may cause Reye's syndrome. For drugs that can be prescribed for children, the dose is usually calculated by weight. Calculating a dose by body surface area is more accurate, but using weight is much more practical (Box 14.3).

BOX 14.3 TIPS FOR SAFE PRESCRIBING FOR CHILDREN

- First, have an approximate idea of what the dose is likely to be
- Then use the BNFC and calculate the dose from the child's weight, making sure it does not exceed the adult dose (if no weighing scales are available or the child is obese, use the ideal weight for age, which can be found in the BNFC online at https://bnf.nice.org.uk/about/approximate-conversions-and-units/)
- Is the dose in line with your expectation? If not, there is likely to be an error in the calculation
- Compare the dose to that given in the BNFC if specified for a given age range
- Note the instruction on how many doses per day
- If there appears to be no suitable formulation to make the dose easy to take (e.g., tiny or large amount of a liquid), recheck the calculation as there is likely to have been an error

R_x

Rounding up or down of a calculated dose may be necessary to make it practical. For example, the BNFC gives the dose of cefalexin for a child aged 5–11 years as '12.5 mg/kg twice daily, alternatively 250 mg three times a day'. Your 8-year-old patient weighs 25 kg, giving a calculated dose of 312.5 mg twice daily, which is more tailored to this particular child at their weight than the stated dose of 250 mg three times a day that covers all children in this age range. An oral suspension is available in a strength of 250 mg/5 ml, so your calculated dose would require 6.25 ml twice daily. Given the alternative in the BNFC, you can appreciate that the 0.25 ml represents an unnecessary degree of precision, so round the dose down to 6 ml twice daily. Avoid assuming that children will always need a liquid (see the later section on Formulations).

Obesity has an influence on this final adjustment of the dose. Most drugs do not penetrate fat well but are distributed within the water of the circulation and tissues. If someone (of any age) has obesity, calculating a dose by weight tends to give a dose that is rather too high, as the weight of the fat is included in the calculation, but most of the drug will be elsewhere. The BNFC advises '… calculation by body weight in the overweight child may result in much higher doses being administered than necessary; in such cases, dose should be calculated from an ideal weight, related to height and age' (BNF, 2023a).

Conversely, a particularly thin person may have a calculated dose that tends to err too low, but no adjustment is usually necessary for this reason alone. Of greater concern is whether they could be thin because they are malnourished, in which case liver metabolism may be less effective, requiring a reduction in dose for drugs eliminated by this route. For example, the BNFC specifies the dose of paracetamol for a 16-year-old to be 0.5–1 g every 4–6 hours, up to four doses per day, but under 'Cautions' alerts prescribers to a higher risk of toxicity in those with a low body weight.

If you suspect an adverse reaction to a drug, vaccine or herbal or complementary product, whether prescribed or OTC, that caused significant harm to anyone under the age of 18 years, report the incident online at https://yellowcard.mhra.gov.uk or through the Yellow Card app. This is particularly useful because experience of use of a drug in children may be limited.

Prescribing in pregnancy and breastfeeding

Every prescriber tries to avoid prescribing in pregnancy, but sometimes the risk from medication is outweighed by a greater risk of leaving a condition untreated, such as a urinary infection or asthma. Independent prescribers can prescribe for medical conditions presenting in pregnancy, so long as they work within their own level of professional competence (RCN, 2021). Before prescribing, always check the relevant section of text for the drug in the BNF that advises on risk in pregnancy or breastfeeding (Box 14.4).

BOX 14.4 FURTHER INFORMATION ON DRUG USE IN PREGNANCY AND BREASTFEEDING

In pregnancy:

UK Teratology Information Service (UKTIS) – https://uktis.org

In breastfeeding:

LactMed (USA) – www.ncbi.nlm.nih.gov/books/NBK501922/

On our website (for minor illness drugs):

www.minorillness.co.uk/content/insights/

An observational study of 96,000 pregnant women in Canada (Muanda et al., 2017) found that women who were prescribed certain antibiotics in pregnancy had an increased rate of miscarriage. There was an increased risk for clarithromycin (odds ratio 2.35, number needed to harm 8) and azithromycin (odds ratio 1.65, number needed to harm 18). There was no increased risk for erythromycin.

There followed a large cohort study in the UK (Fan et al., 2020), which reported a small increase in risk of malformations relating to the heart or blood vessels in babies born to mothers who were prescribed a macrolide in the first trimester of pregnancy. This appeared to be refuted the following year by a nationwide study in Denmark that showed no increased risk of major birth defects (Andersson et al., 2021). This prompted the MHRA to review the evidence; it concluded that there is insufficient evidence to be certain if macrolides taken early in pregnancy cause an increased risk of malformations or miscarriage (MHRA, 2021).

Erring on the side of caution, the NICE antimicrobial guidelines recommend that when a macrolide is needed in pregnancy, erythromycin is the preferred option. Whilst this may be appropriate advice following the Canadian study, be aware of the wording and always consider the even better option of avoiding a macrolide in pregnancy altogether by prescribing a suitable alternative from a different class. When prescribing, remember that, although erythromycin is the preferred macrolide for use in pregnancy, it still has the problems of multiple interactions, prolongation of the QT interval and delayed absorption when using its enteric-coated formulations. It also frequently causes GI side effects. There is an alternative, which is often overlooked because of previous misinformation: cefalexin (see the section on Cefalexin that follows).

Prescribing with multiple comorbidities

Research studies that provide us with the necessary evidence for good prescribing tend to focus on one condition, so that any reported effects of an intervention are easier to attribute to an effect of the condition or an intervention such as a new medication being investigated. Including people with many medical conditions who are taking multiple other medications in trials would make it harder to know the cause of new symptoms or incidents, but such circumstances often reflect what happens in real life outside the research environment.

Guidance in this book, or from a guideline online, may suggest a particular treatment as 'first line', but this doesn't mean it is the best option for everyone. Secondary options are often given in case the first-line option cannot be used because of co-existent conditions, illnesses or medication. For example, the NICE guideline for treating community-acquired pneumonia (NICE, 2019) recommends amoxicillin as first line, but if the person is allergic to penicillins an alternative will be needed. Those suggested as alternatives include doxycycline, clarithromycin and erythromycin. You consider those in turn and dismiss doxycycline because the person is pregnant. The next option is less than ideal because of the suspected small increased risk in pregnancy from clarithromycin. Erythromycin is the preferred macrolide in pregnancy.

This is a straightforward process of considering options in sequence, starting with the usual first-line treatment to arrive at the one suitable for the person with their unique circumstances. Slavishly following a guideline risks missing a conflict between the usual recommended treatment and important details in the social, psychological or medical circumstances, comorbidities or medication history. And, of course, there may be individual factors; they may be vegan, lactose intolerant, unable to swallow tablets or allergic to colourings. Any of these can have an impact on prescribing decisions.

Occasionally an alternative to usual treatment is needed because one drug can benefit more than one condition. For example, someone re-presents with rapidly worsening sinusitis after 10 days, but also mentions coughing up brownish sputum over the past 2 days and there are early signs of a lower respiratory tract infection. Rather than opting for phenoxymethylpenicillin, the 'first-line' antibiotic for sinusitis, you notice the alternatives include doxycycline and co-amoxiclav. The advantage of doxycycline is that it is also a common alternative for treatment of community-acquired pneumonia, whereas phenoxymethylpenicillin is not, and co-amoxiclav is recommended only in combination with a macrolide for severe infection. Getting multiple benefits for someone whilst minimising medication is smart prescribing.

CONSIDERATIONS FOR ANTIBIOTICS

Cefalexin

The first cephalosporin was discovered in a sewage outflow in Sardinia in 1945. Perhaps this inauspicious beginning heralded the bad press these antibiotics later received. The two myths that have propagated through texts and the habits of prescribers are that all cephalosporins have a high risk of causing *Clostridioides difficile*-associated diarrhoea (CDAD), and that because they have a beta-lactam ring like penicillins, they cannot be used if the person is allergic to penicillin.

The first of these myths arose from a dumbing-down of the correct realisation that later generations of cephalosporins, mostly used parenterally for inpatients, do indeed increase the risk of antibiotic-related enteritis. Cefalexin is a first-generation cephalosporin, but it was lumped together with all the rest in well-intentioned but inaccurate dissemination of the information gleaned from hospital care to primary care. The first alerts from the UK regulatory authorities specified a particular risk with third-generation cephalosporins, but this detail was lost in transit to prescribers. The only third-generation cephalosporin likely to be used in primary care in the United Kingdom is cefixime, which is not recommended anywhere in this manual.

While many national campaigns were underway to dissuade prescribers from using any cephalosporin, Quentin Minson and Steve Mok (two American pharmacists) undertook a case–control study that examined the link between

R_x

many different antibiotics and CDAD (Minson and Mok, 2007). They confirmed that third-generation cephalosporins carried a high risk (odds ratio 4.64), but that first-generation cephalosporins such as cefalexin had no association with CDAD (odds ratio 0.8, but the confidence interval included 1). Though the study was small and could be criticised for being underpowered, a subsequent meta-analysis found similar findings (Slimings and Riley, 2014).

Indeed, current advice from NICE (2015) is that the risk seen with first-generation cephalosporins, such as cefalexin, is not statistically significant. Perversely, avoiding all cephalosporins meant that prescribers in primary care were having to choose an alternative antibiotic and, in doing so, they were often using broad-spectrum antibiotics known to be associated with CDAD, such as quinolones or co-amoxiclav.

The second misconception about cephalosporins resulted from a frequency of cross-sensitivity with penicillins of 10% quoted in earlier editions of the BNF, but the rate was falsely elevated by contamination of cephalosporins with penicillin during the manufacturing process used at the time. The presumption was that there would be a cross-sensitivity because both cephalosporins and penicillins share a beta-lactam ring in their molecular structure. There is cross-sensitivity, but now there is strong evidence that it results not from the ring but from the R1 sidechain, which is similar in cefalexin, amoxicillin and ampicillin (Campagna et al., 2012).

Estimates of the rate of cross-sensitivity vary (depending on the research method and type of cephalosporin studied) but a reasonable average is 4.3% (Lee, 2014). The rate of confirmed sensitivity to penicillin in those declaring themselves to have had a mild or moderate reaction to a penicillin is about 5% (Savic et al., 2022). The chance of such a person having a similar response to cefalexin is therefore 0.22%, or 1 in about 450. A very low rate has been found in clinical practice (Blumenthal et al., 2015; Goodman et al., 2001). However, people with a previous episode of immediate hypersensitivity (e.g., anaphylaxis) to penicillin or a cephalosporin should not receive either. Here the sensitivity is definite, and a cross-sensitivity rate of 4% is too high to risk another reaction.

Previous antibiotic treatment

If someone presents with a condition not responding to antibiotic treatment, having already received an adequate course of the first-line antibiotic within the last 7 days, then either the infection is viral or the organism is resistant to the antibiotic. If possible, take a sample for culture to discover which applies.

If a different antibiotic is needed, and there is no information available on sensitivity, then the second course needs to have a different or broader spectrum of antimicrobial activity. Reasonable switches are as follows, bearing in mind that you need to check that the substitute drug is suitable for the person:

- For otitis media or sinusitis – change to co-amoxiclav
- For chest infections – change to doxycycline or add clarithromycin
- For uncomplicated lower urinary tract infections in non-pregnant women – if sensitivities are available from the laboratory, be guided by the results; otherwise use an antibiotic that was not used last time: nitrofurantoin MR, pivmecillinam, trimethoprim or fosfomycin
- For throat infections – in a young person first check there are no other symptoms or signs to suggest glandular fever. If not, consider taking a throat swab and await the result before prescribing a different antibiotic as, in most cases, the infection will be viral

PRACTICAL ASPECTS OF PRESCRIBING

Formulations

Take advantage of the wide range of formulations of drugs. If a person would benefit from a particular medication but there is potential risk or difficulty, consider using the drug via a different route of administration to the usual one, rather than changing to a less appropriate treatment. For example, someone with a previous peptic ulcer with a soft-tissue injury could use a topical NSAID rather than oral treatment.

However, be aware that an unusual formulation may be much more expensive than the usual one. The drug tariff price of paracetamol 250 mg as oral suspension is 16p per dose compared with £2.76 for a paracetamol suppository of the same dose. You can check the NHS price of a drug in the BNF or in Part VIII of the Drug Tariff (NHS Business Services Authority, 2023). Nitrofurantoin liquid is £450 for 300 ml compared with £9.50 for a pack of nitrofurantoin MR tablets. If you cannot find a form of a medicine in the BNF, it may be available but only supplied as a 'special' drug, without a set price, that could turn out to be thousands of pounds.

Clinical computer systems list available formulations of a drug. A frequent decision when prescribing oral medication is to choose between a liquid or a solid tablet or capsule. Avoid assuming that all children will need a liquid; the work of the Canadian paediatrician Bonnie Kaplan showed that children as young as 4 years can be taught how to swallow solid forms easily (Kaplan et al., 2010). If a child is willing to try a solid form and has had experience of bad-tasting liquids, consider offering a solid version of a medication.

Solid medicines have advantages. They are easy for most people to take, portable when travelling, tasteless if swallowed correctly and usually more stable, allowing for a longer shelf life. Prescribing 10 days of phenoxymethylpenicillin for a throat infection is common (despite the change in guidance to suggest that 5 days is acceptable), but prescribers and patients are often unaware that the shelf life of the liquid formulation is only 1 week after reconstitution.

Most standard-release preparations (i.e., not modified or slow release, or gastro-resistant coated) can be taken as powder with soft food after crushing tablets or pulling apart the two halves of a capsule. Many immediate-release tablets will disperse sufficiently in water without the need for crushing (SPS, 2021). This can be very helpful if a child or adult needs a liquid form of medicine but soluble tablets are not available. Advise people to check with their pharmacist when collecting their medication and if needed purchase a tablet crusher/splitter device for a few pounds.

Pack size

For liquid medicines, aim to prescribe an amount that corresponds to a manufactured pack size. This may not necessarily be equal to the amount required for a full course. For example, a prescription for an antibiotic liquid can include an instruction to take it for a certain number of days, but the manufactured pack, which may contain more than is needed, can be dispensed whole, together with the patient information leaflet. The extra supplied can be useful if a dose is spilled or refused by a child.

There is less of an issue for solid medicines, because pharmacists can split a pack more easily. Many of the items prescribed for minor illness are for short courses, when it is appropriate to prescribe the total quantity needed for the course, but if a longer duration is needed, be aware that packs of tablets or capsules commonly contain 28 or 30. The regulations regarding packaging vary across regions.

Dose

Where a medication is suggested in the text for management of a minor illness, the doses given will be appropriate for that illness. Other dosages and formulations may be available for other indications, a point worth bearing in mind when checking the medication in the BNF or another resource.

OTC

Drugs marked 'OTC' are available over the counter and often cost less than a prescription charge. The price depends on the pack size, brand and pharmacy; surprisingly, the cost incurred by the NHS when prescribing such medicines can be greater than the OTC purchase price. In 2018, NHS England released guidance to Clinical Commissioning Groups (now replaced by Integrated Care Boards) aimed at reducing the prescribing of items available OTC, particularly for self-limiting conditions or those lending themselves to self-care. Even if the condition for which the medicine is required is not covered by this guidance, it is always worth enquiring whether the person pays prescription charges and advising them accordingly.

Try to avoid inadvertently triggering an awkward conversation between the person and their pharmacist; only suggest purchasing a medication when it is available OTC for the reason that the person needs it. For example, the antihistamine cinnarizine is available OTC for the prevention of travel sickness, but not for treating the symptoms of vestibular neuronitis. There are also restrictions on the circumstances in which some products can be sold OTC; for example, clotrimazole pessaries cannot be sold OTC to women aged >60. You can check these rules by typing 'PIL' then the name of the medicine into your browser – this will usually take you to the patient information leaflet on the Electronic Medicines Compendium (emc) website.

RISK ALERTS FOR MEDICATIONS

Table 14.4 lists abbreviations found after drug names in the text where there is a significant risk of adverse events. Any drug may have the potential for multiple interactions, but the majority are not clinically significant. The tags provide warnings where there is a significant risk and may vary depending on the context. For example, oral prednisolone is suitable for use in asthma for a pregnant woman where the benefit outweighs the risk, but not when it is being considered as an option to treat hay fever.

Manufacturers often advise against the use of a medication in pregnancy or breastfeeding when there is insufficient evidence of safety. Independent information sources, such as the BNF, UK Teratology Information Service (UKTIS) and Drugs and Lactation Database (LactMed) may advise that there is no evidence of harm. A balance needs to be

R_x

struck to avoid denying pregnant or lactating women helpful medication whilst maintaining adequate safety for the fetus or infant.

It should be remembered that the elimination of many drugs can be affected by renal or hepatic impairment. If the person has either, check the dose of the drug in the relevant section of the BNF/BNFC.

The symbols in Table 14.4 are designed to alert you quickly and simply to prescribing issues which are common and important. They cannot cover all possibilities; further information on prescribing is available in the BNF, the BNFC and the Prescribing Insights in the Members' section of our website.

Table 14.4 Prescribing symbols used in this book

P	**Pregnancy** risk (N.B. the woman may not yet realise that she is pregnant). Use an alternative medication known to be safe in pregnancy. If they are allergic to penicillin, alternatives include erythromycin or cefalexin (as it shares some molecular structure with penicillins, cefalexin should not be used if the person has had an anaphylactic reaction to any penicillin). Erythromycin is preferred to clarithromycin if a macrolide is needed. Information sources: BNF or UKTIS
B	**Breastfeeding** risk. The drug affects breastfeeding or is secreted in milk and is not suitable for the baby. Use an alternative medication known to be safe in breastfeeding. Information sources: BNF or LactMed
C	**Children.** The medication is either harmful to children or has a limited licence; for example, the medicine may only be licensed for children over a certain age. Information source: BNFC
I	**Interactions** likely. For example, macrolides such as clarithromycin inhibit the liver enzymes that metabolise drugs. This can result in an accumulation of another drug to potentially toxic levels. Many drugs can be affected (e.g., amlodipine, colchicine, simvastatin, ticagrelor and warfarin), so always check the BNF for any interaction before prescribing. If a macrolide is needed but clarithromycin is precluded because of interactions, consider azithromycin, which has fewer interactions because it does not interact significantly with the hepatic cytochrome P450 system. Information sources: BNF, emc, Flockhart Table
Q	**QT interval** prolonged. Avoid for anyone with a known long QT interval, or an unknown QT interval plus a family history of unexplained sudden death, or for anyone already taking another drug that prolongs the interval. A long interval between the Q and T waves on an ECG indicates an increased risk of cardiac arrhythmias that can cause sudden death. Information sources: SADS or CredibleMeds

Websites
- BNF: bnf.nice.org.uk
- BNFC: bnfc.nice.org.uk
- CredibleMeds: www.crediblemeds.org
- emc: www.medicines.org.uk
- Flockhart Table: drug-interactions.medicine.iu.edu
- LactMed: www.ncbi.nlm.nih.gov/books/NBK501922/
- SADS: www.sads.org.uk
- UKTIS: www.uktis.org
- NMIC Resource: www.minorillness.co.uk/content/insights/

Every drug mentioned in this book has its own entry in our Prescribing Insights in the Members' section online. The voucher code in the front of this book gives you 6 months' free access. An example entry for nitrofurantoin MR is shown in Figure 14.1.

Nitrofurantoin MR	
Key Info:	Let's get straight to the point. This is a great first-line antibiotic for cystitis but useless for pyelonephritis. Despite this being known as a result of the pharmacokinetics of the antibiotic, many people phone 111 who clearly had, and still have, symptoms inconsistent with uncomplicated cystitis, such as a fever, rigors, vomiting, loin pain, or frank haematuria, who have been prescribed nitrofurantoin. It's as though the prescriber read national guidance[2] as far as seeing that nitrofurantoin is first choice... but failed to see that this only applies to cystitis. Kidneys are very effective at clearing the blood of nitrofurantoin. This is great for cystitis, as the excreted antibiotic is accumulated in the urine inside the bladder - the location of the infection in cystitis, but hopeless for infection in the tissue of the kidney because there is no antibiotic left in the blood. There is another benefit of understanding this. If someone has renal impairment, the antibiotic will be less reliably excreted into the urine and therefore less effective, and blood levels can accumulate, making the risk of side effects greater. Nitrofurantoin may cause nausea (modified release preparations less so). Advise the patient that it colours urine brownish orange, and that they should avoid alkalinising agents (OTC sachets for symptomatic relief) that can disable the antibiotic. The drug is better absorbed if taken with food. The usual prescription is for one 100mg MR capsule twice daily for 3 days, but 7 days are needed for treating cystitis in men or during pregnancy. When it can be used, nitrofurantoin is a good choice; only about 10% of bacteria responsible for UTI in primary care are resistant to nitrofurantoin, and its low systemic levels help preserve the gut biome and reduce the risk of side effects. Nitrofurantoin has to be avoided if the patient has deficiency of the enzyme glucose-6-phosphate dehydrogenase (G6PD), which increases the risk of haemolytic anaemia. This deficiency commoner in males from Africa, Asia, the Mediterranean and the Middle East. For more information and resources see the TARGET Toolkit[3].
Pregnancy:	↪ Nitrofurantoin can be used in pregnancy but not near term when it can cause neonatal haemolysis. While some guidelines suggest avoiding after 36 weeks' gestation, women can start premature labour much earlier than this, so our advice is more cautious and we would avoid nitrofurantoin from 30 weeks onwards.
Breastfeeding:	↪ The same risk of haemolyisis applies if the drug is given to a mother breast feeding an infant in the first 3 months. After this, this risk is low, with the exception that the drug must not be given to infants of any age with G6PD-deficiency.
Children:	↪ Avoid in G6PD-deficiency. If a liquid is needed, the cost is very high.
Interactions:	✔
QT:	✔
Liver:	! Liver damage can result from this antibiotic. The risk may be increased in the presence of pre-existing liver disease.
Renal:	!! Avoid if eGFR <30 and caution (consider using an alternative antibiotic) if eGFR <45.
Cost:	!! Children's suspension costs £450 for one bottle.
OTC:	✘
References:	1:https://bnf.nice.org.uk/drug/nitrofurantoin.html 2:https://www.nice.org.uk/guidance/ng109 3:https://elearning.rcgp.org.uk/mod/book/view.php?id...

Figure 14.1 Nitrofurantoin MR NMIC Prescribing Insights entry.

REFERENCES

Anagnostou, K., and Turner, P.J. 2019. Myths, facts and controversies in the diagnosis and management of anaphylaxis. *Arch Dis Child*; 104(1):83. https://doi.org/10.1136/archdischild-2018-314867 *Use of macrolide antibiotics in pregnancy was not associated with an increased risk of major birth defects.*

Andersson, N.W., Olsen, R.H., and Andersen, J.T. 2021. Association between use of macrolides in pregnancy and risk of major birth defects: nationwide, register based cohort study. *BMJ*; 372:n107. https://doi.org/10.1136/bmj.n107

Avery, T., Barber, N., Ghaleb, M., et al. 2012. Investigating the prevalence and causes of prescribing errors in general practice: the PRACtICe study. (PRevalence and Causes of prescrIbing errors in general practiCe). A report for the GMC. www.gmc-uk.org/about/what-we-do-and-why/data-and-research/research-and-insight-archive/investigating-the-prevalence-and-causes-of-prescribing-errors-in-general-practice

Blumenthal, K.G., Shenoy, E.S., Varughese, C.A., et al. 2015. Impact of a clinical guideline for prescribing antibiotics to inpatients reporting penicillin or cephalosporin allergy. *Ann Allergy Asthma Immunol*; 115(4):294–300.e2. https://doi.org/10.1016/j.anai.2015.05.011

BNF. 2023a. Prescribing in children. https://bnf.nice.org.uk/medicines-guidance/prescribing-in-children/

BNF. 2023b. Prescribing in breast-feeding. https://bnf.nice.org.uk/medicines-guidance/prescribing-in-breast-feeding/

BNF. 2023c. Prescribing in pregnancy. https://bnf.nice.org.uk/medicines-guidance/prescribing-in-pregnancy/

Boggiano, B.G., and Gleeson, M. 1976. Gastric acid inactivation of erythromycin stearate in solid dosage forms. *J Pharm Sci*; 65(4):497–502. https://doi.org/10.1002/jps.2600650406

Campagna, J.D., Bond, M.C., Schabelman, E., et al. 2012. The use of cephalosporins in penicillin-allergic patients: a literature review. *J Emerg Med*; 42(5):612–20. https://doi.org/10.1016/j.jemermed.2011.05.035

Fan, H., Gilbert, R., O'Callaghan, F., et al. 2020. Associations between macrolide antibiotics prescribing during pregnancy and adverse child outcomes in the UK: population based cohort study. *BMJ*; 368:m331. https://doi.org/10.1136/bmj.m331

Faculty of Sexual and Reproductive Healthcare Clinical Effectiveness Unit. 2022. *Clinical guidance: drug interactions with hormonal contraception.* www.fsrh.org/documents/ceu-clinical-guidance-drug-interactions-with-hormonal/

Ghossein, N., Kang, M., and Lakhkar A.D. 2023. Anticholinergic medications. *StatPearls.* www.ncbi.nlm.nih.gov/books/NBK555893/

Goodman, E.J., Morgan, M.J., Johnson, P.A., et al. 2001. Cephalosporins can be given to penicillin-allergic patients who do not exhibit an anaphylactic response. *J Clin Anesth*; 13(8):561–4. https://doi.org/10.1016/S0952-8180(01)00329-4

Herts Valleys Clinical Commissioning Group. 2021. Guidance on crushing tablets or opening capsules in a care home setting. https://hertsvalleysccg.nhs.uk/application/files/7715/8288/4031/HVCCG_Overt_form_for_Crushing_Tablets_or_Opening_Capsules_in_a_Care_Home_Setting_docx_v2.0_-_February_2020.pdf

Kaplan, B.J. 2010. The new method of swallowing. www.youtube.com/watch?v=MXFMZuNs-Fk

Kaplan, B.J., Steiger, R.A., Pope, J., et al. 2010. Better than a spoonful of sugar: successful treatment of pill swallowing difficulties with head posture practice. *Paediatr Child Health*; 15(5):e1–5. https://doi.org/10.1093/pch/15.5.e1

Lee, Q.U. 2014. Use of cephalosporins in patients with immediate penicillin hypersensitivity: cross-reactivity revisited. *Hong Kong Med J*; 20(5):428–36. https://doi.org/10.12809/hkmj144327

MHRA. 2021. Safety of macrolide antibiotics in pregnancy: a review of the epidemiological evidence. www.gov.uk/government/publications/public-assessment-report-safety-of-macrolide-antibiotics-in-pregnancy-a-review-of-the-epidemiological-evidence/safety-of-macrolide-antibiotics-in-pregnancy-a-review-of-the-epidemiological-evidence

Minson, Q., and Mok, S. 2007. Relationship between antibiotic exposure and subsequent *Clostridium Difficile*-associated diarrhoea. *Hosp Pharm*; 42(5):430–4. https://doi.org/10.1310/hpj4205-430

Muanda, F.T., Sheehy, O., and Bérard, A. 2017. Use of antibiotics during pregnancy and risk of spontaneous abortion. *Can Med Assoc J*; 189(17):E625–E633. https://doi.org/10.1503/cmaj.161020

NHS Business Services Authority. 2023. Drug Tariff Part VIII. www.nhsbsa.nhs.uk/pharmacies-gp-practices-and-appliance-contractors/drug-tariff/drug-tariff-part-viii

NHS England. 2018. Conditions for which over the counter items should not routinely be prescribed in primary care: guidance for CCGs. www.england.nhs.uk/publication/conditions-for-which-over-the-counter-items-should-not-routinely-be-prescribed-in-primary-care-guidance-for-ccgs/

NICE. 2015. ESMPB1. Clostridium difficile infection: risk with broad-spectrum antibiotics. www.nice.org.uk/advice/esmpb1/chapter/Key-points-from-the-evidence

NICE. 2019. NG138. Pneumonia (community-acquired): antimicrobial prescribing. www.nice.org.uk/guidance/ng138

NICE. 2020. CG134. Anaphylaxis: assessment and referral after emergency treatment. www.nice.org.uk/guidance/cg134

NICE. 2021. Summary of antimicrobial prescribing guidance – managing common infections. www.bnf.org/wp-content/uploads/2021/07/summary-antimicrobial-prescribing-guidance_july-21-for-BNF.pdf

NICE. 2017–2022. Antimicrobial prescribing guidance. www.nice.org.uk/guidance/published?nai=Antimicrobial+prescribing&ndt=Guidance

Oscanoa, T.J., Lizaraso, F., and Carvajal, A. 2017. Hospital admissions due to adverse drug reactions in the elderly. A meta-analysis. *Eur J Clin Pharmacol*; 73(6): 759–70. https://doi.org/10.1007/s00228-017-2225-3

Planès, S., Villier, C., and Mallaret, M. 2016. The nocebo effect of drugs. *Pharmacol Res Perspect*; 4(2):e00208. https://doi.org/10.1002/prp2.208 *How to minimise nocebo-related risks.*

RCN. 2021. Advanced level nursing practice and care of pregnant and postnatal women. www.rcn.org.uk/Professional-Development/publications/rcn-care-of-pregnant-and-postnatal-women-uk-pub-009-756

Reith, C., Baigent, C., Blackwell, L., et al. 2022. Effect of statin therapy on muscle symptoms: an individual participant data meta-analysis of large-scale, randomised, double-blind trials. *Lancet*; 400(10355):832–45. https://doi.org/10.1016/S0140-6736(22)01545-8 *In people taking a statin, >90% of reports of muscle symptoms were not due to the statin.*

Resuscitation Council UK. 2021. Guidance: anaphylaxis. www.resus.org.uk/library/additional-guidance/guidance-anaphylaxis

Savic, L., Ardern-Jones, M., Avery, A., et al. 2022. BSACI guideline for the set-up of penicillin allergy de-labelling services by non-allergists working in a hospital setting. *Clin Exp Allergy*; 52(10): 1135–41 https://doi.org/10.1111/cea.14217 *A diagnosis of penicillin allergy increases the risk of MRSA,* C. difficile *or VRE infections and death, presumably through increased use of alternatives to beta-lactam antibiotics. It increases the duration of hospital admissions and has significant implications for the cost of healthcare.*

Slimings, C., and Riley, T.V. 2014. Antibiotics and hospital-acquired *Clostridium difficile* infection: update of systematic review and meta-analysis. *J Antimicrob Chemother*; 69(4):881–91. https://doi.org/10.1093/jac/dkt477

SPS (Specialist Pharmacy Service). 2021. Preparing medicines for administration to adults with swallowing difficulties. www.sps.nhs.uk/articles/preparing-medicines-for-administration-to-adults-with-swallowing-difficulties/

Tamma, P.D., Avdic, E., Li, D.X., et al. 2017. Association of adverse events with antibiotic use in hospitalized patients. *JAMA Intern Med*; 177(9):1308–15. https://doi.org/10.1001/jamainternmed.2017.1938

R_x

WEBSITES WITH INFORMATION/EVIDENCE ON A WIDE RANGE OF TOPICS

www.minorillness.co.uk
Our own NMIC website.

There is a voucher in the front of this book with a scratch-off code that will give you 6 months' free access to the Members' section of our website, with online educational materials and email alerts.

Scan this QR code with your smartphone to take you there directly.

www.nhs.uk
A good source of information for patients on common (and uncommon) illnesses.

https://patient.info
Another good source of information including leaflets and self-help groups (if you can cope with the adverts).

www.bbc.co.uk/actionline/
Wide-ranging support and self-help portal.

https://cks.nice.org.uk
Providing fast navigation to evidence-based advice on minor illness. Although under the NICE umbrella, CKS is an independent organisation drawing evidence from a wide range of sources.

www.nice.org.uk
National guidance (for England and Wales) on a wide range of conditions.

www.sign.ac.uk
Clinical guidelines for Scotland; depending on the publication date, they can reflect more up-to-date evidence than guidance from NICE.

https://scholar.google.com/
Google Scholar – this academic version of Google uses the power of Google's algorithms but focuses on academic publications/evidence. Also very useful for finding full-text versions of references. Note that Google will not focus on medical answers to your search; results might come from veterinary, engineering or other backgrounds.

www.tripdatabase.com
Trip finds medical evidence and sorts it according to quality. Top of the tree is 'Secondary Evidence', i.e., evidence that has already been collected, reviewed or evaluated for you. Go to the landing page and watch the 2-minute introductory video. Access is free.

www.cochranelibrary.com
This is an internationally renowned collection of high-quality systematic reviews on a huge variety of clinical topics.

https://thennt.com/home-nnt
Useful information on the NNT: the number of people needed to treat to cause benefit or harm for different medicines or interventions for a wide range of conditions.

https://europepmc.org
Free access to over 42 million life-science publications.

WEBSITES WITH A MORE FOCUSED SUBJECT AREA/REMIT

www.what0-18.nhs.uk
Information for parents, pregnant women and young people, including 'when to worry' guidance for a range of common conditions/minor illnesses. Depending on your location, useful resources for professionals, including Paediatric Pathways, may also be available.

www.medicinesforchildren.org.uk
Advice for parents and healthcare professionals on giving medicines to children, including practical advice on 'Helping your child to swallow tablets'.

https://spottingthesickchild.com
Detailed advice on the assessment of children.

www.whenshouldiworry.com
An evidence-based booklet for parents on respiratory infections.

www.gov.uk/government/publications/health-protection-in-schools-and-other-childcare-facilities/children-and-young-people-settings-tools-and-resources
Information on infectiousness and school exclusion.

www.gov.uk/government/collections/immunisation-against-infectious-disease-the-green-book
Current immunisation schedules and the 'Green Book: Immunisation against Infectious Disease'.

www.gov.uk/government/collections/fit-note
Information about completing fit notes.

www.gov.uk/guidance/notifiable-diseases-and-causative-organisms-how-to report#list-of-notifiable-organisms-causative-agents
List of notifiable diseases.

https://labtestsonline.org.uk
Information about laboratory tests.

www.rcpch.ac.uk/sites/default/files/rcpch/HTWQ/Reference%20ranges%20Jan%2018.pdf
Normal ranges of blood tests for children, which are different from those in adults.

www.pcds.org.uk
Diagnostic algorithms for skin conditions.

https://dermnetnz.org
Images and management of skin conditions.

www.nathnac.net
www.fitfortravel.scot.nhs.uk
www.travax.nhs.uk
Travel advice.

www.bashh.org
The British Association for Sexual Health and HIV provides information and guidelines on sexual health.

www.versusarthritis.org
Information about common musculoskeletal problems. Exercise sheets can be found by using the website's search tool and entering 'exercise sheets'.

www.toxbase.org
Advice on the toxicity of a huge range of substances. Free but registration of your NHS organisation is required.

PRESCRIBING INFORMATION SOURCES

Source	Website
British National Formulary (BNF)	bnf.nice.org.uk *App also available that downloads to a mobile phone, so that information can be accessed when not online*
British National Formulary for Children (BNFC)	bnfc.nice.org.uk *Clear guidance on doses for children*
CredibleMeds	www.crediblemeds.org *Worldwide data on drugs that affect the cardiac QT interval*
DrugBank online	https://go.drugbank.com *Free access to detailed information on half a million drugs*
Electronic Medicines Compendium (emc)	www.medicines.org.uk *Patient information leaflet and SmPC including frequencies of side effects and half-life. For fast access about a specific drug, type into Google the drug name followed by 'emc'*
Flockhart Table drug interactions	https://drug-interactions.medicine.iu.edu *The Flockhart Table. Worldwide database on cytochrome P450 drug interactions*
LactMed	www.ncbi.nlm.nih.gov/books/NBK501922/ *Information on the use of drugs in breastfeeding*
Monthly Index of Medical Specialities (MIMS)	www.mims.co.uk *Up-to-date, succinct information from the pharmaceutical industry with useful tables, e.g., emollients with potential skin sensitisers. Free access for 30 days, after which there is a subscription, but your organisation may already have access*
OTC Drug Information	www.otcdirectory.co.uk
SADS	www.sads.org.uk *UK information on drugs that affect the cardiac QT interval*
Specialist Pharmacy Service	www.sps.nhs.uk *Professional medicines advice*
UKTIS	https://uktis.org *Professional information on the use of drugs in pregnancy, and access to 'Bumps', which gives information for patients*

Many of the best and most up-to-date information sources are on the Internet, either freely available or available with an NHS OpenAthens password via https://openathens.nice.org.uk

CHAPTER 16

Acronyms and abbreviations

5-HT	5-hydroxytryptamine
A&E	Accident and Emergency department
ACE	angiotensin-converting enzyme
ACT	acceptance and commitment therapy
ADR	adverse drug reaction
AKI	acute kidney injury
AMR	antimicrobial resistance
ARB	angiotensin receptor blocker
BASHH	British Association of Sexual Health and HIV
BMA	British Medical Association
BMC	BioMed Central
BMI	body mass index
BNF	British National Formulary
BNFC	British National Formulary for Children
BP	blood pressure
BPPV	benign paroxysmal positional vertigo
BSACI	British Society for Allergy & Clinical Immunology
BTS	British Thoracic Society
BV	bacterial vaginosis
C. difficile	*Clostridioides difficile* (previously *Clostridium difficile*)
CBT	cognitive behavioural therapy
CCB	calcium channel blocker
CCP	cyclic citrullinated peptide (antibody test for rheumatoid arthritis)
CDAD	*Clostridioides difficile*-associated diarrhoea
CKD	chronic kidney disease
CKS	Clinical Knowledge Summaries
CLA	Civil Legal Advice
CNS	central nervous system
COC	combined oral contraceptive
COPD	chronic obstructive pulmonary disease
COVID-19	coronavirus disease 2019
COX	cyclo-oxygenase (enzyme)
CRB-65	scoring system for pneumonia
CRP	C-reactive protein (an inflammatory marker in the blood)
CRT	capillary refill time
Cu-IUCD	copper intrauterine contraceptive device
CXR	chest x-ray
DAMN	medicines which may need to be stopped in dehydration
DDPASS	Prescribing mnemonic: Drug, Dose, Pregnant/breastfeeding, Allergic, Some other drug, System impairment
DMARD	disease-modifying antirheumatic drug
DNA-CPR	do not attempt cardiopulmonary resuscitation
doi	digital object identifier (a stable link to websites)
DVLA	Driver and Vehicle Licensing Agency
DVT	deep vein thrombosis
E. coli	*Escherichia coli*
EBM	evidence-based medicine
EBV	Epstein–Barr virus
EC	emergency contraception
ECDC	European Centre for Disease Prevention and Control
ECG	electrocardiogram

EEG	electroencephalogram
eGFR	estimated glomerular filtration rate
emc	Electronic Medicines Compendium
ENT	ear, nose and throat
ESR	erythrocyte sedimentation rate (an inflammatory marker in the blood)
FBC	full blood count
FIT	faecal immunochemical test (for hidden blood)
FODMAP	fermentable oligosaccharides, disaccharides, monosaccharides and polyols
FPG	fasting plasma glucose
FSRH	Faculty of Sexual and Reproductive Healthcare
GABHS	group A beta-haemolytic *Streptococcus*
GAD	Generalized Anxiety Disorder
GCS	Glasgow Coma Scale
GI	gastrointestinal
GMC	General Medical Council
GP	general practitioner
H. pylori	*Helicobacter pylori*
HARM	heat, alcohol, reinjury and massage
HbA1c	haemoglobin A1c (a marker of blood glucose level in the past 3 months)
HFMD	hand, foot and mouth disease
HIV	human immunodeficiency virus
HLA	human leukocyte antigen (mutations linked to autoimmune diseases)
HPT	Health Protection Team
HPV	human papillomavirus
HRT	hormone replacement therapy
HSP	Henoch–Schönlein purpura
HSV	herpes simplex virus
HVS	high vaginal swab
IBD	inflammatory bowel disease
IBS	irritable bowel syndrome
ICB	Integrated Care Board
Ig	immunoglobulin
iGAS	invasive group A *Streptococcus*
IM	intramuscular
INR	international normalised ratio
ISBN	international standard book number
IUCD	intrauterine contraceptive device
IUS	intrauterine system (progestogen-releasing)
IV	intravenous
kcal	kilocalories
LactMed	Drugs and Lactation Database (USA based)
LFT	liver function test
LMP	last menstrual period
LOVE	load, optimism, vascularisation, exercise
MDI	metered-dose inhaler
MECS	Minor Eye Conditions Service
MED3	certificate of fitness for work
Men B	meningitis B
MHRA	Medicines and Healthcare products Regulatory Agency
MIMS	Monthly Index of Medical Specialities
ml	millilitre
MMR	measles, mumps and rubella
MR	modified release
MRI	magnetic resonance imaging
mRNA	messenger ribonucleic acid
MRSA	methicillin-resistant *Staphylococcus aureus*
MSU	midstream urine

NHS	National Health Service
NICE	National Institute for Health and Care Excellence
NMC	Nursing & Midwifery Council
NMIC	National Minor Illness Centre
NNT	number needed to treat
NSAID	non-steroidal anti-inflammatory drug
ORS	oral rehydration solution
OTC	over the counter
PAIN	scoring system for sore throat (purulence, attends rapidly, very inflamed tonsils, no cough or cold)
PCDS	Primary Care Dermatology Society
PBCIQ	pregnancy, breastfeeding, children, interactions, QT interval
PCOS	polycystic ovarian syndrome
PCN	Primary Care Network
PCR	polymerase chain reaction
PEACE	protect, elevate, avoid NSAIDs and ice, compress, educate
PEFR	peak expiratory flow rate
PEP	post-exposure prophylaxis
pH	measure of acidity
PHQ-9	Patient Health Questionnaire 9
PID	pelvic inflammatory disease
PIL	patient information leaflet
POP	progestogen-only pill
POTS	postural orthostatic tachycardia syndrome (also called postural tachycardia syndrome)
PPI	proton pump inhibitor
PR	per rectum
PRICE	protection, rest, ice, compression and elevation
PRN	as needed
PVL	Panton–Valentine leukocidin (cytotoxin produced by some *Staphylococci*)
QR	quick response code
QT	part of an ECG trace
RA	rheumatoid arthritis
RCGP	Royal College of General Practitioners
RCN	Royal College of Nursing
RCOG	Royal College of Obstetricians and Gynaecologists
RCT	randomised controlled trial
RPS	Royal Pharmaceutical Society
RR	respiratory rate
SADS	sudden arrhythmic death syndrome
SARS-CoV-2	severe acute respiratory syndrome coronavirus 2
SGLT2	sodium-glucose linked transporter type 2
SIGN	Scottish Intercollegiate Guidelines Network
SmPC	Summary of Product Characteristics (of a medicine)
SNRI	serotonin and norepinephrine reuptake inhibitor
SPS	Specialist Pharmacy Service
SSP	Statutory Sick Pay
SSRI	selective serotonin reuptake inhibitor
STEC	Shiga toxin-producing *Escherichia coli*
STI	sexually transmitted infection
TB	tuberculosis
TENS	transcutaneous electrical nerve stimulation
Trip	Turning Research into Practice (database)
TTG	tissue transglutaminase (blood test for coeliac disease)
TV	*Trichomonas vaginalis*
UKHSA	UK Health Security Agency
UKTIS	UK Teratology Information Service
UPSI	unprotected sexual intercourse
URTI	upper respiratory tract infection

Acr

USC	urgent suspected cancer (formerly 2-week wait)
UTI	urinary tract infection
VRE	vancomycin-resistant enterococci
VTE	venous thromboembolism
VZIG	varicella zoster immunoglobulin
WHO	World Health Organization

Index